W9-BRO-320

NUTRIENT TIMING for
Peak Performance

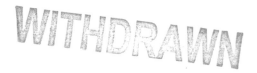

Heidi Skolnik, MS, CDN, FACSM

Andrea Chernus, MS, RD, CDE

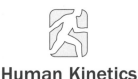

Human Kinetics

Library of Congress Cataloging-in-Publication Data

Skolnik, Heidi, 1961-
  Nutrient timing for peak performance / Heidi Skolnik, MS, CDN, FACSM,
Andrea Chernus, MS, RD, CDE.
      p. cm.
  Includes bibliographical references and index.
  ISBN-13: 978-0-7360-8764-3 (soft cover)
  ISBN-10: 0-7360-8764-8 (soft cover)
  1. Athletes--Nutrition. I. Chernus, Andrea, 1957- II. Title.
  TX361.A8S57 2010
  613.2'024796--dc22

                        2010008325

ISBN-10: 0-7360-8764-8 (print)
ISBN-13: 978-0-7360-8764-3 (print)

This publication is written and published to provide accurate and authoritative information relevant to the subject matter presented. It is published and sold with the understanding that the author and publisher are not engaged in rendering legal, medical, or other professional services by reason of their authorship or publication of this work. If medical or other expert assistance is required, the services of a competent professional person should be sought.

The Web addresses cited in this text were current as of March 2010, unless otherwise noted.

Acquisitions Editors: Laurel Plotzke Garcia and Joe Rodgers; **Developmental Editor:** Laura Floch; **Assistant Editor:** Elizabeth Evans; **Copyeditor:** Patricia L. MacDonald; **Indexers:** Robert and Cynthia Swanson; **Permission Manager:** Martha Gullo; **Graphic Designer:** Fred Starbird; **Graphic Artist:** Tara Welsch; **Cover Designer:** Keith Blomberg; **Photographer (cover):** © Human Kinetics; **Photographer (interior):** © Human Kinetics, unless otherwise noted; **Photo Asset Manager:** Laura Fitch; **Visual Production Assistant:** Joyce Brumfield; **Photo Production Manager:** Jason Allen; **Art Manager:** Kelly Hendren; **Associate Art Manager:** Alan L. Wilborn; **Printer:** United Graphics

Human Kinetics books are available at special discounts for bulk purchase. Special editions or book excerpts can also be created to specification. For details, contact the Special Sales Manager at Human Kinetics.

Printed in the United States of America   10 9 8 7 6 5 4 3 2 1

The paper in this book is certified under a sustainable forestry program.

Human Kinetics
Web site: www.HumanKinetics.com

United States: Human Kinetics
P.O. Box 5076
Champaign, IL 61825-5076
800-747-4457
e-mail: humank@hkusa.com

Canada: Human Kinetics
475 Devonshire Road Unit 100
Windsor, ON N8Y 2L5
800-465-7301 (in Canada only)
e-mail: info@hkcanada.com

Europe: Human Kinetics
107 Bradford Road
Stanningley
Leeds LS28 6AT, United Kingdom
+44 (0) 113 255 5665
e-mail: hk@hkeurope.com

Australia: Human Kinetics
57A Price Avenue
Lower Mitcham, South Australia 5062
08 8372 0999
e-mail: info@hkaustralia.com

New Zealand: Human Kinetics
P.O. Box 80
Torrens Park, South Australia 5062
0800 222 062
e-mail: info@hknewzealand.com

E4997

To Bradley, who is the gravitational force that keeps me in orbit. My heart stretches daily with my love for you. Thank you for being so supportive, cooperative, and patient.

—*Heidi*

To Mom and Dad: Thank you for always being in my corner and telling me to keep my eye on the ball. I'm so appreciative of your encouragement, love, and support.

—*Andrea*

Contents

Preface

"What should I eat before training?" "What's best to eat after a workout? How soon after should I eat?" "How much protein do I need? When should I eat to maximize muscle building?" "Do I need any supplements during a workout?" "How should my eating change on game day?" As sports nutritionists, these are questions that athletes always ask us. So, when writing this book, we envisioned a comprehensive how-to resource that incorporates the latest research on nutrient timing into easy-to-understand concepts and personalized action plans. We show athletes how taking in nutrients at the right time in regard to exercise, in appropriate amounts, will maximize the results of their training and improve their competitive edge.

Many sports nutrition books on the market focus on one type of sport or are geared more generally toward sports nutrition. Ours is unique. We address a specific aspect of sports nutrition: *timing*. This book looks at the needs of all types of athletes—strength athletes, endurance athletes, and those who participate in stop-and-go sports. We focus on not only *what* to eat but also *when* nutrients have their greatest impact on athletes' bodies. No other book contains all the concepts presented here in such a hands-on, usable fashion.

Our aim is to help you, the athlete, formulate an eating plan to meet your goals—whether you are male or female; are a professional, college, or high school athlete; or compete seriously, participate for fun, or are training for health, well-being, and aesthetics. Our book can be used by participants of all sports—runners, soccer players, triathletes, cyclists, football players, swimmers, tennis players, fitness enthusiasts, and those who participate in any sport imaginable. Sports nutritionists, coaches, and trainers may also use our book to help their clients and players eat optimally.

Although it's tempting to start reading the book where we show you how, what, and when to eat, we urge you to start by reading part I, "The Principles." Why? To benefit from the concepts of nutrient timing, it is helpful to know what nutrient timing is and why it's important. We've always found that when our clients understand *why* we recommend a strategy, they are much more successful at adhering to the plan and reaching their goals. The timing of nutrients can have a big impact on an athlete's energy. To be ready to practice or compete at your best, you'll understand why paying attention to when recovery begins will help you restore your capacity for your next hard workout. Did you know that when and how much you eat can help not only with muscle hypertrophy but immune function as well? Additionally, staying well fueled can reduce your risk of injury.

You'll also learn to set goals for yourself that are reasonable and attainable. You'll understand what your body is capable of and what is unrealistic to expect for your age, gender, and body type. There is nothing more frustrating than seeing an athlete who is on track and performing wonderfully only to be upset and discouraged because of unrealistic expectations. We want you to be pleased with your results and stay motivated. In part I, we also explain how exercise affects your body—in everyday language. If you understand these concepts, nutrient timing makes more sense.

Building on this base of knowledge, we introduce the players to all the nutrients involved in part II, "The Nutrients." This part is vitally important because we sort out facts from myths and misperceptions surrounding nutrients. For example, carbohydrate, when eaten at specific times and in specific amounts for your size and energy expenditure, aids in regenerating muscle energy and may help with immune function by freeing up key amino acids; protein ingestion may help push muscle hypertrophy after strength training and may also keep the immune system buzzing; and fat has played a controversial role over the years, but we'll examine how and when it is used as a fuel. Fat can keep your hormones humming, and taking in enough is vital for making testosterone and estrogen, which play important roles in health *and* performance.

Now that you're well versed on the concepts, we'll apply all the knowledge specifically to you and your sport. Part III, "Fueling Strategies, Plans, and Menus," walks you through setting *your* goals, timing *your* intake for training, and understanding how it may differ for competition. We help you determine which type of nutrient timing plan is appropriate for your sport. We show you how to determine your unique nutrient timing and put it all together into a personalized plan for before, during, and after workouts, practices, games, or matches. We have plenty of charts, examples, and sample meal plans to use as guides. We talk about supplements that may be popular in your sport or activity—do they help, or could they harm?

Nutrient timing takes sports nutrition to a new level. It's a targeted and focused way of utilizing science to optimize the effects of diet on sports performance. Nutrient timing can improve both short-term and long-term recovery from the wear and tear of intense workouts, practices, and games to help athletes stay strong and healthy throughout seasons of play. Appropriate timing of nutrients can also help push the muscle-building effects of strength training and help diminish the muscle breakdown that often occurs with heavy endurance training. Immune function and injury prevention are concerns for all athletes. We show you why what you eat and when you eat can influence both your immune function and your chance of injury. What and when you eat can even affect your hormonal levels, which in turn affect everything from body composition to mood. Finally, we show you samples of plans, foods, and strategies you can implement to improve your nutrient timing and that can help you be the strongest, fastest, healthiest athlete you can be.

Acknowledgments

Heidi Skolnik

It takes a village to raise a child while writing book! My gratitude and appreciation to the following families of friends: Kauderer-Abrams, Turitz-Sweifach, Bejar, Silver, and Goldberg. To my support circle: Stacey Freed, Charlee Garden, Melorra Sochet, Michelle Cole, Wendy Best, Stacey Eisler, Robyn Stuhr, the Macdonald Family and Paris Caruolo and Baha.

To have knowledge and never apply it is like having a great recipe that you never prepare or share. Thank you to the organizations and athletes that allow me to apply the science and craft of sports nutrition daily and witness, in action, the benefit it brings: The Football Giants, The Knicks, School of American Ballet, The Juilliard School, and Fordham University. I am honored to be part of a group of extraordinary professionals that get it and keep it going: The Women's Sports Medicine Center at Hospital for Special Surgery, especially Dr. Jo Hannafin, Terry Karl, Polly DeMille, Dr. Beth Shuben-Stein, and a special shout out to Dr. Lisa Callahan for incredible support and belief in me and what I can do. Much thanks to *Men's Health* and their commitment to improving healthy habits through knowledge.

On a daily and more personal level, Jinny Skonik gets the cake for remaining positive and helpful during times of distress (can anyone say "manuscript due"?), unwavering support, and continued belief in achieving one's dreams.

Andrea Chernus

I am thrilled to finally extend my sincerest thanks to all those who expressed interest and supported me through this seemingly endless project. To my friends: Jody Salberg, Barbara Mattera, Larry Wender, Ann Lopez, Lorelei Guttman, Amy Gillenson, Agnes Lee, and Ellen Natter. Thank you for your patience and understanding. I am especially grateful to Maree Lavo and Anne Manning who had just the right words at the right time and helped to save my sanity!

Thanks to Zachary Chernus whose input on high school sports was invaluable; to Spencer and Ryan for being terrific kids, and to Jack and Jennifer whose support and love I cherish.

Thank you to all my fellow athletes at Reebok and to my clients who share their struggles and successes on a daily basis. Lastly, to my companion Baxter, who reminded me on numerous occasions when a 15-hour day was long enough.

In addition, both Heidi and Andrea want acknowledge and thank colleagues, professionals, and experts in their fields who helped research articles, compile information, calculate, and provide answers to their questions:

Craig Turnbull	Kate Huber
Seth Roland	Dr. Lewis Maharam
Jerry Palimeri	Dr. Nicholas Ratamess
Mike Bergeron	Dr. David Rowlands
Nancy Rodriguez	Dr. Robert Wolfe
Jennifer Fox	Dr. Gregory Haff
Cheryl Heaton	Dr. Jose Antonio
Caroline Greenleaf	Dr. Doug Kalman
Mariana Vela Gonzalez	Reyna Franco
Adena Neglia	Lisa Dorfman
Lori Hernberg	Randy Bird
John Gilbert	Sandy Markman
Margaux Harari	Ellen Coleman
James Lucas	Brian Zehetner
Amy Snyder	Mitzi Dulan
Mabel Wong	Lisa Adler

THE
PRINCIPLES

1

The Nutrient Timing Advantage

Have you ever felt dead-legged or worn out during practice? Do you lift and lift and lift yet can't seem to put on an ounce of muscle? Are you frequently getting sick or injured? Maybe you feel great and want to perform at an even higher level than you are right now, but you believe something is missing. What you eat, how much you eat, and when you eat can affect your energy, your training, your immune function, and even your risk of injury.

WHAT IS NUTRIENT TIMING?

Nutrient timing is a strategic approach to how much, what, and when you eat before, during and after training and competition to maximize training effects, reduce risk of injury, maintain healthy immune function, and help with recovery. Nutrient timing is a system of eating meals and snacks in relation to planned exercise. It's a system of working the composition of your food selection, the portions of your food selection, and the timing of intake of your food so that it does the absolute most it possibly can to help your performance. As you read this book, we hope to help you understand how different food components affect your body before, during, and after all types of exercise. Nutrient timing takes advantage of how food influences different chemical reactions inside your body.

Various strategies may be used depending on whether you are cycling, lifting weights, running a marathon or a 100-meter dash; or going to football, baseball, lacrosse, or soccer practices, games, or even tournaments. Nutrient timing helps you understand the principles to fuel your body well—and we give you plenty of examples and tips on planning for real-life athletics.

Essentially, the four most important aspects of sports performance are training, skill development, nutrition, and rest. One cannot make up for another. Training

Timing Tip

Nutrient timing transforms eating into a strategic component of your training, conditioning, and sports performance. By coordinating food intake at the right time with regard to your training, you will be able to take better advantage of the changes in body chemistry that occur with eating and exercise to help with muscle building; to maximize energy storage, which can help generate power and promote endurance; and to facilitate muscle recovery and keep you healthy throughout your training.

harder can't make up for a poor diet, and food can't take the place of appropriate rest. An athlete would never show up for practice without the appropriate gear (soccer cleats, baseball glove, hockey puck, lacrosse stick, and so on), so why would an athlete show up to practice or a game without the proper fuel? Athletes who realize that food is an integral part of training can benefit tremendously. Timing your food intake properly can provide

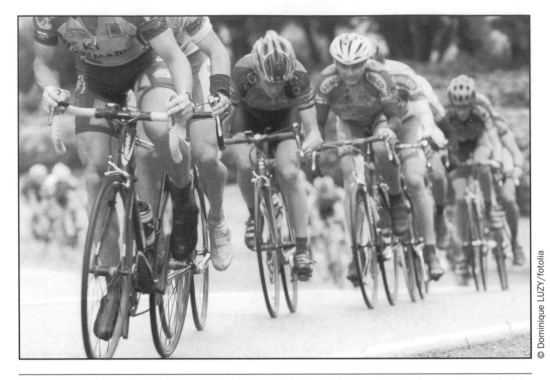

© Dominique LUZY/ fotolia

Whether competing or training for an endurance, stop-and-go, or power and strength sport, following the Nutrient Timing Principles (NTP) can help keep energy consistent.

sufficient energy, help you recover for your next practice or event, keep you strong and healthy, reduce muscle breakdown, aid in muscle building, and even promote hypertrophy (gaining size, not just strength), as well as reduce the risk of injury.

We also realize that for any nutrition plan to work, it has to be realistic and fit into your lifestyle. Athletes often have challenging schedules, and taking time to eat frequently takes a back seat to all of the other responsibilities in athletes' lives. We know that trying to balance training along with work, school, family, social commitments, and other interests or activities can be difficult. Meals can be missed or skipped, or eating gets delayed. Did you know that if you skip dinner, it can severely impact your training the following day? What you ate yesterday affects the energy you will have at the end of today's workout! Since it takes 24-48 hours to stock and restock the energy your muscles need to get the work done, there is a carry-over from one day to the next in terms of energy level. So many athletes tell us that they never thought of that! Are you aware that when you feel shaky during a run it's a sign of inadequate fueling to your central nervous system – which only runs on carbohydrate?

When there are long gaps without food, appetite and eating can become disconnected. Many athletes ask us why they can't stop eating at night—from recreational to college athletes and even some pros. It often happens when you're under-fueled during the day, and when the opportunity to eat presents itself, it's like a dam broke! And it's not all nutritious food that's consumed. In fact, when appetite runs amuck, most likely the foods consumed are done so more in a constant "grazing style," or with a ferocity that pretty much precludes either true enjoyment or sound decision making. It can become a vicious cycle if you overeat at night, awake still full, skip breakfast, and under-fuel again during the day. Having a plan in place and food available when you need it helps avoid these pitfalls. If your day is unstructured, put structure into it by planning the timing of meals and snacks. The best strategy for a practical plan that yields results acknowledges these very real time constraints. Our recommendations will keep this in mind. We will help you determine when to eat, what to optimize training and performance, and to understand how to put the science into real-life eating.

WHAT ARE THE BENEFITS OF NUTRIENT TIMING?

As mentioned earlier, there are several benefits of nutrient timing. These involve maximizing your body's response to exercise and use of nutrients. The Nutrient Timing Principles (NTP) help you do the following:

- Optimize fuel use so that you remain energized throughout your training
- Ensure that you repair and strengthen your muscles to the best of your genetic potential
- Ingest sufficient nutrients to keep you healthy and able to fight off infection, limiting the suppression of the immune system often experienced with intense training
- Recover from your training so that you are ready for your next practice, event, or training session with well-fueled muscles

Energy

When sports nutritionists talk about energy, we are referring to the potential energy food contains. Calories are potential energy to be used by muscles, tissues, and organs to fuel the task at hand. Much of the food we eat is not burned immediately for energy the minute it's consumed. Rather, our bodies digest, absorb, and prepare it so that it can give us the kind of energy we need, when we need it. We transform this potential energy differently for different tasks. How we convert potential energy into usable energy is based on what needs to get done and how well prepared our bodies are; how we fuel endurance work is different from how we fuel a short, intense run. Chapter 2 discusses the science behind energy, but first it is helpful to understand that you must get the food off your plate and into the right places in your body at the right time.

Clients consistently ask us, "What can I eat to give me energy?" For you, "energy" may have different meanings, depending on what you're referring to and how you're feeling. If you're talking about vitality, liveliness, get-up-and-go, then a number of things effect this: amount of sleep, hydration, medical conditions, medications, attitude, type of foods eaten, conditioning and appropriate rest days, and timing of meals and snacks. Food will help a lack of energy only if the problem is food related. You may think that's obvious, but it's not to some. If you're tired because you haven't slept enough, for instance, eating isn't going to give you energy. However, if your lack of energy is because you've eaten too little, your foods don't have "staying power," you go for too long without eating, or you don't time your meals and snacks ideally around practice or conditioning, then being strategic with food intake can help you feel more energetic. What, how much, and when you eat will affect your energy.

Nutrient timing combined with appropriate training maximizes the availability of the energy source you need to get the job done, helps ensure that you have fuel ready and available when you need it, and improves your energy-burning systems. You may believe that just eating when you are hungry is enough, and in some cases this may be true. But, many times, demands on time interfere with fueling or refueling, and it takes conscious

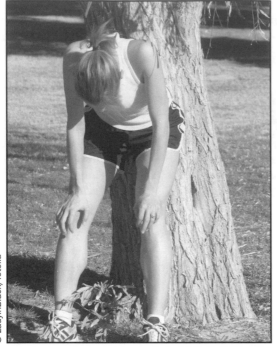

© LadyInBlack/fotolia

What, how much, and when you eat will affect your energy.

thought and action to make it happen. Additionally, appetites are thrown off by training, so you may not be hungry right after practice, but by not eating, you are starving while sitting at your desk in class or at work. Many athletes just don't know when and what to eat to optimize their energy stores.

By creating and following your own Nutrition Blueprint, as you will learn how to do in part III, and incorporating the NTP, your energy and hunger will be more manageable and consistent, whether you are training several times a week, daily, participating in two-a-days, or are in the midst of the competitive season.

Recovery

During the minutes and hours after exercise, your muscles are recovering from the work you just performed. The energy used and damage that occurred during exercise needs to be restored and repaired so that you are able to function at a high level at your next workout. Some of this damage is actually necessary to signal repair and growth, and it is this repair and growth that results in gained strength. However, some of the damage is purely negative and needs to be minimized or it will eventually impair health and performance. Providing the right nutrients, in the right amounts, at the right time can minimize this damage and restore energy in time for the next training session or competition.

The enzymes and hormones that help move nutrients into your muscles are most active right after exercise. Providing the appropriate nutrients at this crucial time helps to start the repair process. However, this is only one of the crucial times to help repair. Because of limitations in digestion, some nutrients, such as protein, need to be taken over time rather than *only* right after training, so ingesting protein throughout the day at regular intervals is a much better strategy for the body than ingesting a lot at one meal. Additionally, stored carbohydrate energy (glycogen and glucose) and lost fluids may take time to replace.

By replacing fuel that was burned and providing nutrients to muscle tissue, you can ensure that your body will repair muscle fibers and restore your energy reserves. If you train hard on a daily basis or train more than once a day, good recovery nutrition is absolutely vital so that your muscles are well stocked with energy. Most people think of recovery as the time right after exercise, which is partially correct, but how much you take in at subsequent intervals over 24 hours will ultimately determine your body's readiness to train or compete again.

Timing Tip

The right mix of nutrients taken just after exercise helps muscles recover, but nutrients must be consumed within the context of an overall well-designed training diet to be most effective.

Muscle Breakdown and Muscle Building

Nutrient timing capitalizes on minimizing muscle tissue breakdown that occurs during and after training and maximizing the muscle repair and building process that occurs afterwards. As you will learn in chapters 3 and 10, carbohydrate stored in muscles fuels weight training and protects against excessive tissue breakdown and soreness. Following training, during recovery, carbohydrate helps initiate hormonal changes that assist muscle building. Consuming protein and carbohydrate after training has been shown to help hypertrophy (adding size to your muscle). The proper amount and mix of nutrients taken at specific times enables your body to utilize them most efficiently—that's one of the Nutrient Timing Principles.

> ### Timing Tip
> Eating a small amount of protein, such as poultry, lean meats, fish, eggs, milk, or yogurt, with each meal and snack will help utilize it effectively for muscle building and repair.

Immunity

Nutrient timing can have a significant impact on immunity for athletes. Strenuous bouts of prolonged exercise have been shown to decrease immune function in athletes. Furthermore, it has been shown that exercising when muscles are depleted or low in carbohydrate stores (glycogen) diminishes the blood levels of many immune cells, allowing for invasion of viruses. In addition, exercising in a carbohydrate-depleted state causes a rise in stress hormones and other inflammatory molecules. The muscles, in need of fuel, also may compete with the immune system for amino acids. When carbohydrate is taken, particularly during longer-duration endurance training (two to three hours), the drop in immune cells is lessened, and the stress hormone and inflammatory markers are suppressed. Carbohydrate intake frees amino acids, allowing their use by the immune system. Carbohydrate intake during endurance training helps preserve immune function and prevent inflammation.

Certain vitamins and minerals also play a role in immunity: iron, zinc, and vitamins A, C, E, B_6, and B_{12}. However, excess intake of iron, zinc, and vitamins A, C, and E can have the opposite effect and in some cases impair the body's adaptation to training. An eating plan incorporating all of these nutrients in reasonable quantities, such as amounts found in food, can help athletes maintain immunity. The quality of the foods selected is very important and needs to be just as much of a priority as the focus on carbohydrate or protein, for example. For instance, eating a bagel for the carbohydrate but also including an orange for the vitamin C is important; drinking a protein shake can be helpful at the right time, but including some lean steak or shellfish for the iron and zinc is also essential.

Injury Prevention

Did you know that dehydration and low blood sugar can actually increase your risk of injury? Avoiding injury due to poor nutrition is absolutely within your control. Inadequate hydration results in fatigue and lack of concentration. Low blood sugar results in inadequate fueling to the brain and central nervous system. This leads to poor reaction time and slowness. Poor coordination as a result can lead to missteps, inattention, and injury.

Additionally, chronic energy drain (taking in fewer calories and nutrients than needed) will increase your risk of overuse injuries over time. Stress fractures are one example; poor tissue integrity can happen when athletes think solely about calories taken in but not the quality of the calories consumed. This is what is behind the phrase "overfed but undernourished." Eating lots of nutrient-poor foods will not provide your body with the building blocks for healthy tissues and overall repair. Inadequate protein will also hinder the rebuilding of damaged muscles during training. If muscles are not completely repaired, they will not be as strong as they could be and will not function optimally. The damaged muscle fibers can lead to soft-tissue injuries. Both protein and carbohydrate along with certain nutrients are needed to help with this repair. For instance, gummy bears may provide carbohydrate, but they don't contain any vitamin E, which is helpful in repairing soft-tissue damage that occurs daily during training. Therefore, the goal is both an appropriate quantity and an appropriate quality in food selection.

The case for nutrient timing has been made, and hopefully you are onboard. In the following chapters, you'll learn about the science behind NTP and how they are applied to athletes' diets by sport. By the end of the book, you'll have all the tools to create your own Nutrition Blueprint and menu plans. Whether you are training for endurance or competing in a sport requiring strength and power or in which intermittent bursts of activity are important, we will help you create an optimal fueling strategy based on the Nutrient Timing Principles.

The Science
Made Simple

Each movement your body makes is fueled by energy that originally comes from foods you've eaten. Whether the movements are small and almost effortless, like tapping your toe, or exhausting, like running a marathon, your body is fueling each action by releasing energy stored in cells for this exact purpose. When you eat, the energy, or calories, in food is digested and then converted and stored in your cells for later use. When you "burn calories," you are using energy to fuel movement or actions in your body. Every single body function—your heart beating, your lungs breathing, your liver and kidneys working—in addition to muscles contracting, requires energy. Nutrient timing is all about matching your energy intake—how, when, and what you eat—with how the body processes food and creates and uses energy. When implemented strategically, nutrient timing can enhance your performance.

To know what and when to eat, let's start with some basics such as how the body breaks down and uses the food we consume for energy, how muscles tap into this fuel, and what role hormones play in helping the body recognize when to use the fuel from food. By understanding these basic functions, we can then match our needs with the right foods at the appropriate time.

HOW OUR BODIES USE FOOD AS FUEL

Did you ever wonder what it is about that bagel or banana that gives your body energy? All foods have to be digested and metabolized (broken down into smaller particles) in order to provide nutrients and energy to your body. Nutrients provide fuel for your muscles to burn as well as play a role in hormone development, immune function, and in the case of protein, provide building blocks that are utilized to build and repair muscles and other structures inside your body. Because of the processes that each nutrient must go through, each provides energy and building blocks at different rates. Understanding how the body moves food from your mouth to your muscles is important when using the NTP. For now, let's focus on the fueling aspect of foods.

Digestion

When food is eaten, it goes through the process of digestion: Food is broken down into much smaller particles that our bodies can use. After you chew and swallow your food, it travels into your stomach where it becomes liquefied. Enzymes, or "helper" substances, break down the food into microscopic pieces, or molecules. As the now liquefied food leaves your stomach, it enters the small intestine. The particles from the food you ate are absorbed at specific points along your small intestine into your bloodstream. From there, the macronutrients, carbohydrate, protein, and fat travel to muscles and organs to be metabolized and converted into energy, which you will learn more about in the next section.

Just as words are made of different letters, food is made of different types of molecules. In the alphabet, we have either consonants or vowels; in food, we have three macronutrients: carbohydrate, protein, and fat; micronutrients, which include vitamins, minerals, and phytonutrients; fiber; and water. Together, they make up all the parts in food.

Carbohydrate

Carbohydrate is found in foods such as fruit, juices, milk, yogurt, grains, bread, pasta, rice, cereals, potatoes, beans, vegetables, and sweets. Regardless of which foods they originally came from, all carbohydrates are broken down into smaller particles called sugars. This is not to be confused with table sugar, though. This form of "sugar" is inside the body and is the simplest carbohydrate structure.

We'll get into more detail about carbohydrates in chapter 3, but for now it is important to know that all the sugars that make up carbohydrates are eventually turned into glucose, which is the universal source of energy for all our body tissues. Glucose is found in the bloodstream (about 5 grams, or 20 calories worth), where it is known as blood sugar; in the brain as fuel; and in muscle and liver, where it is stored for later use in a form called glycogen.

Some carbohydrate foods are broken down quickly and others take more time; some provide fuel only, while others are more nutrient rich. Before, during, and directly after training, quickly-digested carbohydrate is ideal to help with fueling; we are less concerned with nutrient content at this time. There are times when nutrient content overrides the simplicity of fuel only, which is generally at all other meals and snacks. Nutrient timing helps you select which carbohydrate-rich foods to eat and when in order to best provide fuel for the bloodstream, the liver, and the muscles (to stock and restore energy for when it is needed) and to keep the brain and nervous system focused and attuned to the task at hand.

Protein

Protein is found in eggs, beef, fish, chicken, turkey, pork, cheese, beans (especially soy), milk, yogurt, and to a lesser degrees, nuts. Proteins break down into many different molecules called amino acids, or what we call the "building blocks of protein." Just as building blocks can be put together into various formations or structures, there are 20 different amino acids that can form all kinds of proteins in the body. After proteins from food are consumed, they are broken down into amino acids and absorbed into the bloodstream. Most are transported to tissues where they are needed for a variety of functions including repairing or building muscles, forming bone, making new blood cells, growing hair or nails, among other things. Unlike carbohydrates, which are stored for later use, amino acids can't be stored in large amounts. Although certain amino acids can be burned for energy in the muscle or by being transformed into glucose inside the liver, the body prefers to use amino acids for growth, repair, and immune function as opposed to energy by muscle or organs.

Timing Tip

Smaller amounts of protein are digested and used more efficiently than one large amount. Eat small amounts of protein during each meal and snack rather than one large amount at once.

One of the important strategic aspects of Nutrient Timing is to consume the right amount of food at the right time. When it comes to taking in more protein than the body can digest, absorb, and utilize at one time, this is inefficient because you're unable to make good use of the amino acids. Imagine a football game if all the players went on the field at the same time—you can't utilize all the players. Since muscle-building and repair, as well as immune function and bone turnover, are 24-hour processes, protein consumed in small amounts at regular intervals is ideal. Protein as part of recovery is especially helpful to begin the process of reducing breakdown and promoting muscle building. This is just the start of the process. By continuing to consume protein as part of each meal and snack, you can maximize muscle building, minimize muscle breakdown, and help maintain a healthy immune system.

Fat

There seems to be such a knee-jerk reaction to just the word *fat*, but of course, we are talking about dietary fat, which is so essential for athletes. So let's be clear: Body fat and dietary fat are two very distinct entities. What role does dietary fat play? Dietary fat provides fuel and can also affect hormones, health, and a cascade of issues from inflammation to heart disease to bone structure. Fat is found in foods such as oils, butter, nuts, nut butter, salad dressing, mayonnaise, high-fat meats and dairy, most baked goods, ice cream, and fried foods to name a few. The types and amount of fat needed in the diet vary based on health history and activity level. As it relates to nutrient timing, fat consumption is imperative but best left for meals and snacks further away from training. That's because the digestion and usage of fat for energy is different than the other macronutrients.

Fats go through a number of steps in order to be digested and absorbed into the bloodstream. Fats remain in the stomach longer than carbohydrates, and proteins and take longer to enter the bloodstream because of their complicated digestion process. Because of the slow digestion of fat, it is not immediately available to provide energy to muscles, so it is not helpful to eat fat close to training. Once exercise begins, all digestion is slowed, and because fat remains in the stomach longer, it can actually interfere with performance if eaten in excess close to training. Importantly, more of the fat that supplies energy to muscles is either already stored in muscle tissue or is released from adipose (fat) cells.

As you will learn in chapter 5, any type of food—protein, carbohydrate, or fat—can be stored as body fat. We store fat in many places in our bodies: right below the skin, organs, and within muscle tissue. All body fat is potential energy that is stored and must be broken down into smaller particles in order to be burned.

One surprising fact that many athletes may not realize is that stored fat burns on a carbohydrate flame, so carbohydrates are even needed to burn fat as a fuel. Conditioning helps train your body to access and utilize stored fat to fuel the aerobic system, helping you to go longer without fatiguing. Carbohydrate availability will affect your ability to burn fat. We will look at whether one can or cannot manipulate nutrient timing to better access fat stores in Chapter 5.

Metabolism

Metabolism is the process by which you break down nutrients and utilize them to fuel bodily functions: It's the actual use of the nutrient. When you hear people ask, "Do I have a fast metabolism?" they are actually referring to the rate at which foods are broken down and utilized. Digestion can be thought of as the preparation stage, but the nutrient isn't metabolized until it is actually used or broken down further. Think about when you burn wood in a fireplace to supply heat. You may need to find a tree, chop it down, and cut it up into logs. All of these activities are the preparation steps, getting the wood ready to be used. This can be likened to digestion. But not until the wood is actually burned is heat produced and energy used. The logs are metabolized, or burned for energy.

If the potential fuel (wood logs) is not needed immediately, it may be stored for later use, just as we do with nutrients. When the body requires energy for any movement at all—even to breathe—fuel is metabolized, or broken down to supply the energy needed for muscle contraction. When food is metabolized and energy is released, a series of step-by-step chemical reactions occurs, changing the molecule of glucose, amino acid, or fatty acid at each stage along the way. This can take place inside your muscles, heart, liver, or anywhere in your body that uses energy. Your metabolic rate is the speed at which this conversion to energy occurs.

HOW OUR MUSCLES USE FOOD AS FUEL

Muscles store and use food as fuel in specific ways, and in addition, different types of muscle tissue are used for specific functions. Nutrient timing helps ensure muscles have adequate fuel available when needed.

Energy Systems

To use a laptop computer, for example, you might have to run it on a battery (which is stored energy) or plug it into the wall (which is a constant flow). Your muscles have similar systems. Muscles use two main systems to burn fuel and produce energy from the foods you've eaten. These are the anaerobic and aerobic systems.

Anaerobic System

Whether you need to bolt after a bus, steal a base, or run a 100-meter dash, your muscles need a quick burst of energy and power to contract. Working at a high intensity for a short time is fueled by the anaerobic system, which functions without having oxygen as part of the process. Of course, you will keep breathing, but the actual metabolic process of converting the stored energy into fuel happens so fast it does not utilize oxygen in the conversion. To create energy at this high intensity, the only fuel your muscles can use at this moment is glucose, which if you remember, comes from a carbohydrate-containing food or is converted from protein or fat, although these sources are less desirable. Nonetheless, the fuel must be glucose.

The glucose that is stored as glycogen in your muscles is extremely important to have—it's like the gas in a car. It is fuel waiting to be used when the car is in motion. If your gas tank is only partially filled, you won't be able to go as far. Glycogen inside muscles is broken back down to glucose to provide energy to the muscle fibers. Now, glucose must go through an involved step-by-step process where enzymes (the helper substances) cause the glucose to slightly change at each phase. This process of changing the glucose is called glycolysis.

The first part of glycolysis occurs without oxygen, so it's called anaerobic glycolysis. There are two subsets of this process: ATP-Cr System and Lactic Acid System. During some of the steps in the process, a by-product is released into the muscle. This by-product is *very* important because it is the true source of energy your muscles use to contract. It's called ATP, which stands for adenosine triphosphate. The true energy that your muscles use to contract comes from the breaking apart of the ATP molecule. For example, think of pricking a water balloon and how the water gushes out. ATP breakdown is the same—it's a gush of energy. This release or transfer of energy is what allows your muscles to contract. Creatine, a substance that is found in the muscle, helps recycle ATP after it provides the energy so that more energy can be created.

Timing Tip

All those hours spent conditioning will eventually pay off. As you become more fit, the body produces more glycogen-storing enzymes, and you are able to store more glycogen in your muscles. Essentially, your body anticipates an increased need for ready muscle fuel and adapts accordingly.

Just imagine working really hard, exerting a lot of energy. You're fueling your muscles by releasing a molecule of glucose from your glycogen store—and so you start to dip into your "energy savings." Say you take $1 from your savings and you spend part of it, and you get back some change from your dollar bill. You can spend that change for a little longer, but eventually you have only a few cents. All these little pennies can build up and take up space in your pocket without doing much good. Think of this as the lactic acid that is produced as a result of burning glucose at a high intensity. Lactic acid causes muscles to hurt, so you slow down or stop. By decreasing intensity, lactic acid can be converted into more fuel to burn. Thinking of the money example, if you take the time to count up all your pennies, you'll be able to spend them on something. If you want to spend more, you will need to withdraw more from your savings. This is how energy is generated in your muscles. The glucose molecule, as it is broken down or metabolized, gives off a little ATP to keep you going. The ATP stored in your muscles lasts only 8 to 10 seconds at most. The creatine helps recycle ATP for a little while, but once it's used up, more ATP must be created for your muscles to keep working. Burning stored carbohydrate is the only way to supply your muscles with ATP at this very high rate of exercise. You can't use fat to fuel this high intensity. It's similar to putting the wrong size batteries into a flashlight. They just won't provide energy. The bottom line is that high-intensity exercise is fueled by the breakdown of carbohydrate stored as glycogen in the muscles, which is then turned into glucose, and glucose gives off ATP, the bonds of which, when broken, provide energy for high-intensity work.

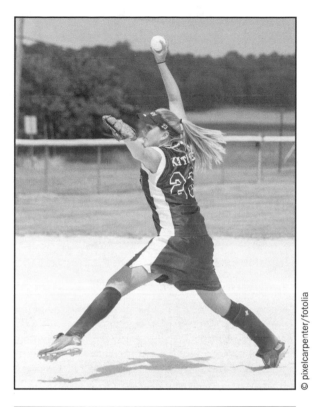

© pixelcarpenter/fotolia

Pitching in softball is an example of an anaerobic movement, using carbohydrate for fuel.

Aerobic System

How does the body provide energy for longer, endurance-based activity? Through the aerobic system. Assume you are training at a moderate pace, just as you would be when you are jogging, cycling, swimming, or rowing. This type of exercise uses the aerobic system to supply energy to your muscles, and it is called such because oxygen is used to help burn fuel. In this system, you do not work as intensely, but you can go for a longer time. Remember in the anaerobic system that there is a step-by-step process to create ATP energy? The process used to create energy during the aerobic system is also step by step, but in the end, it gives off a lot more ATP energy so you can work much longer, even though you have to work at a lower intensity.

Percent Contribution to Energy: Anaerobic and Aerobic

The following table shows the primary energy systems that are used for a variety of sports and athletic events. Notice that most activities rely on more than one system of energy for fuel. Those using primarily anaerobic metabolism are relying on glucose exclusively to fuel the short bursts of energy needed for muscle contraction. Aerobic training relies on a mix of carbohydrate, fat, and even some protein.

Event	Primary energy system used	PERCENTAGE OF SYSTEM USED	
		Anaerobic	Aerobic
100 m dash	Anaerobic	~100%	—
Fencing	Anaerobic	~100%	—
Golf swing	Anaerobic	95%	5%
Gymnastics	Anaerobic	95%	5%
200 m dash	Anaerobic	90%	10%
Ice hockey	Anaerobic	90%	10%
Volleyball	Anaerobic	85%	15%
Soccer	Anaerobic	80%	20%
Basketball	Anaerobic	80%	20%
400 m dash	Anaerobic	75%	25%
Tennis	Anaerobic	70%	30%
Squash	Anaerobic	60%	40%
800 m dash	Anaerobic	56%	44%
200 m swim	—	50%	50%
Boxing	—	50%	50%
2,000 m rowing	Aerobic	40%	60%
1.5K swim	Aerobic	30%	70%
1,500 m run	Aerobic	25%	75%
2 mi run	Aerobic	20%	80%
5,000 m run	Aerobic	12.5%	87.5%
Cross country run	Aerobic	10%	90%
10,000 m run	Aerobic	3%	97%
Marathon (26.2 mi; 42.2 km)	Aerobic	—	100%
Ultramarathon (50 mi; 80 km)	Aerobic	—	100%
24 h race	Aerobic	—	100%

Adapted from Fink, Burgoon, and Mikesky, 2009, p. 359; McArdle, Katch, and Katch, 2007, p. 173; Williams, 2005; and Foss and Keteyian, 2005.

Although some protein may contribute to your aerobic energy needs, fat and carbohydrate are the major fuel sources during aerobic metabolism. Fat is a very concentrated source of fuel but harder to get to than carbohydrate. The body is adept at storing fat—unlike today, in times of famine it was a means of survival. Fat must go through another step before it is ready to be burned for its ATP, so it takes longer. When a person is more fit and able to burn fat at higher intensities, it is because training helps the body adapt by producing more fat-burning enzymes.

Muscle Fibers

The amount and proportion of foods that you are going to need to fuel your muscles depend on the activity required in your sport and your size. Are your muscles working for a long time continuously, or in short powerful bursts, or perhaps a combination of the two? Muscles have specific fibers that are used for each type of activity, and each type of fiber uses fuel differently.

Muscle fibers fall into two main groups: Type I and Type II, with a few subgroups between them. The number and type of fibers that you

> ### Timing Tip
> Conditioning actually helps train your body to recruit and utilize the appropriate muscle fibers more quickly. Conditioning also enables muscle to store more energy and trains the enzymes responsible for releasing energy to do so more efficiently.

have are predominantly determined by genetics and play a role in which sports you are better suited for. Certain body types seem better suited for power and others for long distance. Slow-twitch muscle fibers, or Type I, contract more slowly and are better at working for longer periods of time. Oxidative (aerobic) metabolism fuels these fibers, which allows more energy to be provided for a long period of time. Cross-country skiing, distance running, and long-distance swimming or cycling are all activities where slow-twitch fibers predominate. Clearly, training and conditioning add to the fibers' ability to do their work.

If you are lifting weights, sprinting, swinging a bat or a racket, or heaving a shot, you are using more Type II, or fast-twitch, muscle fibers. They have the ability to contract quickly and provide a burst of energy. Anaerobic metabolism can last from 30 seconds to 2 minutes, utilizing glucose in the ATP-Cr System we learned about earlier, to fuel these fibers in short, intense bursts of activity.

HOW OUR BODIES KNOW WHEN TO USE FUEL

You may be wondering how the body knows what fuel to use when, especially during exercise. Hormones are a big part of the story and influence how our bodies utilize the foods we eat. Hormones are messenger-like substances produced by glands. Glands are cells, groups of cells, or organs inside the body that direct changes that need to happen in the body. The glands produce and send out hormones, which are the "messengers" that act on specific tissues. Some hormones regulate muscle building (anabolic); other hormones act to break down muscle tissue (catabolic). Also remember that not all breakdown is a bad thing. Breaking down is part of the building up process. It is part of the rejuvenation that gets rid of weak or old cells and proteins and replaces them with new and stronger ones. This reinforces the need to eat nutritious foods at regular intervals, providing the body with the materials it needs to get the job done. We need hormones in the right amounts to remain healthy and fit. Our unique hormonal systems regulate how we use the protein, fat, and carbohydrate from the foods we eat. Exercise can tweak our hormonal systems, helping us use food more efficiently.

Low-Carbohydrate Diets and Nutrient Timing

High-fat, low-fat, low-glycemic, DASH, Mediterranean, gluten-free, high-protein, no-sugar, low-carbohydrate. . . the list is long of popular diets out there. It can be confusing because all seem to make claims that are attractive and scientifically based. One important question to keep in mind when evaluating the efficacy of a popular diet is who the diet is intended for. Low-carbohydrate diets may in fact be beneficial for a sedentary, overweight person. However, for an active athlete who is engaging in a regular regime of conditioning, a low-carbohydrate diet can really sabotage best-intended efforts.

Paying attention to when you consume carbohydrate and which carbohydrate foods you consume makes sense for an athlete in training. A low-carbohydrate diet for most athletes (below 40%) does not make sense because it results in suboptimal energy stored in muscle and liver (as glycogen), which is necessary for both aerobic and anaerobic energy production in strength and power, endurance, and stop-and-go activities. The brain and central nervous system need glucose. If not provided through consuming carbohydrate, the body will resort to converting protein and fat for energy. When muscle glycogen is low, proteins are broken down and converted in the liver to supply glucose. Additionally, low glycogen levels cause a release of cortisol, resulting in more protein breakdown and immune system suppression. Fats also need some carbohydrate to burn completely; without them, ketones are formed in the blood, increasing blood acidity.

The absence or even low intake of carbohydrate can not only cause performance to suffer but also lead to injury. Since the central nervous system relies on glucose, coordination and concentration may suffer. Mood may be altered. Additionally, because of the increased muscle tissue breakdown and dehydrating effect of higher-protein diets, healing may be impaired. In metabolizing excess protein, the body excretes extra body water, so often the large weight loss seen when these diets are initiated is mostly fluid. If protein intake seems adequate but total calorie intake is excessively low, much of dietary protein will be burned for energy, and there will not be enough protein to repair the damaged tissue after exercise. It's kind of ironic that even with a proportionally high percentage of calories from protein, one may still not have enough protein available to repair muscle tissues.

Many popular diets proclaim that high-carbohydrate foods provoke an overproduction of insulin, which encourages fat storage. In truth, exercise makes your body more sensitive to the effects of insulin, so your body actually sends out just the right amount to properly handle the carbohydrate you eat. We *do* want to capitalize on the effects of insulin—it helps get the glucose and amino acids into your muscle cells, where they can provide fuel and repair muscle tissue appropriately. Athletes need the appropriate amount of carbohydrate based on their size and the intensity and length of training to stay well-fueled, maintain immune function, reduce risk of injury, and allow for tissue repair and muscle growth. Low-carbohydrate diets do not fit well with the principles of nutrient timing.

Our bodies are fine-tuned to act and react to ever-changing situations. Hormones work in an intricate way to signal hunger and fullness and the need to break down, repair, or build up. Anabolic, or muscle-building, hormones include testosterone, the somatomedins (growth hormone and insulin-like growth factor 1 [IGF-1]), and insulin. Catabolic hormones that break down tissue are glucagon, epinephrine, cortisol, and norepinephrine. We need both types of hormones to regulate and balance signaling within the body.

Testosterone

Testosterone is a hormone that is produced at a higher level in males than females. It has androgenic properties that are gender related, giving males their beards, deep voices, and other masculine features, and anabolic properties that aid in muscle building. Testosterone blocks cortisol receptors, so it has been thought to be anticatabolic (you will learn more about cortisol later). Exercise stimulates the release of testosterone, but the amount is variable between people and type and intensity of training. Dietary fat is required for the manufacture of testosterone. Dietary extremes, such as those too low in fat or too high in fat, have been shown to negatively affect testosterone.

The effect of nutrient timing on testosterone has shown that protein, carbohydrate, or a mixed meal eaten right after resistance training causes a drop in blood levels of testosterone. However, since it has been proven that protein and carbohydrate taken after exercise *increase* muscle building, it is thought that food may in some way help to move testosterone from the blood into muscle, but it is not known for sure at this time.

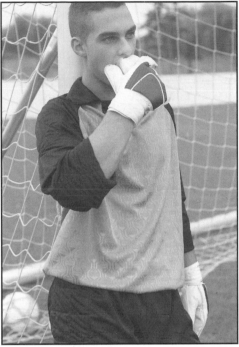

The hormonal system regulates how our bodies use the protein, fat, and carbohydrate from the foods we eat.

Growth Hormone

Growth hormone is an anabolic hormone, meaning it helps build tissues. It stimulates the release of insulin-like growth factor 1 (IGF-1) from the liver, which acts along with growth hormone. Growth hormone acts in two phases. The first is to promote muscle growth by increasing muscle uptake of amino acids and glucose, and it stimulates protein synthesis. The second phase acts on fat tissue to promote fat breakdown.

Growth hormone is stimulated by the hypothalamus in the brain, and many factors affect it: stress, sleep, age, gender, and other hormones. Interestingly, it is released in response to hunger and fasting, as well as after exercise. Sleep and dietary protein also stimulate its release—one more reason sleep is so important for athletes. When increased levels of free fatty acids are present in the blood, growth hormone is suppressed. Exercise seems to be a more potent stimulator of growth hormone than food. Dietary manipulation of growth hormone is not under our direct control.

IGF-1

Insulin-like growth factor 1 (IGF-1) is an anabolic hormone that is made in the liver and by many other tissues as well. It stimulates cell growth and protects against cell death. It acts on many cells of the body, including muscle, cartilage, and bone. It is stimulated by growth hormone and a high-protein or high-calorie intake. Since it is mediated by growth hormone, our dietary manipulation of this hormone is not directly under our control. IGF-1 is responsible for most of the effects of growth hormone on cells.

Insulin

After eating or drinking foods that contain carbohydrate, our blood glucose, or blood sugar, rises. As a result, sensors in the pancreas are stimulated to release insulin, which is considered to be an anabolic hormone, meaning that it builds tissue.

> ### Timing Tip
>
> Insulin inhibits fat burning. How? It works against the hormones and enzymes that are used to mobilize fat stores and metabolize them for energy. It is possible that grazing all day, which can stimulate insulin release, may be counterproductive to weight loss.

Insulin decreases protein breakdown, increases energy storage (glycogen and triglyceride synthesis, or the creation of stored energy from carbohydrate and fat), and increases amino acid (and glucose) uptake by muscle cells. The functions of insulin include the following:

Decreases blood sugar

Transports blood sugar (glucose) into muscle cells

Accelerates the conversion of glucose into glycogen in muscle cells

Helps to incorporate any extra glucose into adipose (fat) tissue (fat storing)

Stimulates protein synthesis (muscle building)

Inhibits the liver from releasing energy (glucose) into the bloodstream (because if insulin is present, then there is already glucose in the blood)

Insulin helps transport energy (glucose) from the blood into muscle and fat cells; interestingly, insulin is not needed to transport glucose into the liver—this is important because it allows our bodies to have an emergency supply of energy even in the absence of insulin. Once inside muscle tissue, energy (glucose) is stored as glycogen and is not released back into the bloodstream, which is why you can get low blood sugar, even if your muscles are stocked with energy, if you have gone too long without eating. The glycogen is used only when the muscle is working and energy is needed.

In addition to moving glucose into fat cells, insulin transports amino acids (proteins that have been broken down into building blocks) into muscle tissue, particularly in the presence of glucose. Maximizing the combination of protein with carbohydrate at specific times to stimulate insulin can be very important and helpful in providing muscle with the ingredients it needs to store energy and build tissue. Depending on when and what you eat, the pancreas will calibrate how much insulin to send out. During exercise, insulin levels drop because exercise helps muscle tissue become more sensitive to the effects of insulin. This means your body can get glucose into muscle, needing smaller amounts of insulin, or even by some other transporters that are called into play during exercise.

Glucagon

Glucagon is a hormone that is not released as a result of eating. Just the opposite, it is released when blood sugar is low, and the muscles are in need of energy. Although it is produced by the pancreas, just as insulin is, it works opposite insulin. Specific sensors in the pancreas detect when blood sugar (glucose) is low and initiate the release of glucagon. Glucagon's job then is to signal the liver. When the liver receives the message from glucagon, it releases some of its stored energy (glycogen) as glucose into the bloodstream, where it can be transported as energy where it is needed, especially for the brain and central nervous system.

Glucagon is considered to be a catabolic hormone—meaning it breaks tissue down. When it signals the liver for energy, the liver either releases glucose from glycogen or, if none is available, signals the breakdown of proteins or fats to make new glucose. The new glucose then is released into the bloodstream. Remember, hormones can also trigger signals of hunger. When energy is low, glucagon sends signals to let you know it is time to eat and to get some fuel into your system.

Epinephrine

Epinephrine and norepinephrine, referred to as the catecholamines, are made by the adrenal glands, which are located just above the kidneys and are responsible for making a number of hormones. Hormones work together, and some have somewhat distinct yet overlapping jobs. During high-intensity exercise, the catecholamines signal the muscles to use glycogen for fuel. If you're starting to run low on muscle glycogen, the catecholamines will act on the liver (similar to glucagon) to release glycogen as glucose into the bloodstream. But, they have other functions because they can also stimulate the release of free fatty acids from fat tissue (adipose tissue). Depending on which source of energy is needed where, epinephrine helps ensure that your muscles and brain have the fuel needed for you to keep going.

There are some more specific differences between glucagon, norepinephrine, and epinephrine. During exercise, norepinephrine is secreted at lower intensities, epinephrine at higher intensities. Another big difference is their relationship with insulin. At rest, after glucagon has done its job and blood glucose levels increase, glucagon subsides and allows insulin to be released. Epinephrine does not permit this—it keeps blocking insulin. That is partly because epinephrine also stimulates fat burning, and insulin inhibits fat burning. Epinephrine keeps our options open to be able to burn fat as fuel.

These hormones play a vital role in the release of energy from the food eaten in advance of exercise that has been digested and stored. Catabolic hormones such as the catecholamines can have important functions. They ensure that fuel is released to feed your muscles and brain, enabling you to keep going. As you will learn, there are times that we need to rely on stored energy and other times we need to supply new fuel as well. The principles of nutrient timing optimize the body's use of stored energy along with taking in additional fuel at strategic times.

Timing Tip

The stored energy in your liver is mostly used up while you are sleeping to fuel breathing, your heart, liver, and kidneys. If you exercise in the morning without fueling first, glucagon will be sending signals to get energy. Since liver stores of energy are low, your body's next stop is to burn protein and fat. Eating even 25 grams of carbohydrate can help you fuel your morning training without breaking down muscle mass to get it done.

Cortisol

Cortisol is another hormone that is produced by the adrenal glands and is often referred to as a stress hormone because it is produced under stressful situations. In terms of exercise, cortisol is usually active during prolonged exercise, which is perceived as a physical stressor to the body. In small amounts, it acts as an anti-inflammatory, helping to reduce the manufacture of cells that cause inflammation. It also helps ensure that you have fuel for your muscles, but when employed in this manner, its effects may not be ideal. That's because its main function is to break down proteins from all cells of the body into amino acids so that the liver can use them to manufacture glucose. Although moderate training boosts the production of immune cells, excess cortisol blocks the creation of some of these beneficial cells.

Cortisol works opposite insulin and also decreases protein formation (it is a catabolic hormone)—something you may not want to happen since most athletes work hard to gain strength and lean mass. Part of the process of building muscle is breaking down and repairing fibers, and with that repair and growth comes strength. Cortisol, however, is not involved in this aspect of breakdown and repair. Think of a house where you might want to replace old flooring. A carpenter comes in and takes off the old floor and replaces it

Immunity and Inflammation

Exercise can have a protective as well as a detrimental effect on immunity. Moderate training helps the body create immune cells that protect against viruses and other unwelcome invaders to the body. Excessive exercise, especially in combination with inadequate nutrition and fueling, can actually decrease our ability to fight off illness. It's been shown that an intake too low in protein or carbohydrate can greatly impair immunity. Numerous studies have shown that carbohydrate taken during exercise can prevent the decrease in immune cells that otherwise occurs when no fuel is taken. Adequate carbohydrate intake allows protein to be used for manufacture of immune cells and prevents the burning of protein for energy. Additionally, beginning exercise with adequate muscle glycogen stores reduces the excess release of cortisol. As we just discussed, cortisol causes muscle tissue breakdown and interferes with formation of immune cells. The timing of your carbohydrate intake can affect how much glycogen you are able to store, which can help protect against muscle breakdown and reduced immunity. Other nutrients play important roles in preventing inflammation, such as the balance between different types of dietary fat (see chapter 5). Certain plant chemicals, known as phytochemicals, influence the body's ability to deal with the effects of exercise and reduce the inflammatory response.

with new flooring. The result is a new and better floor. Now think of termites coming in and breaking down the new floor. Cortisol is more like the termites, not the carpenter. Cortisol is not part of the process of building and repairing muscle; it is only a part of breaking down healthy protein to use as fuel. Preferably, the body would not need to use cortisol to find fuel—the body would rather get fuel from the food you eat and the energy stored in muscle and liver. However, if these stores or blood levels run low and you are still trying to be active, fuel has to come from somewhere. Cortisol is called on to find fuel, and it does this by breaking down protein so it can be converted into glucose. The nutrient timing tips you will find throughout this book are designed to keep you stocked with energy and prevent damaging excess cortisol levels, helping you preserve your hard-earned lean mass.

The foods we eat can provide the fuel we need to train and perform all activities in all sports. Of course, the food needs to be digested, absorbed, and transported to where it's needed in order for it to become usable energy or useful for muscle repair. Even understanding how this occurs begins to give shape and form to when to eat what. The type of activity—sprint work or endurance work—will determine which muscle fibers are called into play. Muscle fibers have the capability to use foods for energy with or without oxygen, depending on how quickly or slowly they need to contract. This in turn determines which energy system is used and how much energy is generated and used up. Hormones help direct fuel use. By understanding the benefits and drawbacks of each, we can time our food in such a way to maximize benefits, such as energy storage and muscle building, and minimize negative effects, such as tissue breakdown.

THE
NUTRIENTS

3

Carbohydrates as the Primary Fuel

No other nutrient elicits the confusion and controversy that carbohydrates seem to in the eyes of the general public. Although some fad diets and dietary extremists shun this class of nutrient, carbohydrates serve vital functions both in sports performance and our overall health. In terms of athletic endeavors, carbohydrates are critical for optimal performance; they are the primary and preferred fuel of all muscle movement. For your brain and central nervous system, carbohydrates are indispensable.

Not everyone realizes the diverse food groups carbohydrates fit into. Here's a true story from Heidi: I was working with some rookie players and playing nutrition tic-tac-toe. We were down to the last square to win, and the question was "Name five carbohydrate sources." The opposing team was outraged; they claimed the question was a giveaway—everyone knows the answer to *that* question. The spokesperson for the team that was up replied, "Pasta." "Good," I said. "Spaghetti," he continued. "Noodles . . . macaroni . . . ziti." I had to give it to him for creativity! He is not alone. Many people, when asked to name carbohydrate sources, immediately go to bread and pasta, forgetting that carbohydrate crosses over food groups: breads, cereals, pasta, potatoes, rice, oats (all grains), fruits and juices, vegetables and vegetable juices, milk, yogurt, legumes (beans), and sweets. In short, carbohydrates provide energy, and most also provide nutrients and fiber to our diets. They can also help us feel full and satisfied from our food.

WHAT IS CARBOHYDRATE?

Complex or simple, processed or unprocessed, whole or refined? To understand which foods to consume when, let's take the first step in understanding which foods supply carbohydrates; what the terms *complex* and *simple* really mean; and in what way carbohydrates may be important for performance, health, and nutrient timing.

As the name implies, carbohydrates (carbo + hydrate) contain atoms of carbon, hydrogen, and oxygen. These atoms are arranged into individual molecules called monosaccharides, meaning single sugars. Single sugars are simple. There are three different monosaccharides: glucose, fructose, and galactose. Each sugar has the same number of carbon, hydrogen, and oxygen atoms; these atoms are just connected to one another a little differently. Glucose and fructose may exist as a single sugar, as in fruit. More often, the monosaccharides pair up to form disaccharides, meaning two sugars:

Sucrose = glucose + fructose

Sucrose is the substance that most people refer to as table sugar. Sucrose is also found in cane sugar, brown sugar, maple syrup, corn syrup, high-fructose corn syrup, molasses, and many fruits; of course, it is also added to many foods.

Lactose = glucose + galactose

Lactose is the carbohydrate form that is found in milk and dairy products (yogurt, cheese, sour cream, ice cream). People who have lactose intolerance lack the enzyme to break apart the glucose from the galactose and therefore cannot digest milk and other dairy products.

Maltose = glucose + glucose

Maltose is made up of two glucose molecules linked together. Maltose does not contribute a large amount of carbohydrate to one's diet. It is found in sprouted grains and the malt found in beer. Barley malt, a sweetener, also contains maltose.

Monosaccharides and disaccharides are simple sugars, or simple carbohydrates. Oligosaccharides, meaning a few sugars, are polymers, or chains of 2 to 20 sugar molecules. These are resistant to stomach acid and enzymes that digest other carbohydrate, so they travel through the digestive tract intact. The implication for athletes is that they are known to cause gas in some people because they are fermented in the large intestine. These may be found in foods such as Jerusalem artichokes, asparagus, barley, beans, garlic, leeks, onions, and rye. Obviously, these are not great foods to take in right before a workout or competition.

So what makes a carbohydrate complex? It is when many single sugars (single glucose molecules) link together to form a long chain, or a polysaccharide. Starch is a polysaccharide. So, starches are actually long chains of glucose. They are found in breads, cereals, pasta, grains, such as rice and oats, and vegetables, such as corn, peas, and potatoes.

It is very important to clarify here that the terms simple and complex carbohydrates may seem straightforward but are often used incorrectly and have created vast confusion around carbohydrates. All starches are complex carbohydrates, even if they are highly processed, such as white bread. The fact that a food is a complex carbohydrate does not influence, in and of itself, how quickly or slowly it is digested, nor does it speak to the food's nutritional value. Fruits are simple carbohydrates since they contain either mono- or disaccharides and yet are among the most nutrient-rich foods available. Table sugar (white sugar) on the other hand, another simple sugar, does not provide any nutrients, only calories. However, there *is* a nutritional difference between complex carbohydrates that are refined or highly processed versus whole grains and less processed foods. Let's talk a little more about this.

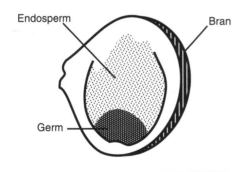

Figure 3.1   The three parts of a grain.

Reprinted, by permission, from L.W.Y. Cheung, H. Dart, S. Kalin, and S.L. Gortmaker, 2007, *Eat well & keep moving: An interdisciplinary curriculum for teaching upper elementary school nutrition and physical activity* (Champaign, IL: Human Kinetics), 584.

What is the difference between refined, enriched, and whole grains?

If you're confused as to the difference between refined, enriched, and whole grains, you're not alone. Grains are from plants that may be eaten as they are, made into flours used for breads and crackers, other baked goods, or made into cereals. The most well-known grains used in the United States are wheat, barley, rye, oats, and rice; less common are amaranth, buckwheat, kamut, millet, and quinoa, among others. All grains are made up of three sections: bran, germ, and endosperm (see figure 3.1), as follows:

- *Bran*. Bran is found in the outer layers of a grain. It contains most of the grain's fiber and some B vitamins.
- *Germ*. Germ is the nutrient-rich part of the grain. It's like the seed of a plant—it contains numer-

ous nutrients. Each grain's germ has a different array of nutrients, which underlies the importance of variety.

- *Endosperm*. Endosperm is the starchy inner part of a grain. Although not as rich as the germ in nutrients, it contains carbohydrates and a small amount of protein.

What do terms such as refined, enriched, and fortified mean?

All three parts of the plant are used in unprocessed, or whole-grain,

Timing Tip

On the Nutrition Facts portion of the food label of a carton of milk, you will see that 8 ounces (240 ml) of milk contains 12 grams of carbohydrate, and listed directly below this, the label shows 12 grams of sugars. All of the carbohydrate in milk consists of the simple sugar lactose (even though milk doesn't taste sweet). The sugars category on the Nutrition Facts lists the amount of simple sugar in a food, but makes no distinction between natural or added sugars. In the case of milk, there is no added sugar, so the 12 grams listed is actually the naturally-occurring lactose carbohydrate that comprises milk.

products. In *refined* products, the germ and bran layers are stripped away, and the flour is made primarily from the endosperm, or starchy part. For certain foods, this is desirable to create a specific taste or texture. Usually, wheat and rice are the most commonly refined grains (e.g., white rice is the result of refining brown rice; white bread and white flour, used in pancakes and baked goods, come from wheat). The result is the loss of most of the grain's fiber and a large proportion of its vitamins, minerals, and phytochemicals.

In the United States, all wheat flour (and much of the white rice) is *enriched*, which means that some of the nutrients that were removed during processing are added back in (but not necessarily in the amount that was initially present in the original form). By law, these five must be added: thiamin (vitamin B_1), riboflavin (vitamin B_2), niacin (vitamin B_3), iron, and folic acid. When you see the term *enriched wheat flour* as an ingredient in a food, that means it is refined wheat flour with some vitamins and minerals added back in. It is not worthless, as some people think, but neither is it as dense in nutrients as whole grains are. Additionally, because a refined food product is typically low in or absent of fiber, it tends not to have the same beneficial effects on stabilizing blood sugar and helping with satiety (feelings of fullness). *Fortified* foods have nutrients added that may not be naturally found in that food (e.g., adding calcium to orange juice).

Should I stay away from all processed foods?

People often think of processed foods as junk or not nutritious. This isn't necessarily true; processing merely makes a food ready for eating. For example, all flour used to make bread is processed (you can't really eat a stalk of wheat). Just because a food is processed does not mean it is inherently bad for you; it depends on what is added and what is taken out of the food. For example, potato chips and instant mashed potatoes have had all of the fiber removed that was originally found in the natural potato; the vitamin C might be destroyed in the processing, and a lot of sodium is added. So those processed foods are not as nutritious as the potato naturally is.

The main goal is for the majority of your intake to come from foods providing beneficial nutrients with less emphasis on foods that have had nutrients removed or unhealthy ingredients added. The training diet of athletes is best made up of mostly whole, unrefined foods that retain their nutrients and fiber. There may be some times when eating refined foods makes the most sense so that food is digested and energy can get to muscles quickly. Right before, during, and after training, we think of fueling more than nutrition. For all the rest of the meals, we think more about nourishing.

Timing Tip

The "gas" associated with eating higher-fiber food, such as beans, comes from the body's inability to break down all the sugars completely. By eating fiber-rich foods more frequently, the body manufactures more of the enzymes and healthy bacteria that digest and break down the sugars and fibers, resulting in less gas production. Athletes who are used to eating higher-fiber foods may experience less discomfort than a teammate who is not accustomed to consuming such foods. Just as you work other muscles in your body, your intestinal muscles need to be worked.

Why should athletes care about fiber content?

Fiber is a component of some carbohydrate-containing foods that cannot be digested or absorbed in our intestinal tracts. Fiber is present in two forms that act somewhat differently inside our bodies:

Insoluble fiber

Insoluble fiber is found in the outer layer of grains and gives plants their structure. Wheat bran is particularly high in insoluble fiber, as are nuts, broccoli, asparagus, carrots, and spinach. Insoluble fiber can't be dissolved in water, so it remains kind of bulky, can help you feel full, and helps alleviate constipation.

Soluble fiber

Soluble fiber can dissolve in water and add thickness or viscosity. When you make oatmeal, the white gummy part you see when you stir it is the soluble fiber. Other foods containing soluble fiber include barley, legumes (beans), citrus fruits, berries, apples, pears, broccoli (foods can contain both soluble and insoluble fibers), brussels sprouts, carrots, and potatoes. Soluble fiber is associated with lowering cholesterol, especially LDL, the "bad" cholesterol.

Fiber is an important part of our diets because it helps keep the intestinal tract healthy. High-fiber foods, which stay in the stomach longer, tend to slow digestion and release glucose into the bloodstream more slowly than do carbohydrates without fiber. Fruit may contain some soluble fiber and fructose, which delay digestion somewhat. Some athletes find fruits with higher soluble fiber don't sit as well with them as those with lower amounts. For example, a pear may not be as comfortable as, for instance, a ripe banana just before exercise. Meals with adequate naturally occurring fiber tend to help us feel full, tend to be nutrient rich, and tend to allow blood sugar levels to be more even, preventing spikes in insulin. In people who don't exercise, spikes in insulin are associated with arterial damage and increased risk for diabetes. However, athletes will use this knowledge to be strategic about when they want insulin levels to rise and when they might not.

What's the difference between getting my fiber from a pill or powder and getting it from food?

It's far better to get your fiber from foods rather than fiber pills and powders or even one large dose of a high-fiber cereal. That's because all the foods that contain fiber naturally provide vitamins, minerals, and numerous plant compounds, termed phytochemicals (Greek *phyto*, meaning plant). Phytochemicals are naturally occurring plant chemicals of which thousands exist in nature. You've probably heard of beta-carotene, and there are many, many more that work together to keep us healthy in terms of immunity and overall health. Often they are present in all plant foods and may be distinguished by their colors. Just as beta-carotene is found in orange produce, others are found in red, blue, yellow, purple, or white foods. That's why nutritionists often suggest picking your produce according to the rainbow, as shown in figure 3.2. Consuming a variety of these foods supplies a wide range of nutrients and fiber, whereas fiber pills or fiber-fortified food supply only fiber. Even fiber added to foods has not been proven to provide the same health benefits as those foods that inherently provide fiber.

FIGURE 3.2
Phytochemicals and their functions in foods

Color	Phytochemical	Foods	Functions
Red	Lycopene	Tomatoes, pink and red grapefruit, watermelon	Antibacterial and antifungal properties; antioxidant; protects cells against DNA damage
Red, blue, and purple	Anthocyanins	Apples, red peppers, blueberries, blackberries, plums, prunes, purple grapes, red cabbage, cherries, cranberries	Neutralizes reactive oxygen molecule; anti-inflammatory; reduces damage to DNA
Orange	Alpha- and beta-carotene	Apricots, cantaloupe, carrots, mangos, pumpkin, acorn and winter squash, sweet potato	Antioxidant; protects skin against sun damage; can be formed into vitamin A as needed
Yellow and orange	Limonoids	Yellow grapefruit, nectarines, oranges, tangerines, lemons, limes, all other citrus	Detoxes carcinogens from the liver
Yellow and green	Lutein and zeaxanthin	Avocado, yellow and green peppers, collard greens, corn, cucumber, green beans, honeydew melon, kiwi, peas, spinach, zucchini, mustard and turnip greens	Antioxidant needed for vision and prevention of age-related vision loss; prevention of sun-related skin damage; anti-inflammatory
Green	Indoles, sulforaphane, and isothiocyanate	Bok choy, broccoli, brussels sprouts, cabbage, cauliflower, kale, Swiss chard	Antioxidant; stimulates production of enzymes that detoxify carcinogens
White	Allicin and quercetin	Garlic, onion, shallots	Antioxidant; antimicrobial; cardiovascular health; possible anti-inflammatory

HOW OUR BODIES USE CARBOHYDRATE

Whether it is brown rice or gummy bears, all carbohydrate is digested into its simplest form and absorbed into the bloodstream as glucose. Both quick- and slow-digested carbohydrate take the same route, but they release glucose at different rates. Here's what happens to glucose after it is digested and absorbed into the bloodstream:

> Some remains in the bloodstream (about 5 grams, or 20 calories worth) as blood glucose (also known as blood sugar).
>
> Some is stored in your liver.
>
> Some goes to fuel the brain and other organs.
>
> Some goes to your muscles, where it is stored for later use (kind of like a rechargeable battery: We store it, use it, and restore it).

Stored glucose is called glycogen. When energy is needed by a muscle to contract, specific enzymes break glycogen back down into individual molecules of glucose (glucose to glycogen back to glucose for energy). The carbohydrate you may take right before training will "top off your tank," so to speak; the foods eaten in advance of exercise, say four hours or more, will have time to be digested, absorbed, and transported to your muscles, where they can be stored as glycogen. The other nutrients (vitamins, minerals, and phytonutrients) also have time to be absorbed. Muscles need a ready supply of glucose to contract, and it is readily available as stored glycogen in muscle tissue.

Did you know that when the body is at rest, carbohydrate is the *only* source of fuel for the brain and red blood cells? Muscles and other organs use some carbohydrate; however, they also use fat to fuel basic body functioning, but at a much slower rate than jogging, for example. Mostly, when at rest, we conserve carbohydrate stored as glycogen in muscles so that it's available as fuel when we need to run, jump, throw, hit—any movement that requires a burst of energy.

As the intensity of our movements increase, so does our reliance on carbohydrate to fuel muscle contractions. During lower-intensity exercise that may last a long time, when your muscles use oxygen to burn fuel (aerobic metabolism), such as race walking, cycling, cross country track, lap swimming, or rowing, a combination of carbohydrate, fat, and protein will provide the energy to allow muscle fibers to contract. During very high-intensity exercise involving short, powerful bursts of action, such as the 100-meter dash, a baseball pitch, or a bench press, carbohydrate (glucose) is the only fuel your muscles *can* use to contract.

As we describe in chapter 2, carbohydrates are stored as potential energy, or glycogen, in muscles and the liver and exist in the bloodstream as glucose (blood sugar). Initially during exercise, muscles rely on the glycogen stored within them. As the duration of exercise continues, muscles take up glucose (sugar) from the blood. The blood contains a very small amount of glucose at any one time. As it is used to fuel exercise, the liver releases some of its glycogen as glucose into the bloodstream so that blood glucose, also known as blood sugar, does not drop too low.

Since the body's stores of carbohydrate are extremely limited (we can store approximately 450 to 475 grams of carbohydrate), the timing of intake is very important for endurance and sports performance. In figure 3.3, we show how an average male stores energy, both glycogen and fat. As you can see, carbohydrate stores are much more limited than fat. If we need glucose for so many activities, why don't we store more? Each molecule of glucose requires three molecules of water, so glycogen takes up a lot of space. If we stored all our energy as glycogen, we'd be so heavy we couldn't move. However, if an athlete consumes a high-carbohydrate diet, his body will manufacture more glycogen-storing enzymes, meaning that the upper capacity for a very active athlete who consumes a high-carbohydrate diet could reach about twice the amount shown.

FIGURE 3.3
Where an average male stores energy

Body composition	
Height: 5 ft, 8.5 in (174 cm) Weight: 70 kg (154 lb) Lean body mass: 61.7 kg (88%) (136 lb) Muscle mass: 31.3 kg (44.7%) (69 lb)	
Body fat	**Glycogen**
Storage fat: 8.4 kg Essential fat: 2.1 kg (located in bone, spinal cord, brain and organs)	Muscle: 375 g (1,500 calories) Liver: 75-100 g (300-400 calories)
Total body fat = 94,500 calories	Total glycogen = 475 g or 1,900 calories (about the calories utilized during 18 mi [29 km] of running); Blood glucose is about 4.5-5 g (18-20 calories)

Body composition and body fat data adapted from McArdle, Katch, and Katch, 2008, pp. 400-401, and other sources.

HOW CARBOHYDRATE IS USED DURING EXERCISE

Carbohydrate is vital for optimal performance in all types of athletic pursuits. Strength and power, endurance, and stop-and-go athletes use carbohydrate for muscle contraction, to prevent excessive muscle damage, and to facilitate hormonal responses that aid in muscle repair. Strategic timing of carbohydrate intake—before, during, and after training—serve specific purposes. Since we've spoken about the different types of carbohydrate, we can now discuss which are best to have at specific times and why.

The Glycemic Index and the Glycemic Load of Foods

The glycemic index (GI) is a ranking of carbohydrate-containing foods in order of how quickly or slowly they raise blood glucose, or blood sugar, as compared to a standard food, such as white bread or pure glucose. To determine the GI, tests were performed that meaesured blood glucose two hours after the subjects ate one specific food in a quantity that amounted to 50 grams of carbohyrate. If their blood glucose went up exactly the same as it did for white bread, the test food had a GI of 100. If it went up half as much, the food had a GI of 50, and so forth. Foods are generally categorized as high, medium, or low on the glycemic index. Foods that have no carbohydrate will slow digestion, reducing the glycemic effect. So a well-rounded meal that includes fat, protein, and carbohydrate will have a much lower GI than carbohydrate consumed by itself. The main concept behind using the GI in sports nutrition is capitalizing on the *rate* blood glucose rises with regard to training and competition. It does not speak to the nutrient richness of a food.

The GI has a number of drawbacks. How your body responds to a particular food can be different from what the charts predict because of variance in rates of digestion and absorption. Other factors that change GI include the way a food is cooked (pasta al dente is lower than when cooked soft); particle size also makes a difference (instant oatmeal that is chopped up in small pieces is high and steel-cut oatmeal is low, yet both are whole grains). The ripeness of a fruit or vegetable can influence the rating, as can eating any food with something acidic—lemon juice and vinegar slow the digestion of carbohydrate, for example.

The most confusing part is that quantity makes no difference. For example, one jelly bean has the same GI as an entire bag of jelly beans, but obviously there is a difference in how much your blood sugar rises. To better address portion size, a more specific ranking was developed with regard to quantity: glycemic load (GL). GL reflects the expected increase in blood glucose taking portion size into consideration.

Probably the most useful application of GI is choosing what to eat before, during or immediately after activity. The general guideline is to select lower GI foods further in advance and higher GI foods immediately before, during, and immediately after exercise. When consuming carbohydrate alone, meaning not mixed in with a full meal of carbohydrate and protein, athletes can use GL to strategically select foods that can get right into the bloodstream, say, in between tennis matches or swim meets. See figure 3.4 for GI rankings for common foods. For a more complete list of both GI and GL, visit www.glycemicindex.com or www.mendosa.com.

FIGURE 3.4
GI ranking for common foods

High GI foods	Moderate GI foods	Low GI foods
White or whole-wheat bread	White or whole-wheat pasta	Apples
Bagels	Oatmeal	Plums
Corn Flakes	Sweet potatoes	Cherries
Crackers, all types	Peas	Pears
Rice cakes	Corn	Beans (lentils, navy, kidney)
White or brown rice	Oranges	Peanuts
White potatoes	Grapes	Milk (cow's)
Beets	Wild rice	Plain yogurt
Pancakes	Grapefruit	Barley
Raisins	Blackberries	All-Bran cereal
Watermelon	Corn tortilla	Soy milk
Bananas	Kiwi	Strawberries

Adapted from K.Foster-Powell, S.H.A. Holt, and J.C. Brand-Miller, 2002, "International table of glycemic index and glycemic load values: 2002," *American Journal of Clinical Nutrition* 76(1): 5-56.

Carbohydrate Before Exercise

Preexercise meals and snacks come at all different times. The *true* pregame meal begins 24 hours before competition, while "topping off the tank" happens within 15 minutes of taking the field, court, course, track, or water. Each presents its own set of recommendations and guidelines, and we will illustrate plenty of examples for each in part III of this book. The main intent of preexercise meals and snacks is to be sure you're well fueled before training and competition. But, it is equally important that you don't eat something that could *hurt* performance. This could include gastrointestinal problems (e.g., like eating spicy food that has the potential to "repeat").

However, do note that when considering the 15-minute window before a workout, paying more attention to the glycemic index makes more sense. This is when choosing pure carbohydrate foods only is practical. For strength and power, endurance and intermittent sports, such as soccer, hockey, football, basketball, rugby, and tennis, carbohydrate needs are important. Many of these sports require short high-intensity bursts of energy, which are fueled by carbohydrate. In soccer, Leatt and Jacobs (1989) found that taking in 35 grams of carbohydrate in a beverage 10 minutes before a soccer game and again at halftime resulted in a substantial (39 percent) *sparing* of muscle glycogen. Since glycogen levels have been shown to deplete rapidly in soccer, carbohydrate intake before, during, and after is a must. Although other sports haven't been studied as intensively, most stop-and-go sports are likely to benefit as well. In endurance training, Tomakidis and Karamanolis (2008) found runners lasted 12.8 percent longer with a preexercise carbohydrate beverage (1 g/kg body weight) taken 15 minutes prior with no additional fuel during.

Significant amounts of muscle glycogen are used during resistance training. Studies have found a decrease of glycogen content during multiple repetition schemes at moderate intensity, as are found during the hypertrophy phase of many weightlifting protocols. Carbohydrate consumed before resistance exercise can also influence muscle building by

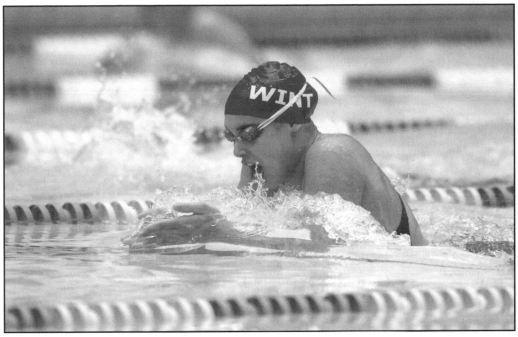

Consuming a mixed meal 3-4 hours before activity seems to be the best choice for fueling.

providing fuel to lift weight and by assisting with amino acid transport into the muscle, which is needed for muscle repair. This leads to increases in size (hypertrophy) and strength. Although some lactate may be recycled into glycogen during recovery, day after day of training without taking in enough carbohydrate can reduce glycogen stores significantly, compromising performance even over a one-week period. Starting out on day 2, you may feel fine with 50 to 60 percent of your glycogen stores, but that may drop down to 20 percent or less on your third day of training. That's why you may feel wiped out, and performance suffers. Taking in carbohydrate before training can help spare glycogen from being depleted and help you complete more exercise than if you consume nothing.

Additionally, carbohydrate elicits a release of insulin, and together these can improve hormonal effects. When insulin is present, and when glycogen stores are high, cortisol levels are reduced. Cortisol, a hormone that is released as a consequence of muscle contraction, contributes to muscle protein breakdown, and excess amounts are not desirable for muscle building. Insulin is an important anabolic hormone and can help prevent muscle tissue breakdown, limiting muscle damage during resistance exercise. If the food or beverage also contains protein or amino acids, insulin will facilitate their entry into muscle tissue, further enhancing muscle building. We will discuss this in greater detail in chapter 4.

Carbohydrate During Exercise

Carbohydrate intake during exercise has repeatedly been shown to improve performance in all types of exercise. Taking in carbohydrate while running or cycling, for example, has been shown to spare muscle glycogen because the muscles take up glucose from the blood and utilize it for fuel instead of using stored energy. Sparing glycogen is desirable because glycogen depletion causes fatigue, and saving it ensures that there is energy in reserve (e.g., for a sprint to the finish). For stop-and-go sports, taking in carbohydrate during helps

Carbohydrate Intake and Immunity Protection

Did you realize that something as simple as taking in carbohydrate during exercise may also help with immunity? Your immune system is a very complex network that the body deals with invading organisms that may be a threat to your well-being. Numerous substances made in the body use a variety of mechanisms to detect, attack, and destroy invaders that pose a threat to your health. Although it has been shown that moderate exercise has a positive influence on fighting off bacteria and viruses, continuous intense training can potentially have the opposite effect. For many athletes during intense training, multiple stressors can impair immunity: lack of sleep, mental stress, inadequate nutrition, weight loss, and inflammation from exercise.

In terms of nutrition and immune function, a number of factors may be involved; however, inadequate carbohydrate in particular can contribute to decreased immunity and increased possibility of getting sick. Lancaster et al (2005) found that taking in 30 to 60 grams of carbohydrate per hour during 2.5 hours of high-intensity cycling prevented the decline of an important virus-fighting substance, interferon-y. A number of other researchers found improved levels of various antibodies when carbohydrate was taken during exercise.

Hormonal changes that affect immunity are also influenced by carbohydrate intake. When exercising in a carbohydrate-depleted state, contracting muscle cells cause a release of cortisol, which was discussed in chapter 2. Although cortisol has anti-inflammatory effects, it also can suppress the immune system, and herein lies the reason we *want* to have carbohydrate during exercise. We want to avoid the negative consequences of excess cortisol: muscle tissue breakdown and suppression of the immune system. Carbohydrate consumption may also free up key amino acids to help with immune function.

This is an emerging area in exercise science, and much more has yet to be learned about the effects of carbohydrate on immunity. However, consuming carbohydrate during and after exercise seems to help lessen the suppression of immune function.

to preserve sports skills, timing, speed, concentration, acceleration and reduce risk of injury. For power sports, carbohydrate helps preseve protein. Even a mouth "rinse" with carbohydrate has shown to stimulate the central nervous system and improve performance (Chambers 2009).

So what type of carbohydrate is best to take in during training? Not just anything will do. Fructose by itself is known to cause stomach upset, particularly in sports where the body is jostled (like running, sprinting, jockeying, cheerleading), so it is not recommended to drink juice during workouts. Although juice is a great addition to any training diet, it is not a sports drink for consumption during an event. Although it is very common for athletes to eat orange slices at halftime, from high school all the way up to the pros, you won't see them drinking cartons of juice, and for good reason. Eight ounces (240 ml) of juice has twice as much fructose as a piece of fruit.

Timing Tip

It is important to include carbohydrate during the post woukout window. Carbohydrate does more than just restore energy; it also helps with immune function and decreases the amount of muscle breakdown.

Glucose is absorbed quickly, yet there is a limit to how much of any one single sugar the intestinal tract can absorb at a time. This is what we call "rate limited." Think of five lanes of traffic trying to enter a one-lane tunnel—it backs up. The same thing happens if you take in too much of one form of sugar during exercise. It will remain in your stomach or intestinal tract too long and can cause nausea or pain and discomfort, which of course impairs performance. All the carbohydrate that you think you are supplying to your muscles is not being absorbed at the rate you expect. A mixture of sugars is best. However, a similar situation can happen with beverages that are too concentrated, even if they are a mixture of sugars, such as soda. These are combinations of glucose and fructose, but they are so concentrated that they can cause stomach problems if you drink them too close to or during training.

The solution is at least twofold: (1) Consume a mixture of different sugars in less concentrated forms, and (2) consume smaller quantities more frequently than a large intake at once. Jentjens et al (2004 and 2006) have repeatedly shown that a mixture of carbohydrates (i.e., sugars) improves absorption and allows for greater energy availble for muscles to use than does glucose alone. Studies show athletes able to burn 78 grams carbohydrate per hour when taken from mixed sugars. If only glucose was taken, only 60 grams per hour was the maximal amount burned. Many studies done with glucose-sweetened beverages showed that athletes could absorb 1 gram of carbohydrate per minute, or 60 grams per hour. Later studies found that combinations of different sugars taken every 15 minutes allowed for the greatest amount of carbohydrate absorption—up to 78 grams per hour. That's why sports drinks usually contain a few different types of sugars. Although it's mainly recommended to keep carbohydrate intake during training to between 30 and 60 grams per hour, some athletes can tolerate more. Try experimenting to see what foods and beverages you tolerate during training. Solid foods stay in the stomach longer than liquids.

Carbohydrate After Exercise

Recovery begins as soon as you leave the field, court, river, beach, water, track, slopes—you get the idea. Everyone has heard about the three Rs in school. In sport, the three Rs are different: refuel, rehydrate, and rest. The intent behind the three Rs in sport is, at a minimum, to help the athlete be prepared for the next training session or competition, to reduce some of the muscular damage that occurs with intense training, and to help keep the immune system as strong as it can be.

Ensuring that muscles are well supplied with glycogen is one of the most important nutrition strategies that an athlete can easily focus on. If muscles lack carbohydrate, performance suffers—particularly high-intensity exercise. Feeding your muscles just after a workout is one of the best ways to prepare for your next workout. That's when the hormones and enzymes that are involved with storing glycogen are at their peak.

The first two hours after exercise is when you store glycogen at the fastest rate. Over time, you continue to store glycogen just at a slower rate. If your main goal is to restore energy, it's most effective to start with a high-GI food or beverage as soon as possible. Right after exercise, you quickly digest and absorb carbohydrates, which are swiftly delivered as glucose into your bloodstream. Insulin is very responsive at this time also, helping to get the glucose into your muscles for prompt storage, where the enzymes are primed to get going, just like your teammate in a relay race. All the players are pumped and ready to get the job done. As time goes on, these functions slow down. It can take up to 24 hours to fully replenish glycogen stores that have been depleted. If you have a couple of days in between workouts, timing is not as critical as long as you take in sufficient carbohydrate on a daily basis. However, if you are training hard the next day, or sooner, time is of the essence.

Both the timing and the type of carbohydrate you eat are important. After exhaustive exercise, glycogen is replaced at the rate of approximately 5 to 7 percent per hour, which means it could take 15-20 hours to replace glycogen. In the case of muscle damage or eccentric exercise where you are going against gravity, such as resistance training or running downhill, glycogen restores more slowly. For immediate recovery, consume high-GI carbohydrates in the amount of 1.0-1.5 g/kg body weight as soon as possible after exercise

Overreaching and Overtraining

Have you ever felt dead-legged, stale, just not into your training? Many factors can contribute to this—inadequate rest, excessive training, inadequate nutrition, and psychological and other stressors. Physically, inadequate caloric intake is the number one cause of "burnout." It is not uncommon, because of the demands of training, to skip meals and snacks. When in heavy training, it is easy to create an energy deficit, even without losing weight. This energy deficit can take a huge toll on the health and well-being of any athlete. From mood disturbances to hormonal imbalances to increased risk of stress fractures, eating too few calories over time is detrimental to performance and health.

Intense training combined with inadequate recovery in the shorter term is referred to as overreaching, and if it persists, overreaching turns into overtraining. Overreaching can typically be turned around relatively quickly, but overtraining can sideline you for a year or more. Overtraining can result in injury, but it can also create a chronic feeling of fatigue and depression. Hormonal systems may become unbalanced. Some athletes can become so emotionally drained and exhausted, they may lose their desire to train and compete. Training day in and day out without sufficient caloric intake fails to restore glycogen, and even over the course of a week, energy levels will progressively decline. It is difficult to restore glycogen to a fully stocked state every day. This is just one more reason to build in at least one rest day per week and organize training into hard and easy days. Over time, the strategies to ensure adequate fuel and rest keep you in the game.

and repeat in two hours. Paying attention to recovery nutrition just after exercise is one part of the athlete's needs; consuming enough total carbohydrate over the course of the day, based on body weight, training intensity, and duration, will ensure total recovery and adequate energy to meet daily training needs.

For athletes training more than once per day or competing in meets or tournaments, recovery between events is crucial. Performance is impaired in the second event if glycogen stores are inadequate. Even during play, between periods or halves, carbohydrate intake can mean the difference between winning and losing. Kirkendall (1993) found that soccer players who took a carbohydrate supplement during halftime engaged in 30 percent more running "at speed" during the second half. Muckle (1973) found that carbohydrate intake during soccer resulted in more goals scored and fewer conceded, especially in the second half. Without supplementation, there was a 20 to 50 percent reduction in the number of ball contacts and involvement in play occurring during the final 30 minutes. If time permits, have a high-GI carbohydrate snack of 1 gram per kilogram right after the first event and again two hours before the next event (see table 9.5 on page 110 to figure out how many grams you, specifically, would need). Again, depending up scheduling, additional snacks may be taken in between, immediately before, and during the second event.

Timing Tip

Recovery nutrition beginning in the first 15 minutes postexercise is essential to get a jump start on replenishing depleted muscles. Still, athletes need to eat at regular intervals after that to get in all the carbohydrate and nutrients needed in a 24-hour period.

Carbohydrate's Role in Resiliency

There is a difference between recovering from one training session to the next and having the resiliency to go day in and day out over a week, a month, a season, several seasons, a career. Resiliency refers to the athlete's ability to bounce back each day despite the wear and tear of training and competition.

Typically, when we talk about fueling or recovery nutrients, we focus on amounts of carbohydrate and protein but not so much on the quality of the food taken in. This is for good reason. For example, a white bagel with honey will be absorbed quicker and be easier to digest than a plateful of beans with spinach in tomato sauce. The bagel and honey are digested and absorbed quickly, supplying glucose to the muscles, so it is a good fuel source. However, it is not nutrient-rich and provides little for long-term sustenance.

Just before and right after exercise, it is important to have glucose readily available to muscle without having food to interfere with performance by remaining in the stomach too long. The beans with spinach and tomato sauce, while nutrient rich, would take longer to digest because of the fiber and protein in the beans. The acidity of the tomato sauce could cause some athletes discomfort, and if spicy, might even repeat on them. Obviously, athletes intuitively would choose the bagel over the beans before a workout or a practice. But too often, even at meal times hours away from practice or training, we see athletes choose quick and easy foods that are lacking in nutrients. The bean dish will provide the body with carbohydrate as the bagel does, but it also will provide lutein, vitamin C, B vitamins, iron, potassium, lycopene, and protein (the list is long). Clearly it is healthier than a bagel with honey, even though a bagel with honey has its place in a training diet. For short-term fueling or recovery, go with the bagel. For long-term resiliency, choose dishes like the beans and spinach that provide your body with an array of nutrients to keep you healthy and strong.

Long-term resiliency requires high-quality, nutrient-rich food intake to provide tissues and bones the nutrients they need for repair and the immune function nutrients to thrive on. Unprocessed or minimally processed carbohydrate will restore muscle glycogen stores and fuel other systems in the body, such as immune function, over time. So we care about nutrient quality at most meals and snacks—we just don't emphasize it around the time of activity. At that time, we are more concerned about fuel.

C H A P T E R

4

The Protein Profile

Did you know the word *protein* comes from late Greek, meaning "of the first quality," as it was believed to be essential for life? The ancient Greeks were right. Protein certainly is essential for life. Protein has been a topic of interest to athletes, seemingly forever. Will a high-protein diet enhance performance? Increase strength? We will investigate all the current and most relevant evidence, regarding protein; help you understand the truths and myths surrounding this nutrient; and help you determine the ideal protein intake in the optimal amounts at the right time to help with muscle repair and building, hypertrophy, immune function, and performance.

WHAT IS PROTEIN?

Protein forms a wide range of structures in the body and plays a crucial role in a number of body functions. Protein accounts for 15 to 20 percent of the body, and it is not all found in muscle, as you might initially assume. Only 15 to 20 percent of your muscles are made of protein—the rest is water, stored carbohydrate, fat, and minerals. One pound (.5 kg) of muscle contains only 2.4 to 3.2 ounces of protein. Proteins comprise other structures in the body including muscles of the heart, GI tract, eyes; tendons and ligaments, collagen, and forms skin, hair, and nails. Proteins are part of metabolic, hormonal, immune, and transport systems. They carry out these vital functions:

- Form red blood cells, known as hemoglobin, which transports oxygen in blood, and myoglobin, which transports oxygen in muscles.
- Form hormones, which are substances that cause an effect or change the activity of another cell.
- Create enzymes, which are "helper" substances that cause or help a chemical reaction to take place, including metabolism, and the storage and usage of dietary carbohydrate, protein, and fat.
- Help regulate fluid balance by directing where fluids are kept inside the body. Proteins serve as a pump that moves particles into or out of a cell, and fluid then follows.
- Regulate the acid and base quality of body fluids. For example if a fluid, such as blood, becomes more alkaline or acidic than the body tolerates, proteins may be used as a buffer to bring the pH to the required level.
- Create antibodies, which are substances that attack invaders in our bodies, thereby helping the immune system.

Let's see how the proteins in our body are created from the dietary protein that we consume from food. Dietary proteins are digested and broken down into their component parts, amino acids. These amino acids are then put back together by and within our bodies, just like pieces of a puzzle, to create different proteins our bodies need to function—the structural or functional proteins we just described.

Timing Tip

Protein is necessary for growth during infancy and childhood. Once growth stabilizes, proteins in the body turn over, meaning some are broken down (degraded) and rebuilt, which is required to rid the body of older, worn out protein and rebuild newer, stronger, healthier protein. It's like a never-ending remodeling project. Our bodies need a constant supply of dietary protein to remain healthy.

All proteins are made up of amino acids. They are molecules, or building blocks, composed of carbon, hydrogen, oxygen, nitrogen, and occasionally sulfur. At one end is an "amine," which contains nitrogen, and at the other is an "acid," hence the name, amino acid. If the body doesn't need some of the amino acids, such as when we eat too much protein, the nitrogen-containing amine can be removed and formed into urine, leaving the middle part of amino acids, which contains molecules similar to carbohydrates. There are 20 different amino acids in nature, and they combine in various ways to form the different proteins needed by the body. In addition, three amino acids have side chains that look like a branch, so they're called branched-chain amino acids (BCAAs). The three branched-chain amino acids are leucine, isoleucine, and valine. While the other amino acids are metabolized in the liver, the branched-chain amino acids bypass the liver and go straight to the perphery (i.e., muscles located away from the core). BCAAs can be used as an energy source or for repair, maintenance, or building of muscle tissue.

HOW OUR BODIES USE PROTEIN

The body doesn't have a large storage depot for protein, as it does for carbohydrate and fat. The protein we eat from food has to be handled as we eat it. Like rookies sitting on the bench waiting for their chance to play, the amino acids in the pool are ready and waiting to be utilized. Either the amino acids are used within a limited time to build a body protein, or they are transformed.

If amino acids in the pool aren't needed to become a protein, the body is equipped to reconfigure them either back to glucose to be used as energy or into fat. To transform an amino acid, the liver strips off the nitrogen, which may then be incorporated into DNA, RNA, or a nonessential amino acid. Excess nitrogen may also be incorporated into urea, or ammonia, both of which are excreted in the urine. In order to eliminate these, water is needed, so a high protein intake can result in excess fluid loss. The remaining part of the stripped-down amino acid may be reconfigured into glucose, and it is burned for energy.

How much protein do we need?

As you can see, our bodies can do a lot of things with the protein we eat. The recommended dietary allowance (RDA) for protein for people over the age of 18 is not a huge amount—.8 gram per kilogram or .36 gram per pound. For younger people who are still growing, ages 4 to 13, it's .95 gram per kilogram or .43 gram per pound; and for ages 14 to 18, it's .85 gram per kilogram or .39 gram per pound. These amounts represent the average daily dietary intake level sufficient to meet the nutrient requirements of about 97 percent of people in these age groups. However, athletes need more.

How much protein should be recommended is a hotly debated subject among some because, although the previous recommendations will supposedly maintain health, they do not necessarily represent the *optimal* intake or cover the needs of an athlete in training. Muscle damage does occur as a result of exercise, and additional protein is needed for repairing tissue. Optimal protein intake for athletes not only maintains health but also supports muscle growth, preserves bone integrity, and in certain instances helps with weight management. The type and intensity of training, duration, frequency, your fitness

Essential and Nonessential Amino Acids

Of the 20 amino acids, we must get 9 of them through food because our bodies do not make them. We call these essential, or indispensable, amino acids. The other 11 nonessential, or dispensable, amino acids are present in food but can also be made inside the body. Here is a breakdown of the essential and nonessential amino acids:

Essential amino acids	Nonessential amino acids
Histidine	Alanine
Isoleucine	Arginine
Leucine	Asparagine
Lysine	Aspartic acid
Methionine	Cysteine
Phenylalanine	Glutamic acid
Threonine	Glutamine
Tryptophan	Glycine
Valine	Proline
	Serine
	Tyrosine

Foods that contain all the essential amino acids in the proportions we need for creating structural or functional proteins in the body are called *complete* proteins. Any protein that is derived from an animal source is a complete protein. Plant foods also contain amino acids, but the only complete plant protein is soy; the others have insufficient levels of one or more amino acids (i.e., they are incomplete). They still contribute to our protein needs, and you may meet your protein requirements without animal foods (as vegetarians can and do with proper planning); however, a variety of plant food proteins need to be ingested so that the incomplete proteins, when combined, can provide all the essential amino acids. An example of an incomplete protein is the kidney bean. It is low in methionine. It just so happens that rice, a food commonly eaten with beans, contributes enough methionine to form a complete protein. You do not necessarily have to eat them together, as once thought. The body breaks down dietary protein and creates an amino acid "pool" inside the body. As long as all essential amino acids are consumed within a 24-hour period, the body will pull amino acids from the pool to create structural or functional proteins as needed.

See the following chart for food combinations that make up complete proteins. Over the course of a day, vegetarians do need to eat foods that will provide all the amino acids so that their bodies can create proteins as needed. Grains combined with legumes (beans) form complete proteins, as do grains and dairy and legumes and seeds/nuts. Although dairy foods are complete proteins, they also contain extra amino acids to complete the missing amino acids in grains.

Grains and legumes	Rice and beans, pea soup and whole-grain crackers, peanut butter sandwich, pasta fagioli soup (pasta and beans), vegetarian chili and rice, hummus (chickpea spread) and pita bread, pinto beans and corn bread, couscous and black beans, tortilla chips and chili, black bean soup and a whole-grain roll, lentil curry and rice, lentils and bulgur, tortillas and refried beans
Grains and dairy	Cereal and milk, oatmeal and milk, granola and yogurt, macaroni and cheese, pasta with cheese, grilled cheese sandwich, cheese ravioli or tortellini, graham crackers and milk, cheese and crackers, cottage cheese on toast, yogurt and wheat germ
Legumes and seeds/nuts	Salad with kidney beans, slivered almonds, and sunflower seeds; lentil soup with walnut loaf; trail mix including cashews, walnuts, chickpeas and tanini (sesame paste), almonds, sunflower seeds, pumpkin seeds, and peanuts

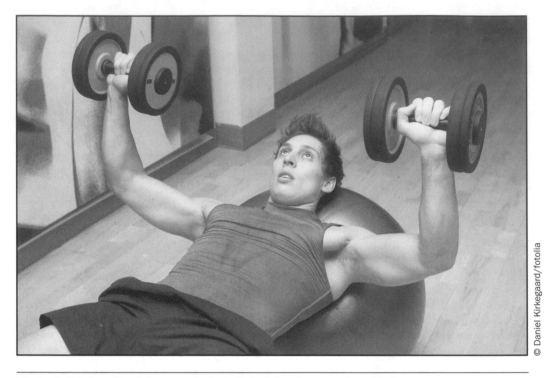

© Daniel Kirkegaard/fotolia

Strategic intake of protein around strength training improves lean body mass.

level, and your weight will all be considered when determining your protein needs (we will discuss this in more detail later).

What happens with excess protein intake?

Athletes do need more protein than their sedentary counterparts, but there still is a limit to how much can be used. Often when people consume excess protein, the ammonia formed as a by-product of protein metabolism cannot be eliminated through urine. So it is lost in sweat. If your sweat has an ammonia odor, your protein intake may be higher than your body needs. In healthy people, the body will employ protective mechanisms so that ammonia doesn't build up to toxic levels. The rate that food leaves the stomach slows as a way to try to protect the body from ammonia overload. That's why very high protein intake can sometimes make people feel nauseated.

Additionally, staying hydrated is a challenge for many athletes, and an excessive amount of protein intake requires fluid to break down amino acids and rid the body of nitrogen. If protein is consumed too close to practice, there is an increased demand for oxygen by working muscles and organs that process protein. In research published in the *British Journal of Sports Medicine* (Wiles, 1991), subjects thought the exercise was harder one hour after having a high-protein meal compared with those having only water; their Rate of Perceived Exertion (RPE) was higher. If your protein intake is very high, it is also likely that you are not taking in adequate carbohydrate, which will negatively affect performance. As is the case with many nutrients, too much of one can displace enough of another and cause imbalances. Power athletes can handle a lower percentage of calories coming from carbohydrate (as low as 42 percent, perhaps, although not necessarily ideal); however, some power athletes eat protein almost exclusively. The main point is that while athletes do need more protein than inactive people, excessive amounts can hurt performance.

How much protein can our bodies use?

Our bodies cannot use more than about 2 or 2.5 grams per kilogram of protein per day efficiently and may need less (1.6-1.8 g/kg). According to Robert Wolfe, PhD, a clinical investigator and noted protein expert, the maximal effective dose of protein at one time to support muscle repair, maintenance, and growth is between 20-35 grams of high-quality protein, such as found in animal-based proteins. This would amount to about 3-5 ounces (150 grams) of meat, poultry, or fish and contain approximately 9-15 grams of essential amino acids. Note that a 3-ounce (90 grams) serving of meat or poultry is about the size of a deck of cards—it is certainly not uncommon for athletes to consume portions much greater than this at each meal. Many commercially prepared protein drinks and mixes provide 40 or more grams of protein per serving and are often too low in carbohydrate for adequate fuel or recovery. Realize that for muscle building, it is absolutely essential to have a positive caloric intake and perform lots of hard work. Rasmussen et al (2000) showed that significant urea was produced when 40 grams of whey protein was ingested at once, indicating it wasn't entirely taken up by the body. We will show you many examples of better recovery options in part III beginning on page 101.

Consensus in the sport science field recommends that protein needs be determined by weight, not percentage of calories. As your caloric needs increase, so, too, do your carbohydrate needs to provide fuel for the greater physical output. Endurance, strength and power, and stop-and-go athletes appear to need 1.2 to 1.8 grams of protein per kilogram of body weight. We will show you in part III, when you formulate your Nutrition Blueprint, how to determine the right amount of protein you need, depending on your sport, your size, and whether you are trying to change your body composition.

How quickly do our bodies absorb protein?

Absorption rates vary for different types of protein. The digestive tract permits only a certain amount of amino acids to enter the bloodstream at a time, which varies by protein source. For example, many athletes find that eggs seem to keep them very full when eaten for breakfast. This is because on average, we absorb only 2.8 grams of cooked egg protein per hour (one egg has 6 grams of protein, so it would take four hours to digest and absorb two eggs).

Many athletes think that the fastest absorbed proteins are the best; however, that may not be the case. Muscle protein breakdown occurs for a time after exercise is over, and so does muscle repair. As a matter of fact, initial muscle repair may continue for 24 to 48 hours postexercise. The time-release quality of some proteins is very helpful because although muscle protein breakdown is necessary, excessive amounts may take away from positive protein balance. By consuming a mixture of proteins, both slow-acting and fast-acting amino acids are available for muscle repair. Of course, real gains in muscle size and strength occur over time with persistent resistance training and nutrition.

> **Timing Tip**
>
> Eating foods with varying absorption rates can be very helpful as the window for nutrient intake doesn't close. In fact, continued nutrition every few hours is equally important. If the postworkout window is missed, all is not lost. Make sure you eat small amounts of protein along with carbohydrate and fat at each meal, and snack to maximize protein absorption and muscle building and repair.

Are certain types of protein better than others?

Protein quality refers to how well the amino acid makeup of the food fits into the pattern needed by our bodies to contribute to growth, repair, and maintenance. Different systems have been established that rate how well proteins from various sources are digested and used inside the body. The one adopted by the Food and Agriculture Organization/World Health Organization (FAO/WHO) and frequently referred to is called the Protein Digestibility-Corrected Amino Acid Score (PDCAAS). It takes into account digestibility and how well the food supplies all nine essential amino acids. It ranks cow's milk and egg protein the highest with beef and soy following closely after. Another assessment of protein quality is biological value, which estimates how the food contributes to our overall nitrogen balance—an indicator of how well the body uses the food. Foods of high biological value include eggs, milk, soy, meat, poultry, and fish, for example.

It is important to obtain protein from a variety of foods. Including animal-based proteins ensures that you will take in all the essential amino acids and not have to worry about individual amino acid needs. However, if being vegetarian is important to you, be sure to seek out the correct information to determine how to meet your protein needs. Often, vegetarian athletes may need more protein to make up for the missing essential amino acids abundant in animal protein sources.

HOW PROTEIN IS USED DURING EXERCISE

Let's use all the protein basics we just covered and apply them to how and when our bodies need protein when you are training. If you are engaged in endurance training or stop-and-go sports, your protein needs will be different from when you are engaged in resistance training.

Protein During Endurance Training

During prolonged endurance exercise, muscles take up amino acids from the bloodstream to become part of a pool of individual amino acids within muscle tissue. It has been shown that when carbohydrate stores are low, muscle tissue may burn amino acids for energy, especially the BCAAs, and usually more leucine than isoleucine or valine.

This discovery raised interest in a possible benefit of BCAAs as an aid in performance to provide an additional source of fuel to working muscles. When carbohydrate stores are low, muscles rely on alternate sources of fuel—fat and/or protein. When there are many steps in a process, if one step is delayed or does not work, the whole process slows down or stops (we call this "rate limited"). In the case of supplying BCAAs to muscle as fuel, the limiting factor is the enzymes needed to burn BCAAs for energy. Muscles don't have a lot of these enzymes, so this slows the rate that BCAAs can supply energy to muscles. Just taking more of the amino acids doesn't guarantee that they will be used in the body as you intended. In this case, the *rate* at which they can be burned is *limited* by the fact that there aren't enough enzymes to help use these amino acids.

If adequate carbohydrate is present, then there is less demand for converting protein into fuel. Is there any reason to take in protein during endurance training? Let's investigate a bit further by answering a few common questions.

Can protein intake during exercise improve stamina?

There are a few studies that looked at the inclusion of protein in a sports drink on time to fatigue. Studies show that when enough carbohydrate is present, adding protein provides no benefit to speed or endurance. Protein alone does not seem to enable endurance athletes to improve performance by going faster or longer before fatigue sets in.

However, one study that showed a positive outcome of protein intake during exercise had a major flaw: The caloric level provided in the protein drink was higher than either the carbohydrate-only or placebo drink. So the result in this one study, that protein did limit fatigue, may be attributed to a higher caloric level versus protein's presence. Additionally, Ivy (2003) pointed out that the better stamina experienced when protein or amino acids are added to a carbohydrate beverage consumed during activity may be an entirely different

Protein Supplements: Does It Matter Which You Take?

Sometimes in light of convenience and appropriate timing, athletes prefer to take some of their protein in the form of a supplement or shake. Protein supplements are usually in the form of whey, casein, soy, or albumen (egg protein) in powders, mixes, or bars. So, which should you take when?

Whey

Whey protein is found in milk. It may be present as whey protein isolate (the highest form of whey protein), which is 90 percent or more protein and contains very little else (typically lactose free), or as whey protein concentrate, which is 29 to 89 percent protein and contains lactose and fat.

Whey protein is considered a fast protein in that it is digested and absorbed quickly. Its amino acids are delivered to muscle tissues—more specifically, peripheral muscle tissues, meaning those away from the center of the body. Leucine, a BCAA found in whey protein, may also be burned for energy if need be.

Casein

Casein is the other protein found in milk. Casein is a slow-digesting protein. It helps prevent muscle protein breakdown, which results in retaining muscle mass. When whey and casein are used together, muscle building and a lessening of protein breakdown occur.

Both casein and whey protein may be hydrolyzed (partially broken down), which helps them to dissolve better when mixed in liquids. Hydrolyzed casein reduces its ability to prevent muscle protein breakdown. Before buying, look at the labels to ensure that the protein powder being used is *not* hydrolyzed casein. Casein and whey are best taken together. Nonfat dry milk is a great, low cost substitute for high price protein powders.

Soy Protein

Soy protein isolate is a powder that is 90 percent protein; most of the fat and carbohydrate have been removed. Soy protein concentrate is only 70 percent protein and about 23 percent fiber, which may cause stomach discomfort if taken before training. When soy protein is compared to whey protein (both are considered fast proteins), studies have shown that both may contribute to increases in lean body mass. When soy is compared to milk, which contains both casein and whey, milk leads to greater increases in lean body mass, possibly because casein protects against muscle protein breakdown. The net effect is a greater increase in muscle protein synthesis with milk than with soy, although soy is still effective.

Albumen

Albumen, the protein found in egg, is a complete protein and among the most digestible. Eggs are high in the BCAA leucine and provide an excellent source of protein for incorporation into muscle tissue. Albumen is not usually found on its own. It is often incorporated into bars along with other sources of protein.

mechanism driving the improvement in performance. Some of the breakdown products of protein can actually be taken up and used during the carbohydrate metabolism process that produces all the ATP energy, providing more fuel to the muscles.

Very little science has been done on protein or amino acid inclusion in a sports drink. There are no definitive recommendations at this time. The challenge remains in creating a drink that is palatable, will not slow gastric emptying or interfere with hydration, and provides a performance edge.

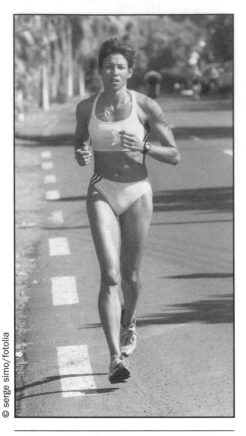

© serge simo/fotolia

Endurance athletes can reduce muscle soreness by adding protein to their post-training recovery snack.

Can protein help prevent muscle damage and soreness?

Typically during endurance training, there is a fair amount of soft-tissue damage and muscle breakdown that is inevitable. A number of studies have evaluated both performance changes and muscle tissue breakdown when endurance athletes added protein (mostly in the form of amino acids) to their training fuel. Many of the studies found a decrease in blood markers of muscle tissue breakdown in the protein-supplemented groups, showing that the protein was helpful in that vein.

Although protein or amino acid intake may help to reduce muscle soreness, there is no consensus as to the optimal amount of protein. Additionally, it is not yet clear if consuming protein during training is more effective in reducing muscles damage and soreness than including protein as part of recovery.

Protein and Endurance Training for Recovery

Recovery from endurance training includes restoring used energy (glycogen replenishment), reducing muscle wasting or breakdown, and, depending on the intensity and distance, limiting the suppression of the immune system. Let's take a look at how protein intake following endurance training affects these variables. Additionally, we will explore how soon after training or competition one should begin nutrient recovery.

Protein and Glycogen Replenishment

As far as nutrient timing goes, the period after exercise has become one of the hottest topics and most researched time frames in the sports nutrition world. Clearly, after an exhaustive training bout, replenishing energy used (carbohydrate) helps prepare an athlete for the next training session. Hormones and enzymes that are essential for nutrient metabolism are very sensitive just after exercise. Researchers have thought that it might be helpful to add protein to the mix at this time in case it, too, will hasten muscle recovery and immune protection.

Protein and Muscle Repair

It is encouraging when we look at protein and muscle repair. Most athletes polled in research studies felt less sore and some less tired when receiving protein as part of their recovery supplement. In some studies, blood markers of muscle breakdown were lower when protein was added during recovery.

In other studies, athletes felt less sore with protein although blood markers of breakdown were not lower. Although the research is not 100 percent clear on this point, it does seem that including protein along with carbohydrate for optimal recovery after endurance training results in less muscle protein breakdown and reduced soreness. In addition, prevention of additive muscle damage may help performance in the long run. This may be a more practical approach that achieves the same results as taking in protein during endurance training. Exact protein amounts have not been established, although some research has shown .1 to .2 gram per kilogram body weight to be helpful. We recommend including this amount in your recovery food or beverage along with adequate carbohydrate when you develop your Nutrition Blueprint in part III.

Protein and Resistance Training

Short of bodybuilding and weightlifting as a sport, most athletes participate in a resistance training program as part of a conditioning plan; they lift to get stronger and perhaps to get bigger. The act of lifting weight is a stimulus that initially causes a breakdown of muscle fibers and then a rebuilding of the breakdown, resulting in stronger fibers and muscles. To build size and strength, the repair of muscle proteins must occur. This repair and building actually occurs between training sessions. Without exercise, our bodies still go through cycles of protein losses and gains, called negative or positive protein balance, but we do not see the strength, size, or toning that occurs with resistance training. Basically, we stay in a relative state of net balance, maintaining what muscle we have as long as we consume adequate calories and appropriate amounts of protein. Later in life, we tend to lose muscle. See figure 4.1 for a summary of negative, net, and positive protein balances.

To build strength and increase size, protein synthesis must be greater than breakdown for a prolonged period of time—it takes weeks to months of positive protein balance, along with the stimulus of resistance training, to really see results. It's a slow process because, according to Koopman (2007), contractile proteins turn over at a slow rate—only about 1 percent per day.

Engaging in the proper exercise to stimulate protein synthesis is essential. Consuming adequate calories is just as important. Adequate carbohydrate and fat are needed to spare protein for muscle repair. It has been thought that if the breakdown that occurs during training could be minimized by eating, the synthesis that occurs after training would have more of an effect on positive protein balance in the muscle tissue. Is this true? Can strategic eating before or during exercise help and have a positive effect on the rate of muscle building? If so, what type and how much?

FIGURE 4.1
Protein balances

Negative protein balance	Muscle protein breakdown is greater than muscle protein synthesis; there is a loss of muscle protein tissue.
Net protein balance	Muscle protein breakdown is offset by muscle protein synthesis; there is no gain or loss of muscle protein tissue.
Positive protein balance	Muscle protein synthesis exceeds muscle protein breakdown; there is an increase in muscle protein tissue.

Timing Tip

Remember, a food does not advertise or list on its label its amino acid content, but protein foods are made up of amino acids. Supplements focus on the amino acid content because that is what they are selling. In fact, most whole, real foods have a much greater amino acid content than an amino acid supplement.

Protein Before Resistance Training

Taking in a protein and carbohydrate supplement before resistance exercise has been shown to be beneficial. Tipton et al (2001 and 2007) found greater protein synthesis when subjects had a supplement containing 6 grams of EAAs (essential amino acids) and 35 grams of carbohydrate immediately before resistance training rather than after. When these researchers investigated using whole protein, in the form of whey, they saw no difference in amino acid uptake by leg muscle whether the supplement was taken immediately before or one hour after exercise. All participants in both studies had fasted, except for the supplement given to half before exercise (see figure 4.2 for a comparison of amino acid content in a supplement versus low-fat yogurt). Why didn't they see the same results with the whey protein? Tipton and his researchers drew the conclusion that part of the reason the EAAs worked so well was because they were absorbed quickly into the bloodstream, and during exercise, when blood flow to the muscle was increased, the amino acids were able to get into the tissue more efficiently than if taken afterward. In addition, the insulin response stayed higher longer after pre-exercise consumption than after post-exercise consumption. As you have already learned, insulin is an inhibitor of protein breakdown and so improves protein balance.

It's interesting to note that the Tipton study was done in a fasted state. If you train at any point in the day after having eaten, these results may not be relevant because, hopefully, you'll have a filled amino acid pool from the foods you've eaten. Would food have worked equally as well if eaten earlier and digestion time was allowed for? Perhaps, but we don't know for sure. Eating right before training seems advantageous. How crucial amino acids are if you have eaten and the difference between food consumed further in advance versus amino acids taken right before training all remain to be determined with more research.

FIGURE 4.2

Comparison of amino acids in supplements and food

ESSENTIAL AMINO ACID CONTENT FOR BCAA SUPPLEMENT (6 CAPSULES PER SERVING)		ESSENTIAL AMINO ACID CONTENT FOR LOW-FAT YOGURT (1 CUP PER SERVING)	
Amino acid	Quantity (mg)	Amino acid	Quantity (mg)
Isoleucine	630	Histidine	319
Leucine	900	Isoleucine	701
Valine	270	Leucine	1,296
Total	**1,800**	Lysine	1,124
		Methionine	380
		Phenylalanine	701
		Threonine	529
		Tryptophan	73
		Valine	1,063
		Total	**6,186**

Protein During Resistance Training

Many of the studies investigating protein intake during resistance training also administer the supplement before and/or after as well as during training, making it difficult to evaluate the specific value of taking protein during resistance training. Bird et al (2006) looked exclusively at protein intake only during resistance training. Subjects took a 6 g amino acids and 6 percent carbohydrate beverage during resistance training and found a decrease in muscle tissue breakdown and decreased cortisol levels as compared to carbohydrate alone. Actual measurements of muscle protein synthesis were not performed. Beelen et al (2008). found an increase in protein synthesis when subjects were given a beverage containing 10 g protein and 10 g carbohydrate both before and during resistance training. While protein intake during resistance training seems promising for reducing muscle tissue breakdown, we can't say whether it is superior to taking protein either before or after training or if it should be combined with one of these for maximum effectiveness.

Protein and Resistance Training for Recovery

When participating in resistance training, remember there are at least two things going on: One is muscle tissue breakdown—a necessary step in signaling repair, building, and growth. The second is the repair and growth. The third is energy utilization from the anerobic energy system. The damage to muscle tissue that occurs during resistance training needs to be repaired in order for muscles to become stronger and bigger. Without food, muscle protein breakdown will occur, and muscle protein balance will not increase and may even become negative. Imagine all that hard work for nothing! Consuming a recovery snack can not only help limit the muscle tissue breakdown but also promote muscle building.

Nutrient Timing in Action

A client of Heidi's, a New York Giants veteran receiver, was concerned that he was not seeing results from his off season program. Heidi took a look at his day-to-day routine—he typically slept in and got to the stadium just in time to work out. He would lift, then run and go through drills, get treatment, hang out, shower, and go home, all while having eaten close to nothing all day. Some days he might grab a granola bar or something of the sort, but nothing substantial. Once home, he would have a feeding frenzy and pass out for a nap.

Together, we took steps to correct his patterns. I bought him a Captain Marvel lunch box and filled it with foods he could eat on the go, such as granola bars, fruit leathers, beef jerky, orange juice, trail mix, mixed nuts, applesauce, raisins, Gatorade, chocolate milk, string cheese, and hummus with pretzels, so he could consume calories earlier in the day. Essentially, he was in breakdown mode when he was lifting because he had not eaten anything since the night before. No wonder he was not seeing the benefit of his work. Needless to say, the veteran player got a great amount of grief from his teammates about the Captain Marvel lunch box (they all wanted one of their own), and he began to see improvements in his body composition, energy, and quality of training once he began to distribute his calories more evenly throughout the day, providing fuel for work and energy for repair before and after training.

Additionally, glycogen has also been used, and so replenishing used-up carbohydrate still applies. It's well established that your muscles are primed to take in nutrients at this time. You want to maximize the period that your muscles are repairing and rebuilding protein, and there must be sufficient raw materials available to do the job. Imagine gathering a bunch of people to build a house. Everyone's ready and waiting, but no one brought the tools or lumber; you're out of luck. That's how it is if you don't eat after your weight training session.

Carbohydrate stimulates the release of insulin, which helps prevent muscle tissue breakdown, and the addition of protein or amino acids further enhances its response. Insulin helps incorporate amino acids into muscle tissue after exercise. Studies repeatedly have shown a small amount of protein (10-15 grams) taken right after training along with carbohydrate promote muscle gain and prevent excessive protein breakdown. Don't wait until you get home, or until your next meal. Immediately after is best; two hours later delays the process and reduces the effect.

5

Smart Fat in the Diet

By now you recognize the importance of protein and carbohydrate for training and performance. Although it often gets a bad rap, fat serves vital functions in your health and exercise regime. For example, did you know that a diet too low in dietary fat can inhibit muscle building? Dietary fat is necessary for providing calories, particularly for those athletes who require a lot. Dietary fat is also needed for the production of hormones, such as estrogen and testosterone, and for the absorption of important nutrients (such as beta-carotene and vitamins A, D, E, and K). Both when we consume fat and how much affect performance directly (e.g., too much right before working out can slow you down) and indirectly (e.g., too low an intake can inhibit testosterone production and therefore muscle building and strength).

To determine the right time to consume fat in terms of performance, it is important to understand that digesting and using fat is a multistep process. Unlike carbohydrates, fats go through a series of transformations before they supply muscles with energy. Let's start at the beginning, however, and first describe what fat is.

WHAT IS FAT?

Just as proteins and carbohydrates are made of smaller components, so are fats. Most of the stored fat in our bodies (body fat) and fat found in food (dietary fat) exist in a form called triglycerides. These are made up of three individual fatty acids that are connected together by another molecule, glycerol.

Also, you may often hear the terms *saturated*, *monounsaturated*, and *polyunsaturated* in relation to fat and wonder what they really mean. The saturation refers to the chemical bonds of the fatty acid molecules. Saturated fats tend to be a bit more solid at room temperature and are found in many animal foods, such as higher-fat cuts of beef, lamb, veal, pork, and poultry; butter; cream; full-fat and 2 percent milk; cheese; and full-fat yogurt. Saturated fat, in a more liquid form, also occurs in coconut and palm oils. Our bodies can handle saturated fat; however, eating too much may increase inflammation throughout the body and blood cholesterol levels. High saturated fat intake is associated with other health problems, such as diabetes and some forms of cancer. The American Heart Association allows for 7 percent of total calories to come from saturated fat (16 grams in a 2,000-calorie diet).

Monounsaturated fats are found in foods such as olive oil, canola oil, peanuts and peanut oil, most nuts (except walnuts), and avocados. Sometimes they are also referred to as omega-9 fatty acids. People refer to monounsaturated fat as a "good" fat because it plays a role in keeping our hearts healthy.

Polyunsaturated fats are further designated by their structures: omega-3 and omega-6 fatty acids. The omega-3 fats are found in many varieties of fish and also in some plant foods: flaxseed, walnuts, and canola oil. Omega-6 fatty acids are found in safflower, sunflower, corn, soybean, cottonseed, and sesame oils. Just as there are essential amino acids that the body needs but cannot make, there are essential fatty acids. The specific omega-6 fatty acid that is essential is named linoleic acid. The omega-3 that is essential is called alpha-linolenic acid. These fats are required to make substances called eicosanoids, which are hormonelike substances that affect blood pressure, immunity, inflammation, contraction of smooth muscle tissue (such as your heart), and more. A small amount of each of the polyunsaturated fats are needed daily.

Trans fat is a type of fat that occurs naturally in small amounts in meats and dairy; there is also a man-made trans fat, which is the type we know to be most harmful to health. The naturally occurring trans fat may actually be handled by the body differently than trans fat found in partially hydrogenated oils, which are artificially created. Partially hydrogenated oils are made when hydrogen is added to oil, which causes it to become solid; examples include margarine and shortening. Originally designed to increase shelf life and add stability to processed foods, we have since learned that trans fats are not healthful and cause good cholesterol (HDL, or high-density lipoprotein) to go down and bad cholesterol (LDL, or low-density lipoprotein) to go up. Artificial trans fat may increase inflammation and has a negative heart health consequence. Unlike saturated fat, there is no need for any artificially created trans fat in the diet. The American Heart Association recommends no more than 1 gram a day of trans fat.

Sterols are substances present in the fatty tissue of plants and animals that have a ring structure instead of a chain. The most well known sterol is cholesterol, which is found only in animal-based foods. Different sterols have different effects in the body. Some sterols in plant foods have actually been isolated and added to salad dressings, made into spreads, and used to fortify drinks to help lower cholesterol. Too much cholesterol in the body may not be healthy, but cholesterol is vital to our well-being. It is necessary to form steroids in

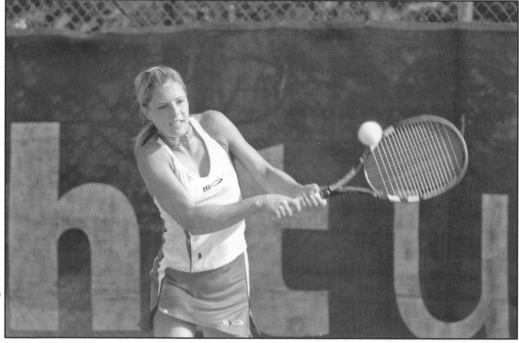

© Lovrencg/fotolia

Sufficient dietary fat and body fat are both needed for all athletes to perform optimally and remain healthy.

the body (the hormones estrogen, androgen, and progesterone as well as the adrenocortical hormones), bile (which is needed to digest fat), and vitamin D. Cholesterol is also in the membranes of all cells in our bodies. Much of the cholesterol we need can be made by our bodies. It is only when we produce too much cholesterol that it becomes problematic to our well-being. Dietary saturated fat consumption has a greater influence on increasing the levels of cholesterol in our blood than does the actual cholesterol content of food. Figure 5.1 shows which foods are sources of the different fats. Many foods contain more than one type of fat; we listed each food under the fat that predominates.

It's important to make the distinction between dietary fat and body fat. Fat that is eaten serves important functions in the body and is a source of calories. However, dietary fat does not necessarily turn into body fat. Including enough fat in the foods we eat helps food taste good and helps satisfy our appetites. Dietary fat provides nine calories per gram compared with four calories per gram of carbohydrate or protein, so it is a dense source of calories. Exceedingly high-fat diets can crowd out, or not allow us to get enough of, the other macronutrients, protein, and carbohydrate.

Having adequate body fat is also essential for health and performance. Regulating weight is a big concern for many athletes, as is achieving the right ratio of lean mass to fat weight. Although an overfat athlete may feel sluggish, too little body fat can impair hormone production, leading to inadequate muscle building and demineralization of bone. Let's first look at dietary fat and then follow that discussion with one about body fat.

FIGURE 5.1
Dietary fats and their sources

MONOUNSATURATED	POLYUNSATURATED		SATURATED
	Omega-3	Omega-6	
Avocado	Chia seeds	Margarine, trans-fat free	Bacon
Nut butters, trans-fat free: almond butter, cashew butter, peanut butter (smooth or crunchy)	Fish: anchovies, black caviar, bluefin tuna, herring, mackerel, oysters, sablefish (black cod), salmon, sardines, shad, whitefish	Mayonnaise	Butter
Nuts: almonds, Brazil nuts, cashews, filberts, hazelnuts, macadamias, pecans, pistachios	Flaxseed, flaxseed oil	Oils: corn, cottonseed, grapeseed, hemp, safflower, sesame, soybean, sunflower, walnut	Coconut
Oils: avocado, canola, olive, peanut		Pine nuts, walnuts	Cream, half and half
Peanuts		Salad dressings made with oils listed above	Cream cheese
		Seeds: hemp, pumpkin, sesame, sunflower	Lard (pork fat)
		Tahini (sesame paste)	Oils: coconut, palm, palm kernel, fractionated poly kernal oil
			Tallow (beef fat)

Dietary Fat

A diet too low in fat can be detrimental to males as well as females because fats are an integral part of certain hormones, such as testosterone and estrogen. Without sufficient dietary fat, your body may not produce adequate levels of these essential hormones. Without enough estrogen, females' menstrual cycles are interrupted, which can have a severely negative impact on bone health, resulting in stress fractures and other complications affecting both short-term and long-term health. Estrogen is also required for reproductive health, so a diet too low in fat may impair fertility. Without adequate calories and dietary fat, males may not manufacture enough testosterone, which can inhibit muscle development, strength, growth, bone health, and the development of secondary sex characteristics such as facial and body hair, deepening of the voice, and more. Fats also are used to formulate eicosanoids, which are hormonelike substances that affect inflammation, blood pressure, and even the viscosity, or thickness, of your blood.

Dietary fats have other benefits; one is satiety. Foods containing fat stay in our stomachs longer than protein and carbohydrate foods, so they contribute to our feeling full. The timing of dietary fat needs to be considered with regard to training and competition. A higher-fat meal should be given ample time, four hours or more, to digest, particularly for stop-and-go and endurance athletes. If you're a strength and power athlete and will do strength training first, then conditioning exercises, fat can be consumed closer to your workout. Although there is no exact guideline for fat quantity and timing, your own individual tolerance will play a role—some athletes can handle more than others. For example, some athletes enjoy having a peanut butter sandwich before training because it stays with them yet isn't a large quantity of food. Here are a few considerations regarding preexercise foods, fat, and fullness (satiety):

- The food should not interfere with your training.
- The food should help prevent you from becoming hungry during training (so that you can concentrate and not just be thinking about food).
- High-fat foods should not take the place of high-carbohydrate foods, which are needed to fuel your muscles.

Body Fat

Body fat is different from dietary fat. In the body, fat serves many functions. Fats in the body are stored not only as adipose (fat) tissue but also in muscle tissue, where they are burned for fuel during submaximal (mid to lower) intensity training. Very important, fats are also part of cell membranes, nerve sheaths, hormones, and other structures and substances that influence body functioning. Every cell of the body contains a small amount of fat. In addition, our nerves contain a coating called a myelin sheath that also contains small amounts of fat. Organs must have a layer of fat surrounding them to protect and insulate them. Even the back of your eyes, the bottom of your feet, and palms of your hands have fat pads that cushion and protect them.

Within the body, energy stored as fat provides a concentrated source of fuel. Fat is stored virtually without water and is more compact than carbohydrate, so we can store a lot more energy in the form of fat than we can carbohydrate. Calorically, fat is energy rich. One gram of protein or carbohydrate provides four calories; fat provides nine, so it is more than twice as concentrated. A person weighing 154 lb (70 kg) who has 17 percent body fat would have about 107,000 calories worth of potential energy to burn. Even elite athletes with very low body-fat percentages still have a substantial reserve of calories. However, accessing that fat has its limitations, which you will learn about later.

Fat is stored in different places throughout our bodies. Its location serves specific functions. Although many people think fat is a dormant body tissue, it actually is quite active, contributing to energy needs, temperature regulation, and in some cases, release

Body Fat and Athletes: Is Low Always Best?

An athlete with the lowest body fat is not always the best competitor. In and of itself, low body fat doesn't make you stronger or faster. For some athletes, trying to maintain a low body fat may result in insufficient fuel, and performance consequentially suffers. Additionally, by taking in fewer calories than needed on a chronic basis to maintain an artificially lower body-fat level, the body adjusts, and metabolic rate slows. Muscle strength, speed, and skill are all developed through training, not necessarily through a reduction of body fat only. However, it is true that excess body fat may slow an athlete down, cause excessive stress on joints, and hinder cooling.

There is no one ideal body composition number that is universal for all athletes to obtain in order to perform at their peak. Most athletes go through the balancing act of finding the best body-fat level that lets them eat to compete and fuel adequately without being restrictive. It's a process that requires mindful food selections. Focus on performance goals (strength, speed, power, stamina), acquiring skills, conditioning, and fueling yourself appropriately. Where body composition falls is then most likely going to be in line with the most realistic body weight and composition for you.

of inflammatory substances. So you see, not all body fat is the same; there are actually different kinds of body fat.

White Fat

The majority of body fat is white fat. Although all cells can store some fat, most of our body fat is stored in cells designed solely for fat storage. These cells are called adipocytes—more commonly known as fat cells. They specialize in making and storing body fat in the form of triglycerides. Although white adipocytes don't burn much energy, they aren't dormant either. As energy is required by working muscles during exercise, they release individual fatty acids into the bloodstream. One negative consequence of white enlarged fat cells is the manufacture and secretion of substances that cause inflammation and insulin resistance.

Brown Fat

This type of fat is very different from white fat. When activated by cool temperatures, brown fat burns a lot of energy because it produces heat. Babies have quite a bit of brown fat because they are unable to shiver, so brown fat helps keep them warm in cool temperatures. As we age, we lose some of it. Younger people tend to have more than older people, and women have more than men. It is found in the upper back, on the side of the neck, between the collar bone and shoulder, and along the spine. The calorie-burning ability of brown fat increases in cooler environments, but we do not yet know how the calorie-burning ability is affected by exercise.

Subcutaneous Fat

Subcutaneous fat is the fat layer just below the skin and is mostly comprised of white fat; about 50 percent of our body fat is subcutaneous. Subcutaneous fat helps conserve body heat in colder temperatures—it's a natural form of insulation. People who have a lot of subcutaneous fat may have difficulty releasing body heat that is generated during exercise in very hot weather. Because the body has a more difficult time dissipating body heat through conduction (one of the routes of regulating body temperature), core body temperature can rise and cause heat stress or, in severe cases, heat stroke. The body may produce excess sweat in an attempt to cool off, increasing risk of dehydration.

Visceral Fat

Visceral fat is the deeper body fat that surrounds organs and is made up of white fat. Although it is important to have visceral fat to protect organs, excessive amounts are unhealthy. Accumulation of fat around one's midsection, particularly this deeper fat, is more detrimental to health than accumulation of fat in other areas, such as around the hips and thighs. Why? Deep visceral abdominal fat cells are large and very active—they release free fatty acids into the bloodstream along with inflammatory substances that may contribute to the development of diabetes and heart disease. Unfortunately, we are genetically programmed as to whether the shape of our bodies is more like an "apple" (fat around the middle) or "pear" (fat around the hips and thighs). The good news is that exercise has a powerful effect on preventing or reducing the accumulation of visceral body fat in the abdominal area.

Intramuscular Fat

Intramuscular fat is the fat that is stored inside muscle tissue, where it is available to provide energy to muscles during exercise. The technical name for this fat is intramyocellular triacylglycerol, abbreviated IMTG. Many factors influence when and how much of this fuel is burned for energy. IMTG is burned during moderate-intensity endurance exercise. Moderate-intensity exercise lasting one to three hours utilizes 20 to 40 percent of IMTG. Extremely well-trained athletes may utilize even more because of hormonal changes as well as increased development of Type I (oxidative) muscle fibers. As athletes increasingly utilize intramuscular fat as fuel, the muscles have the ability to "remember" to store more fat so they will have access when needed. It's been shown that with low-fat diets (25 percent of calories or less), athletes have lower stores of IMTG, and it takes longer to replenish them. With very high-fat diets (40 to 65 percent of calories from fat), athletes have greater stores of IMTG. However, there are also shortfalls with such a high intake, such as a shortage of other important nutrients. An intake midway between may provide adequate fat and room for sufficient protein and carbohydrate. The greatest advantage of IMTG is during moderate-intensity exercise lasting more than one hour.

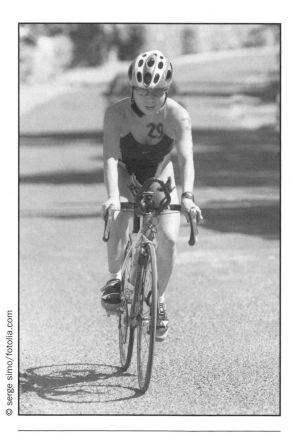

© serge simo/fotolia.com

Fat supplies energy to the oxidative muscle fibers utilized by long distance athletes.

HOW OUR BODIES USE FAT

Rival teams sometimes don't get along very well, but they need to coexist to compete. The same can be said of fats inside our bodies. That's because fats are not soluble in liquids, and most athletes' bodies are 50 percent water or more. Digestion of fats is a bit more complicated than it is for other nutrients because of this. Basically, when we eat food that contains fat, it's in the form of a triglyceride (three connected fatty acids). In the digestive tract, the triglycerides are broken down into individual fatty

> ### Timing Tip
>
> If an athlete eats a large amount of fat just before exercise, it can cause discomfort and possibly impair performance. Choose dietary fat at meals and snacks further away from training.

acids, similar to how proteins and carbohydrates are broken down into smaller, simpler molecules. Fatty acids aren't absorbed directly into the blood, as amino acids or sugars are. That's because oil and water don't mix well (think of how Italian salad dressing separates). Since fats we eat don't travel well in the blood all by themselves, they are repackaged into molecules that can carry them to where they are needed. These are called chylomicrons. The chylomicrons are released into the lymphatic system, then into the blood. The chylomicrons travel through the blood and release fatty acids directly into muscles or adipose (fat) tissue. Why does this matter? Because the fats we eat are not immediately available for fuel during exercise. Fat digestion is slow; by the time the fatty acids reach muscle and can be burned for energy, they have been broken down from triglycerides and put back together a few times.

How do we burn fat for fuel?

Muscle cells need energy to contract, which they may get from carbohydrate or fatty acids when they are metabolized (broken down). As we discussed in chapter 2, fat needs to have oxygen present in order to go through the stages of metabolism to create ATP (quick energy). Fat is burned for fuel only during aerobic metabolism, or anything more than three minutes. Fat is not burned in power or anaerobic work. When muscles burn fat, it may come from the fat stored inside muscles (IMTG), from the fatty acids that are released from adipose cells and travel to the muscle, or from chylomicrons.

Remember the game Mouse Trap, which was set up so that a series of events was triggered once the ball was released at the top of the structure? Well, fat metabolism reminds us of that game. When you are just sitting around or resting, adipose (fat) cells release fatty acids into the bloodstream. As you begin to exercise, the body releases catecholamines (epinephrine, norepinephrine) along with growth hormone and glucagon. These hormones activate enzymes needed to break apart the triglycerides that may be inside muscles or fat tissue. Larger amounts of fatty acids are released into the bloodstream from adipose tissue (fat stores) and are carried by blood flowing to the working muscles.

The muscle can burn either the fat it already has stored (its "veteran" fats) or the newly delivered ("rookie") fatty acids to fuel exercise. Which does it choose? That depends on the intensity and duration of the exercise and the fitness level of the athlete. At very low intensities, and at the beginning of exercise, the muscles choose the rookie free fatty acids from the blood, mostly because they are in such great supply. As intensity picks up, and a little further into the workout, the veteran stored fat (IMTG within the muscle) is used. This contributes more energy during moderate-intensity exercise lasting about two hours; after that, the muscles go back to burning mostly free fatty acids from the blood. There is an inverse relationship between the muscle's burning of free fatty acids from the bloodstream and the stored IMTG. It seems that when there are a lot of free fatty acids, the IMTG "allows" them to be burned so they don't build up even more in the blood. As athletes enter a high-intensity workload, however, less fat and more carbohydrate is burned.

Numerous studies indicate that well-trained athletes are able to burn more fat at higher intensities than untrained individuals. Trained athletes show this adaptation to their exercise by releasing lower levels of catacholamines, resulting in fewer fatty acids in the blood. They become better able to tap into their stored IMTG. Trained individuals have

Myth and Truth About Carnitine

It is a common myth that carnitine, taken in supplement form, will help fat burning. People think this because carnitine carries fatty acids inside cells to be burned for energy.

Truth: Carnitine is plentiful in the body. It is found in meats but is also made inside the body from two amino acids. Our bodies are adept at recycling carnitine, so healthy people have a good supply, even vegetarians. Because using fat for fuel is a multistep process, adding one component, such as carnitine, will not speed up or enhance the fat-burning process (it is rate limited). Carnitine itself does not limit the amount of fatty acids that can be brought into muscle tissue, so taking more will not increase the transfer of fat into the muscle to be used.

also been shown to have a greater storage capacity for IMTG in their muscles, possibly due to increased usage and increased manufacture of enzymes that store and burn these fats.

Inside the muscle, once the free fatty acids are released from the triglyceride (IMTG), they must be activated by a coenzyme and then carried into the mitochondria (energy factory in the cell) by a substance known as carnitine, which is plentiful in muscle tissue (carnitine knows the route to get into the muscle). If free fatty acids enter muscle tissue from the blood, they, too, need carnitine to enter the mitochondria. Once in the mitochondria, fatty acids undergo two separate processes to release energy. As you can see, this is quite an extensive course of action to release energy.

Can medium-chain triglycerides (MCTs) enhance fat burning or spare glycogen?

Medium-chain triglycerides (MCTs), made from coconut oil and palm oil, are shorter in length than other fats. They are digested and absorbed much more quickly than other fats, are absorbed directly into the bloodstream instead of being formed into chylomicrons like the longer-chain fats, are delivered directly to the liver and burned for energy rather than being stored in adipose tissue, and enter the mitochondria more quickly than other fatty acids because they don't require a carrier to get in. Investigators thought these characteristics might provide an advantage to endurance athletes since it appears that MCTs provide energy much more quickly than other fats and could potentially spare glycogen. In reality, the amount of MCTs that athletes can tolerate (25 to 30 grams or less) doesn't seem to make much of a difference. Larger amounts cause abdominal cramps, gas, and bloating in many athletes and even vomiting in a few cases during endurance training. The bottom line is that MCTs were not shown to spare glycogen, burn additional fat, or improve performance.

What interferes with fat burning?

There are circumstances inside the body that reduce our ability to burn fat. Once fatty acids enter the muscle, they need to enter the mitochondria in order to be burned for energy. At very high exercise intensities, they are denied entry. It's like when you have a ticket to go to a ball game; you may be able to get into the arena, but if you don't have a ticket for the stadium club, you can't get into that area. It's not known exactly what keeps the fat out of the mitochondria, but at high intensities, carbohydrate, not fat, is burned for energy.

Other substances prevent fatty acids from being released from adipose tissue. Lactate, ketones, and insulin block release of fatty acids from adipose tissue and inhibits the stored triglycerides from being broken down inside muscle tissue.

HOW FAT IS USED DURING EXERCISE

It is well established that fat provides the fuel to muscles at low intensities and continues to supply most of the energy up to a point, when carbohydrate begins to supply energy. What is the point of maximal fat burning? Can we make our muscles burn fat past that point? Can fat burning improve performance? Let's take a look.

As we mentioned, when you are sitting around, not doing much of anything, your muscles are burning fat. However, since just sitting around doesn't require much energy, you don't burn a huge quantity of fat. As you begin to exercise, caloric demands increase, and the additional energy required by muscle is supplied mostly by burning more fat and some carbohydrate. As exercise intensity increases, there's a point where the scales tip and the body begins to burn more carbohydrate and less fat. We will learn how that happens, but first we have to understand a bit more.

In talking about exercise intensity, we use the term $\dot{V}O_2max$ to describe the maximum amount of oxygen a person is able to use. One way intensity is measured is as a percentage of $\dot{V}O_2max$. The highest intensity possible while working aerobically is 100 percent of $\dot{V}O_2max$. Of course you are still breathing and taking in oxygen when working above your aerobic threshold, crossing over into your anaerobic threshold. However, at this point, the oxygen you are taking in is not being utilized to burn the carbohydrate used to fuel such intensity.

When muscles contract, there is a release of the hormone epinephrine, which causes fat cells (adipose tissue) to release more free fatty acids into the bloodstream. At low exercise intensities, say 25 percent of $\dot{V}O_2max$, muscles get most of their energy from fatty acids in the bloodstream. As the intensity increases, muscles use more of their own fat stores—the IMTG (intramyocellular triacylglycerol) and fewer free fatty acids from the bloodstream because their release from adipose tissue is slowed. Slow-twitch muscle fibers (used predominantly in aerobic endurance exercise) contain more fat-burning enzymes than do fast-twitch muscles (which produce more power and are used in high-intensity activity), so that could influence the ability of the muscle to burn fat at different exercise intensities. Even if you are still using aerobic metabolism, at higher levels, fat burning drops off.

Can a high-fat diet improve performance?

Your muscles are very smart. They remember all your fitness efforts, and they adapt very well to exercise so they are able to burn more fat than the muscles of your untrained friends. The more you exercise, the better your muscles become at burning fat for fuel. How? You actually build more "energy factories"—mitochondria (the cells that burn energy inside muscles)—and you make more fat-burning enzymes. Athletes who engage in regular endurance training increase their level of fitness and, in time, are able to burn fat at higher intensities than when they were just starting out. The benefit of burning fat at higher intensities is that you don't deplete your glycogen stores as easily, and you're able to exercise for longer periods before becoming fatigued. If you can burn more fat, does that mean you should eat more fat?

Some studies have shown that when fat makes up half of one's intake, that's too high. Heart rate may be higher with high-fat diets because of increased levels of epinephrine and norepinephrine. Your rate of perceived exertion (RPE), or how hard you feel you are exercising, is often higher when taking in 50 percent or more of your calories from fat.

In a review of studies on athletes who consumed prolonged high-fat diets (more than 40% of calories from fat for more than 10 days), it was concluded that endurance performance may be maintained but most likely not improved. There is no evidence to recommend a diet that provides more than 40% of calories from fat, especially since most athletes we know train to improve performance, not merely stay the same. We believe that anywhere from 25 to 35 percent calories from fat can make up a healthy, balanced intake for train-

The Fat Burning Zone: Does It Really Exist?

You may have heard that the fat-burning zone is between 65 and 85% HRmax (heart rate max), and to burn the most fat you should exercise in this zone. Here's the real story: At lower levels of exercise, muscles primarily utilize a greater percentage of fat for fuel. Mostly Type I (oxidative) muscle fibers are at work, and they can produce energy slowly from fat. As intensity picks up, you continue to use the Type I but also begin to use Type IIb muscle fibers (crossover fibers)—because you need to exert more power to work harder. These fibers use both fat and carbohydrate. So although you may not be using as high a percentage of fat, you are working harder and burning more total calories and, possibly, more total fat. Achten et al (2004) found the highest rate of fat burning to be at 64% $\dot{V}O_2$max, which corresponded to a 74% HRmax in their study. They also found that at a wide range of intensities, subjects were within 10% of the peak fat-burning zone, so at anywhere from 55 to 72% $\dot{V}O_2$max, subjects were burning a good amount of energy from fat. This corresponded to a heart rate of 68 to 79% HRmax in their subjects. The levels in these studies were determined after a 10- to 12-hour overnight fast.

Ingesting carbohydrate before or during exercise may result in decreased fat burning but increased ability to work harder longer. Being able to work out harder or longer will result in more total calories burned, which ultimately is more helpful toward weight loss efforts. In fact, you won't improve your fitness or fat-burning abilities if you intentionally exercise at a very low intensity to maximize fat burning (which is different from planning hard and easy days). That just doesn't make sense. Working at a higher intensity improves your ability to burn fat at a higher percent $\dot{V}O_2$max or a higher percent HRmax, ultimately improving fitness, performance, and fat burning.

ing. Some athletes do well at this level, some with a slightly lower intake. Athletes who consume a very high calorie load may need to keep fat at 40 percent to maintain weight. The challenge of course is being sure to take in adequate protein and carbohydrate as well.

Should I exercise without eating so I burn more fat?

Although exercising without eating might seem advantageous, the intensity of your workout will most likely suffer. Remember that if you train in the morning, you'll have low liver glycogen, and you can quickly deplete muscle glycogen. A number of studies have shown that training without preexercise fuel leads to decreased performance and early fatigue. In Tokmakidis' (2008) trial, athletes were able to run 12.8 percent longer with pre-exercise fuel as opposed to in a fasted state. What you might gain in fat burning, you lose in increasing your fitness and your ability to burn fat at higher intensity levels all the time. Additionally, working out at a lower intensity to burn more fat actually means you will most likely burn fewer calories, a short-sighted plan at best.

Does dietary periodization help enhance fat burning?

Another concept that has gained much attention is to train low and compete high, meaning train with low carbohydrate intake (high fat intake) and compete with high glycogen stores (carbohydrate in muscles). In athletic circles, it's also called dietary periodization. This type of design involves athletes training while taking in high-fat diets for a period of time. Then, right before competing, the athletes load up on carbohydrate just for a day or so. The idea is that the muscles will have adapted to burning fat, at the same time, glycogen will be present when athletes need it for quick bursts of speed. Sounds great—but does it work?

It's been shown that athletes can adapt their metabolic machinery to shift to fat burning by consuming a high-fat diet for five days. Endurance athletes, even those who work pretty much at steady state, still need to tap into carbohydrate at times during competition. Real-life sports performance requires bursts of energy, such as climbing hills or sprinting to the finish of an endurance race, so carbohydrate is still needed (and remember, fat burns on a carbohydrate flame). Relying only on these high-fat diets might compromise the athletes' ability to go all out. Finding a way to have the best of both worlds would be great. The reality? Although athletes certainly could keep burning fat at low to moderate exercise intensities, even when restoring glycogen stores, most times it hasn't translated into improved performance. It seems as if these high-fat diets are sparing glycogen, but, in reality, the body's ability to use glycogen becomes impaired. When glycogen is needed at high intensities, these athletes can't get to it because of decreases in an enzyme that breaks it down (Stellingwerff 2006). Although cyclists following a 10-day high-fat/3-day high-carb diet experienced improved performance, they also experienced insulin resistance when they went back to eating carbohydrate (Lambert et al 2001). As you know, high insulin impairs fat burning and persistent high levels lead to health problems.

Omega-3 Fatty Acids

Omega-3 fatty acids are found in a variety of plant foods and fish. The specific fatty acids that are found in fish (eicosapentaenoic acid, EPA) and (docosahexaenoic acid, DHA) have beneficial effects on our health and may confer benefits to athletes under certain circumstances. When these are consumed, they take the place of omega-6 fatty acids in certain blood and liver cell membranes, improving the functioning of each cell membrane (without the harmful eicosanoids that excess omega-6s give off). The result is an anti-inflammatory effect on blood vessels and reduced "stickiness" of our blood.

Exhaustive exercise, as can be undertaken during intensive training, can cause the production of damaging molecules as a by-product of metabolism. In addition, some elite athletes are prone to a narrowing of their airways during or after intense aerobic exercise. Fish and fish oil containing EPA and DHA have been shown to inhibit the production of these inflammatory eicosanoids. Although we need the fatty acids derived from omega-6 fats (soybean, safflower, sunflower, corn, soybean, cottonseed, and sesame oils; mayonnaise and many salad dressings), Americans take in a disproportionately high amount of these fats. These fats, in excess, are pro-inflammatory and at the same time inhibit the positive anti-inflammatory action of the omega-3 fatty acids. It is recommended, therefore, to limit the omega-6 fats and increase intake of omega-3s for optimal anti-inflammatory benefits. Omega-3 fatty acids do not provide an immediate effect on performance. Their inclusion in an athlete's diet over time is what allows the body to shift from being pro-inflammatory to anti-inflammatory. Remember, not all inflammation is bad—our bodies needs inflammation to protect and promote healing. It is the excessive intake of omega-6, saturated, and trans fats that can overload the balance and tilt the body's defense mechanisms too far to an inflammatory state that is the concern.

We're not implying that you analyze each morsel of fat that passes your lips, but rather be aware and strive for balance because all fat is needed for optimal health. Vary the sources of fat you consume—choose fish, canola oil, olive oil, nuts, seeds, and avocado, along with some of the other plant and animal sources listed earlier in this chapter on page 51.

Havemann et al (2006) conducted a well-designed study in which athletes worked similarly to real-life competition. The study included training rides throughout the week and ended with a 100-kilometer (60 mile) time trial including sprints. The cyclists followed a high-fat diet for 6 days followed by 1 day of carbohydrate loading. The researchers measured a number of indicators to better understand how these diets affected the subjects' perception, nervous system regulation, use of fuel, and, of course, performance. They found a decrease in high-intensity sprint power performance. Those following the high-fat diet felt the sprints were harder, and their heart rates were higher than those on the high-carbohydrate diet. No benefit to performance was found for the high-fat group. This is an extremely important point. Although fat loading sounds like a good idea, there just doesn't seem to be conclusive evidence of performance benefits. High fat diets make competition seem harder (plus many athletes do not feel good while fat loading).

Can dietary fat improve performance if eaten before exercise?

Another idea has come up to improve performance, as there is no limit to new ideas on this subject. An alternate way to preserve glycogen stores and carbohydrate metabolism could be to maintain a normal training diet and add a meal or large dose of dietary fat just before exercise. The premise is that blood levels of fatty acids would increase and be available as a source of energy for muscles during submaximal exercise. However, studies have not been able to prove a benefit of this strategy either.

Earlier in this chapter, we described the multi-step process for fat digestion; triglycerides in food are broken down, put back together, and repackaged into chylomicrons. During exercise, muscles obtain fatty acids mostly from their own stored fuel source (IMTG) or from fatty acids released from adipose tissue. A high-fat meal prior to training is digested slowly and provides no performance advantages. Remember, the body adapts and becomes more fit as a result of training. We can use fat more efficiently and utilize oxygen longer through fine-tuned muscles and improvements in the hormone and enzyme systems. It is these adaptations, over time with training, that produce results. All that hard work has benefits!

6

Essential Vitamins and Minerals

Vitamins and minerals are found in food, but now they are also abundant in all sorts of products, such as vitamin waters and other beverages, vitamin-fortified bars and protein powders, and fortified cereals. The real question for athletes relating to the NTP is: Does when you consume any vitamin or mineral from food or supplement offer a performance benefit? It is true that vitamins and minerals cannot be made by the body and so must be consumed. We need vitamins and minerals as well as antioxidants and phytonutrients for health and well-being, but is there a performance edge from their consumption? This chapter will describe what they are, highlight foods that provide specific nutrients, and give some insight into how activity impacts our bodies' need for selected nutrients.

WHAT ARE VITAMINS AND MINERALS?

As you know by now, carbohydrate, protein, and fat, also termed maronutrients, supply energy for training and the raw materials necessary for tissue repair and recovery. Vitamins and minerals, and other plant chemicals (phytonutrients and antioxidants) are referred to as *micronutrients* because we need them in such small amounts—milligrams or micrograms, which are hundredths or thousandths of a gram (.01 or .001 gram)—as opposed to carbohydrate, say, of which you need *hundreds* of grams per day.

Vitamins and minerals do not provide energy by themselves; rather, they enable the release of energy from food—that is, they act as catalysts, or "starters" if you will. Some vitamins and minerals are involved in oxygen delivery to muscles and other tissues. Others are incorporated into body structures (such as bone) and serve vital functions in healing or protecting tissues against damage that may occur during training and competition. Ingesting certain antioxidants and phytonutrients through food may affect the health of tissues and cells. However, unlike the macronutrients carbohydrate and protein, the timing of vitamin and mineral intake does not seem to be as important. Whether there are any specific timing benefits to including these before, during, or after exercise has not yet been shown. Since their functions are not hormonally dependent for delivery (as glucose is, for example, via insulin), the timing of intake with regard to exercise is not critical, except for sodium and its role in fluid balance and hydration status.

Although their timing may not be critical, many vitamins and minerals influence performance, and they all are needed for good health. How they affect *immediate* performance is overstated in some circles of sports nutrition. For example, the B vitamins (of which there are 8) are involved in releasing energy from food—some of them are actually used in the step-by-step process of metabolizing (or breaking down) carbohydrates, fats, and proteins; some are part of an enzyme or coenzyme that gets a chemical reaction going. The body stores B vitamins and uses them as needed. The marketers of many products create the impression you need a certain vitamin during exercise which is just false.

For optimal health and performance, nutrients should be replaced on a daily basis. That's because we want to replace the small amounts that are used during training and normal body functioning. Although we are not going to become deficient in a day or even a week, our bodies still need nutrients on a daily basis to function optimally. Additionally, micronutrients are absorbed better in smaller quantities throughout the day rather than in one big dose. That's one more reason why eating balanced meals that provide foods from at least three food groups is healthier than eating, say, all starch, which may provide some micronutrients but is less likely to provide as great an array. Furthermore, many micronutrients work better as part of a team than individually, so eating mixed meals is better than taking isolated supplements. For example, if vitamin C is present, you do not need as much vitamin E.

Foods supply vitamins, minerals, and antioxidants that work well together—synergistically, kind of like the way a winning team functions. When nutrients are obtained from foods, most often they are in amounts that are reasonable rather than excessive—some supplements and fortified or enhanced foods can supply such high amounts that, when consumed on a regular basis replacing a balanced and well-rounded diet, can cause imbalances or even reach toxic levels. Another point is that "bioengineered" foods often contain some but not all nutrients. Many of the active compounds found in food have just been identified over the last 20 years or so—and there may be even more constituents that have yet to be discovered. Relying too heavily on bars, gus, gels, shakes can actually leave you short on some yet unidentified nutrient.

Fruits, vegetables, and whole grains contain all types of phytochemicals, which are naturally occurring plant chemicals that can have health-promoting and antioxidative properties. It's not advisable to take these in supplemental form because when isolated and concentrated, some have been shown to have harmful effects. For example, vitamin

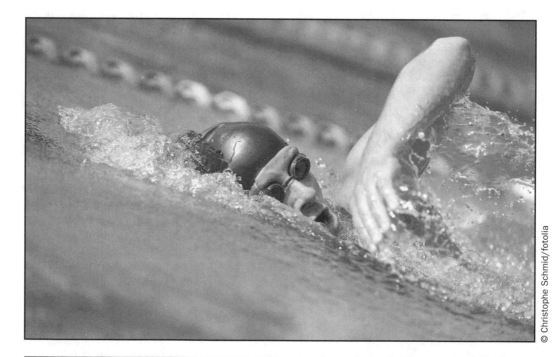

© Christophe Schmid/fotolia

Vitamins and minerals may be used in the process of releasing energy from food; the food supplies the actual fuel for muscles.

Dietary Reference Intakes and Values

You may be familiar with the term *RDA,* which stands for recommended dietary allowance. This value refers to the amount of each vitamin and mineral that is sufficient to meet the needs of 97 to 98 percent of healthy people in each age and gender group. The levels are set to prevent deficiency and avoid certain diseases. On a food or supplement label, you will see a percent daily value (DV) column. This represents the percentage that one serving of the food or supplement contributes to one's daily need. All these values are part of a larger set of recommendations called DRIs (dietary reference intakes). Also part of the DRIs are tolerable upper limits—amounts that, if routinely exceeded, can result in health problems. Although some of each vitamin and mineral is necessary for good health, too much can be harmful. All these values are set by the Food and Nutrition Board of the National Academies' Institute of Medicine, and they are based on a review of all the available scientific evidence at the time these levels were established.

C taken in high doses can become a pro-oxidant. In fact, current research concludes that supplementation with certain antioxidants (beta-carotene, vitamins A and E) resulted in an *increase* in mortality rates (Bjelakovic et al 2007). There are no such negative outcomes from eating more fruits, vegetables, and whole grains.

Have you ever heard the term "overfed but undernourished"? Think of it this way: if you consumed a pound of sugar, you would not die of starvation, but you may suffer malnutrition. Quanity does not equate to quality. Deficiencies can very well impair performance by limiting oxygen delivery and reducing the energy supplied to muscle cells, both of which can lead to early fatigue. Even athletes who consume adequate calories may be at risk. However, nutritionally inadequate diets traditionally have been prevalent in weight-conscious athletes, including wrestlers, dancers, gymnasts, jockeys, some crew members, and divers. This disturbing trend has expanded into every sport, including team sports where weight is not a criterion for participation and uniforms are ample (e.g., field hockey, softball). Runners often strive to be as light as possible or to reduce body fat even though there is no evidence showing a universal improvement in performance at a given weight or body-fat percentage. If maintaining a low weight requires chronic dieting, nutritional adequacy may suffer.

When calories, calcium, vitamin D, protein, or fat intake is too low, stress fractures can occur. Iron-deficient diets impair endurance because of the limited oxygen-carrying capacity of blood. Lack of vitamin C may impair wound healing. The effects of nutrition deficiencies may be compounded by low-calorie diets. Although taking in sufficient vitamins and minerals is important, a supplement alone does not fix the problem unless the athlete also consumes enough protein, fat, carbohydrate, and calories.

ESSENTIAL VITAMINS AND MINERALS

In this section, you'll learn why each essential vitamin and mineral is needed; what, if any, impact it has on training and performance; its supplemental forms; and the food sources it is found in. But, first, let's explain what each of the two types of vitamins are and what minerals are.

- *Water-soluble vitamins.* Water-soluble vitamins require only water to be absorbed, unlike fat-soluble vitamins, which need dietary fat. Although excess intake may be excreted in the urine, it doesn't mean large doses are harmless. Water-soluable vitamins include Vitamin C and the B Vitamins.

- *Fat-soluble vitamins.* Fat-soluble vitamins require dietary fat to be absorbed. They also may be stored in body fat, and some can build up to toxic levels if taken in excess. They are not excreted as easily as water-soluble vitamins. Fat-soluble vitamins include vitamins A, D, E and K.

- *Minerals.* Calcium, phosphorous, sodium and magnesium are considered macrominerals because they exist in the body in large quantities. Other minerals, known as trace minerals, exist in the body in extremely small amounts. Regardless of the size of their presence in the body, all the minerals serve vital roles in our health.

Figure 6.1 outlines the main function, deficiency symptoms, and foods sources of each vitamin and mineral. Recognize that, although not listed, there are toxicity symptoms that can occur with supplement overload.

FIGURE 6.1
Vitamin and Mineral Guide

Vitamins	Function	Deficiency	Food Sources
A (retinol)	Supports vision, skin, bone and tooth growth, immunity and reproduction	Loss of appetite; dry, rough skin; lowered resistance to infection; dry eyes	Mango, broccoli, butternut squash, carrots, tomato juice, sweet potatoes, pumpkin, beef liver
B_1 (Thiamin)	Supports energy metabolism and nerve function	Muscle cramps; loss of appetite	Spinach, green peas, tomato juice, watermelon, sunflower seeds, lean ham, lean pork chops, soy milk
B_2 (Riboflavin)	Supports energy metabolism, normal vision and skin health	Cracks and sores around the mouth and nose; visual problems	Spinach, broccoli, mushrooms, eggs, milk, liver, oysters, clams
B_3 (Niacin)	Supports energy metabolism, skin health, nervous system and digestive system	Dermatitis, depression, dementia	Spinach, potatoes, tomato juice, lean ground beef, chicken breast, tuna (canned in water), liver, shrimp
B_6	Amino acid and fatty acid metabolism, red blood cell production	Anemia, irritability, patches of itchy skin	Bananas, watermelon, tomato juice, broccoli, spinach, acorn squash, potatoes, white rice, chicken breast
Folate	Supports DNA synthesis and new cell formation	Impaired cell division; anemia; diarrhea; gastrointestinal upsets	Tomato juice, green beans, broccoli, spinach, asparagus, okra, black-eyed peas, lentils, navy, pinto and garbanzo beans
B_{12}	Used in new cell synthesis, helps break down fatty acids and amino acids, supports nerve cell maintenance	Rare except in strict vegetarians	Meats, poultry, fish, shellfish, milk, eggs

Vitamins	Function	Deficiency	Food Sources
C (Ascorbic Acid)	Collage synthesis, amino acid metabolism, helps iron absorption, immunity, antioxidant	Muscle weakness, bleeding gums; easy bruising	Spinach, broccoli, red bell peppers, snow peas, tomato juice, kiwi, mango, orange, grapefruit juice, strawberries
D	Promotes bone mineralization	Bone softening in adults; osteoporosis	Self-synthesis via sunlight, fortified milk, egg yolk, liver, fatty fish
E	Antioxidant, regulation of oxidation reactions, supports cell membrane stabilization	Anemia, muscle necrosis	Polyunsaturated plant oils (soybean, corn and canola oils), wheat germ, sunflower seeds, tofu, avocado, sweet potatoes, shrimp, cod
K	Synthesis of blood-clotting proteins, regulates blood calcium	Defective blood coagulation	Brussels sprouts, leafy green vegetables, spinach, broccoli, cabbage, liver
Minerals	**Function**	**Deficiency**	**Food Sources**
Sodium	Maintains fluid and electrolyte balance, supports muscle contraction and nerve impulse transmissions	Cramping	Salt, soy sauce, bread, milk, meats
Chloride	Maintains fluid and electrolyte balance, aids in digestion	Muscle cramps, muscle fatigue	Salt, soy sauce, milk, eggs, meats
Potassium	Maintains fluid and electrolyte balance, cell integrity, muscle contractions and nerve impulse transmission	Nausea, anorexia, muscle weakness, irritability	Potatoes, acorn squash, artichoke, spinach, broccoli, carrots, green beans, tomato juice, avocado, grapefruit juice, watermelon, banana, strawberries, cod, milk
Calcium	Formation of bones and teeth, supports blood clotting	Rickets in children; osteomalacia (soft bones) and osteoporosis in adults	Milk, yogurt, cheddar cheese, Swiss cheese, tofu, sardines, green beans, spinach broccoli
Phosphorus	Formation of cells, bones and teeth, maintains acid-base balance	Rare	Meats, fish, poultry, eggs, milk
Magnesium	Supports bone mineralization, protein building, muscular contraction, nerve impulse transmission, immunity	Nausea, irritability, muscle weakness; twitching; cramps, cardiac arrhythmias	Spinach, broccoli, artichokes, green beans, tomato juice, navy beans, pinto beans, black-eyed peas, sunflower seeds, tofu, cashews, halibut
Iron	Part of the protein hemoglobin (carries oxygen throughout body's cells)	Skin pallor; weakness; fatigue; headaches	Artichoke, parsley, spinach, broccoli, green beans, tomato juice, tofu, clams, shrimp, beef liver
Zinc	A part of many enzymes, involved in production of genetic material and proteins, transports vitamin A, taste perception, wound healing, sperm production and the normal development of the fetus	Slow healing of wounds; loss of taste; retarded growth	Spinach, broccoli, green peas, green beans, tomato juice, lentils, oysters, shrimp, crab, turkey (dark meat), lean ham, lean ground beef, lean sirloin steak, plain yogurt, Swiss cheese, tofu, ricotta cheese

(continued)

FIGURE 6.1   *(continued)*

Minerals	Function	Deficiency	Food Sources
Selenium	Antioxidant. Works with vitamin E to protect body from oxidation	Unknown	Seafood, meats, grains
Iodine	Component of thyroid hormones that help regulate growth, development and metabolic rate	Hypothyroidism; fatigue, weight gain, cold intolerance, dry skin, constipation, depression	Salt, seafood, bread, milk, cheese
Copper	Necessary for the absorption and utilization of iron, supports formation of hemoglobin and several enzymes	Rare in adults	Meats, water
Manganese	Facilitates many cell processes	Unknown	Widespread in foods
Fluoride	Involved in the formation of bones and teeth, helps to make teeth resistant to decay	Increase risks of having dental caries, osteoporosis	Fluroidated drinking water, tea, seafood
Chromium	Associated with insulin and is required for the release of energy from glucose	Contributes to glucose intolerance and unhealthy blood lipid profile	Vegetable oils, liver, brewer's yeast, whole grains, cheese, nuts

Courtesy of Lisa Dorfman, MS, RD, CSSD, LMHC.

Following are some interesting facts about selected vitamins and minerals as they relate to the athlete.

Vitamin B$_1$ (Thiamin)

Exercise may slightly increase an athlete's needs. Including enriched and whole grains in the diet is a good way for athletes to meet energy and thiamin needs. Supplementing when an athlete already has sufficient thiamin levels does not improve high-intensity performance or result in an increased rate of metabolism.

Frequent sushi eaters should note that raw freshwater fish and shellfish may contain certain enzymes that can destroy thiamin, leading to a deficiency. Cooking fish destroys these enzymes.

Vitamin B$_2$ (Riboflavin)

An increased need for riboflavin was found in studies of women who were exercising moderately, dieting, or exercising and dieting, by amounts of 30 to 65 percent above the RDA. As yet, there are not enough data available to quantify what adjustments should be made. Very little excess riboflavin is stored—whatever is not needed is excreted in the urine. Note that excess riboflavin is responsible for the bright yellow color of urine when taking large doses of vitamins. Also, excess riboflavin in the urine can interfere with certain drug testing.

Vitamin B$_3$ (Niacin)

Increased needs of niacin have not been found for athletes. Studies show that taking 1 gram (1,000 mg) of niacin actually inhibits performance because niacin inhibits free fatty acid release from adipose cells (Murray et al, 1995; Heath et al, 1993).

Vitamin B$_6$ (Pyridoxine)

Some studies show an increased need for B$_6$, while others do not, as exercise itself may cause a retention of B$_6$. A definitive conclusion as to an increased need of B$_6$ by athletes has not been made. The current RDA is expected to cover most people's needs. Remember that an increased need is different from experiencing an ergogenic (performance enhancing) benefit from supplementation. One study that had athletes consume an amount far exceeding the RDA (20 mg/day) found no improvement in exercise endurance (Virk et al 1999). Also note that blood levels of B$_6$ fluctuate; most of the body's B$_6$ levels are found in muscle. Blood tests do not appear to be an accurate way to determine B$_6$ status.

Vitamin B$_{12}$ (Cobalamin)

There is no evidence that exercise increases the need for B$_{12}$; however, inadequate intake can lead to megaloblastic anemia (characterized by large and dysfunctional red blood cells), which causes fatigue and impairs performance. Typically, poor absorption may occur with aging or a high intake of antacids (you need stomach acid to absorb vitamin B$_{12}$). A deficiency in B$_{12}$ will hurt performance, but extra B$_{12}$ in well-nourished athletes (with no absorption problems) *will not* improve endurance or any other metabolic function.

Vitamin B$_{12}$ has gained the reputation of boosting energy. This misconception likely came about after people who lacked energy and may have been deficient in B$_{12}$ felt a boost after taking the vitamin. B vitamins in and of themselves, B$_{12}$ included, do not provide a pick-me-up for people with adequate stores. Shots of B$_{12}$ may be used for people unable to absorb it, but the shots provide no benefit to otherwise healthy people. Excess folic acid can mask a vitamin B$_{12}$ deficiency. Supplemental B$_{12}$ is necessary for vegans or anyone omitting animal proteins. It has been suggested that certain algae contain B$_{12}$; however, the measurement of B$_{12}$ in these sources may not be accurate.

Vitamin C (Ascorbic Acid)

Vitamin C is needed for collagen, which forms connective tissue in cartilage, tendons, skin, and bones. It is also needed for wound healing; the production of carnitine, hormones and neurotransmitters, particularly epinephrine; and the absorption of nonheme iron. Vitamin C is an antioxidant, it inactivates damaging molecules known as free radicals. Although it had been touted to prevent colds, we now know that it can decrease their duration by about a day and the severity of symptoms, but it does not prevent catching a cold. Interestingly, the absorption of vitamin C is dose dependent: Only 50 percent is absorbed with dosages of 1,000 mg, and this decreases with larger doses. The maximum pool of vitamin C in the body is 2,000 mg—stored in tissues and the blood. Although studies have shown that 200 mg per day saturates blood plasma, body tissues and immune cells are saturated at the RDA levels (90 mg/day for men and 75 mg/day for women) (Food and Nutrition Board 2000).

Although not conclusively proven, athletes may need slightly more vitamin C than do sedentary people because of its role in repairing oxidative damage and healing. Endurance exercise increases blood levels of vitamin C in the 24 hours after exercise. Supplemental vitamin C can have both a positive and negative impact on athletes. Ultra-marathon runners experienced a decreased incidence of upper respiratory tract infections for two weeks postrace when 600 mg of vitamin C were taken for 21 days before the race. It has also been shown that athletes exercising in the heat have decreased body temperatures when taking 250 mg of vitamin C. On the flip side, a study from Spain showed that athletes supplemented with 1,000 mg per day for eight weeks reduced adaptations to exercise, resulting in decreased endurance. Another study out of Germany showed similar results with a combination of vitamins C (1,000 mg) and E (400 mg). There may be a threshold level above which vitamin C does more harm than good by becoming a pro-oxidant (Gomez-Cabrera 2008; Davidson 2007; Ristow 2009; Peters 1993; Kotze 1977).

Vitamin D

Vitamin D is both a vitamin and a hormone. Due to its role in calcium absorption, a deficiency can impair bone health. Because Vitamin D receptors exist throughout the body, it is suggested by some researchers to have more widespread effects on our health than have been proven so far. Some experts believe that vitamin D may be protective of hypertension, diabetes (types 1 and 2), certain forms of cancer, multiple sclerosis, fibromyalgia, and more. Its relevance to performance known at this time is mainly in the area of bone health, as it is vital for absorbing calcium and maintaining proper levels in bone; a lack of vitamin D results in improper bone strength and density and an increased risk of fractures. Deficiency has also been associated with muscle weakness and pain; however, increased intake when blood levels are adequate does not result in increased muscle strength. Still, many athletes may benefit from getting vitamin D levels checked because they may have insufficient intake.

The recommendations for D may increase to as much as 1,000 international units (IU) per day the next time new RDAs are determined. Currently, it is 400 IU. Vitamin D testing is not standard and must be requested by the patient or a physician. However, a blood test may reveal a deficiency for which supplementation would be warranted. In addition, vitamin D is the only vitamin that can be formed in the body from sunlight, and so it is sometimes called the sunshine vitamin. However, when sunscreen is used, the body cannot make vitamin D. During winter months in northern climates, sunlight may be insufficient to provide adequate vitamin D.

Vitamin E

Vitamin E is an antioxidant. Specifically, it protects the fats located within cell membranes from damage (lipid peroxidation), thereby maintaining the health of many cells in the body. It inactivates harmful free radicals (free radicals are instable cells that can cause damage to other healthy cells), similarly to vitamin C. Since some free radicals are produced as a by-product of exercise, it has been thought that vitamin E may be protective against muscle damage, soreness, and reduced strength and endurance. The studies done to date have had very mixed results: some have shown an increase in antioxidant activity with supplemental vitamin E, some have shown no benefit, and others have shown a protection of red blood cells while exercising at high altitudes (5,000 and 15,000 feet; 1,500 and 4,500 m). A team of researchers from a German medical school and Harvard Medical School found that vitamins C and E taken together in a supplement negate the positive effects on insulin sensitivity that exercise produces (Ristow 2009).

Vitamin K

Ingesting large amounts of sugar, vitamins A and E, above the upper limit and antibiotics can all decrease intestinal bacteria, decreasing vitamin K production. Adequate vitamin K intake is necessary for bone health. However, studies with endurance-trained female athletes have shown conflicting results of supplemental vitamin K on improvements in low bone mineral density.

Calcium

Calcium is required for bone and tooth formation, and it mediates the constriction and dilation of blood vessels to help maintain a healthy blood pressure. It is also involved in muscle contraction, nerve transmission, and glandular secretions. Ninety-nine percent of calcium in the body is found in the bones and teeth. The remainder is found in extracellular fluid (including the blood), muscle, and other tissues. Its absorption is dependent on vitamin D. Blood levels of calcium are tightly regulated to remain within a specific range. If they drop, a series of hormonal actions signal the bones to release calcium into the bloodstream. Over time this can cause a demineralization of the bone, increasing the risk of fractures.

Adequate calcium is important for all athletes to keep bones strong. It is extremely important for female athletes with amenorrhea (cessation of the menstrual cycle) or the female athlete triad (energy deficit, amenorrhea, and osteoporosis). These conditions cause reduced calcium absorption, and bone formation occurs at a lower rate than in menstruating females. Exercise-induced amenorrhea also results in reduced calcium retention and lower bone mass, putting the athlete at increased risk for fractures. Note that calcium intake above recommended levels does not improve performance by otherwise healthy athletes.

It is also worth mentioning that calcium inhibits the absorption of iron and zinc. This is not a major concern for well-nourished athletes; however, it may have an impact on athletes who keep their calories low and have inadequate intake of these minerals. If calcium supplements are taken, it is usually recommended to separate them from multivitamin, multimineral, or iron supplements by four hours. Also, caffeine can have a modest effect on calcium excretion. For each 150 mg of caffeine consumed, 5 mg of calcium is excreted in the urine. Adding a couple of tablespoons of milk to your coffee can offset the loss.

Magnesium

Since magnesium regulates the flow of calcium in soft tissue, low levels may contribute to muscle cramps. If too much calcium is allowed in, muscle contraction occurs, possibly leading to cramping. Although some athletes take magnesium for cramps, adequate dietary intake can help avoid this in the first place. Note also that supplemental magnesium may cause diarrhea.

Iron

Iron is the oxygen-carrying component of blood and is part of many enzymes that make things happen in the body. About two-thirds of the body's iron is present in the hemoglobin of red blood cells. Hemoglobin carries oxygen from the lungs to muscles, organs, and other body tissues. In muscle tissue, iron is present as myoglobin and is stored as protein compounds called ferritin. Iron is also part of molecules in the mitochondria and other oxidative enzymes. There are two forms of iron in food: heme iron (attached to the blood; only in animal sources) and nonheme iron (found in animal, plant, and fortified foods). The absorption of heme iron is much higher and not affected by foods consumed at the same time. Nonheme iron is not absorbed as easily. To boost absorption of nonheme iron, eat it with a food containing vitamin C; cook it with an acidic food in iron pots and pans; or consume it with meat, fish, or poultry.

Since iron is vital to the transport of oxygen, athletes need adequate amounts, particularly those engaged in aerobic training. Causes of low blood levels include: low dietary intake, losses through sweat and GI bleeding, female menstrual losses, and ruptured red blood cells from footstrike force. Low iron levels are common in runners but have also been detected in female basketball players, field hockey players, and crew members. Long-distance cyclists have experienced reduced iron levels caused by GI bleeding as blood is shunted to muscles and away from the intestinal tract, resulting in inflammation and bleeding. Rowers and weightlifters have been shown to suffer from handgrip hemolysis—the force of holding equipment ruptures red blood cells. Other athletes at risk are those with low calorie intakes and vegetarian diets.

Iron deficiency occurs slowly, and in stages:—first iron stores (ferritin) will drop. Next, blood levels of iron are reduced. As the situation worsens, anemia develops. Iron-deficiency anemia occurs when the body has trouble making hemoglobin, the protein in the blood that carries iron and oxygen. At this point, both iron and hemoglobin blood levels are low. Larger doses of iron are required by supplement than can be provided by diet alone. Typically an athlete needs to be monitored by a medical professional, as it is not recommended to take iron supplements for extended periods of time without medical supervision. Note that excessive intake of tannins found in coffee and tea can inhibit iron absorption. Athletes with low iron levels or anemia should drink tea and coffee in between meals as opposed to with meals to keep the tannins from reducing iron absorption.

Potassium

Potassium is an electrolyte that conducts electrical impulses across cell membranes, particularly in nerve and muscle tissue (including the heart). Potassium has a positive charge and is chiefly located inside cells. It helps regulate fluid balance along with sodium and chloride, which are located outside the cells. Potassium also helps with the transport of glucose into muscle cells and the storage of glycogen.

The body regulates serum potassium levels rather tightly. If there is an excess, hormones signal the kidneys to excrete potassium; if levels are low, the kidneys will conserve it. During fasting, diarrhea, vomiting, or use of diuretics, very low levels can occur, termed hypokalemia. This can result in muscle weakness and even heart attack because of potassium's role in electrical conduction in the heart. Potassium supplementation is not recommended and in fact can be dangerous, as it can disturb the natural rhythm of the heart. Supplements should not be taken without medical supervision. Although a small amount of potassium is lost in sweat, it can be easily replaced with food.

Sodium

Sodium is an electrolyte that works along with potassium to regulate fluid balance. Outside the cells, it maintains plasma volume and blood pressure. The body maintains sodium levels in the blood within a range that is hormonally controlled. If a large intake occurs, the body will excrete more sodium in the urine; conversely, if little is ingested through diet, very little will be excreted.

During exercise, however, we lose sodium through sweat. The renal (kidney) feedback mechanism may be overridden if losses through sweat are large. As described in chapter 7, increased intake of sodium is required for athletes competing for many hours, especially novice marathoners who may overdrink, thus diluting their blood sodium, and so may become hyponatremic (low blood sodium). However, if you have high blood pressure, talk to your medical provider about your exercise and the right level of sodium intake for you.

Zinc

More than 100 enzymes need zinc to catalyze (spark) reactions, affecting numerous bodily functions. It is involved in protein synthesis and breakdown; it's incorporated into proteins involved with vitamin A and D receptors; and it's needed for DNA and RNA synthesis, taste acuity, immunity, acid–base balance, collagen formation, wound healing, insulin functioning, and testosterone production. Zinc is also part of an important antioxidant, superoxide dismutase. It is clear that zinc is essential for many functions of training.

Some studies have shown that zinc blood levels increase initially after endurance training and significantly decrease two to four hours later. After exercise, zinc may be redistributed away from contracting muscle and into the blood from which some is sent to the liver and the rest is excreted in the urine, possibly leaving decreased levels in muscle tissue. Some studies have shown rather sizable urinary zinc losses after endurance exercise. Therefore, zinc-rich food should regularly be part of an endurance athlete's diet, particularly in post-competition meals. Excess zinc (from supplements) decreases good (HDL) cholesterol and can interfere with copper absorption.

Chromium

Chromium helps insulin work effectively and is required in the body's use of glucose, fats, and amino acids. Early studies with supplemental chromium picolinate indicated a role in body fat loss and increased lean mass. This was later disproven because the early studies did not measure whether or not the athletes were deficient in chromium. Plasma and urine are not good indicators of chromium status. Since it is concentrated in the liver, spleen, soft tissues, and bone, it is difficult to measure.

Excess intake does not improve performance or body composition in untrained or well-trained athletes. Although chromium has a role in glucose metabolism and adequate amounts are necessary, taking more will not cause your blood sugar to go down or move glucose into muscle cells faster.

Iodine

Iodine plays a role in protein synthesis, enzyme activity, and is important for the manufacture of thyroid hormone, which regulates metabolism, or the speed of reactions throughout the body. Thyroid hormones act on the brain, muscles, heart, kidneys, and pituitary gland. Inadequate iodine results in reduced thyroid hormone levels, and some studies show that inadequate iodine may impair immunity. Selenium deficiency can impair the action of thyroid hormone, and deficiencies of vitamin A and iron can make the effects of an iodine deficiency worse. Since the actions of thyroid hormone are widespread throughout the body, adequate iodine is essential for athletes. Note that excess iodine will not speed up metabolism.

Iodized salt is the main source of iodine in the American food system (although also found in seafood and seaweed). Note that the popular sea salts and Kosher salt do not necessarily contain iodine.

Selenium

Selenium regenerates vitamin C, aids in regulation of thyroid hormone, and acts as an antioxidant within the body; it is incorporated into the enzyme glutathione peroxidase, which scavenges free radicals, so it aids the body's defense against oxidative stress. Since athletes may create more free radical molecules than sedentary people, having an adequate antioxidant defense system is thought to be helpful. Increased selenium intake has not proven to be performance enhancing.

Note that both food and supplements can be toxic at high intake levels, unlike some other nutrients. Symptoms include hair and nail brittleness (popular complaint), gastro-intestinal disturbances, skin rash, nervous system abnormalities, fatigue, irritability, and garlic breath odor.

Copper

Copper is a component of several enzymes. It contributes to the functioning of hemoglobin (in blood) and helps iron with oxygen metabolism. It is needed for collagen synthesis and for creating connective tissue. Athletes have been shown to increase their manufacture of copper-containing antioxidants without requiring additional intake. Supplements may cause nausea, vomiting, and diarrhea, so they are not advised. High intakes of zinc impair copper absorption.

Timing Tip

The body uses B vitamins (thiamin, B_{12}, B_6, and folic acid) to process alcohol. B vitamins play a crucial role in energy metabolism. After a night of drinking, you may feel lackluster. Magnesium and vitamin C used to metabolize alcohol can leave your immune system and recovery process more vulnerable. Additionally, alcohol can contribute to dehydration and can alter blood sugar regulation.

Vitamins, minerals, and phytonutrients are topics of interest and concern among the athletes we see. They are always wondering how they will know if they are getting enough vitamins and minerals in their diets and whether they should take supplements. The truth is that vitamins, minerals, and phytonutrients are essential for good performance because good health is essential for good performance—at least if you are in it for the long haul.

Science is still sorting out just what each nutrient really does within the body. The more we find out, the more evident it is: Nutrients work together to keep us healthy, and many body functions are interdependent.

Sometimes athletes are used to being able to eat so many calories that they may not be conscious of the quality of the food they consume. This is a short-term approach to well-being. To get the most out of your body, get the most out of your food. Choose nutrient-rich foods that will provide an array of vitamins, minerals, and phytonutrients for the foundation of your diet. A multivitamin doesn't make up for a nutrient-poor diet because all the beneficial substances we find in food cannot be found in one pill. There are times when vitamin supplementation is indicated, but there is no specific need to spend extra on vitamin drinks or bars based on claims of their vitamin, mineral, or antioxident content.

7

The Role of Fluids

An athlete called the office and said, "I have a quick question. How much water should I drink each day?" That might be a quick question, but it doesn't have a quick answer! If you're thinking, *Doesn't everyone need eight glasses of water every day?* The answer is: *not necessarily*. Hydration needs vary not only from person to person but also in the same person from day to day and under different conditions. We'll discuss all of these factors and explain how to be sure you're properly hydrated. Optimal fluid intake is as important as any other aspect of nutrition for sports performance. Drinking too much or too little can be harmful to health and performance.

HOW OUR BODIES USE FLUIDS

Did you know that at least half of your body is made of water? Overweight people might be close to 40 percent water, while elite athletes could be nearly 75 percent. Much of the body's water is in muscle tissue and blood. Every day we lose water through breathing, digestion, waste elimination, and sweat—which is the largest route. When you burn calories, you actually create heat within the muscle. This heat has to be released from the body. How does this happen? During exercise the heat you create is carried in your bloodstream from your core to just below the surface of your skin. This heat activates sweat glands, which release salty water onto your skin. When your sweat evaporates, it cools the blood just under your skin. That's how your body regulates its temperature. If sweat does not evaporate, as on a humid day, it becomes more difficult to cool off and harder to work at the same intensity. If the heat produced from exercise isn't released from your body, heat illness could develop with dire consequences. When you dehydrate, some fluid is lost from blood, making it thicker and resulting in reduced blood volume. This causes you to work harder to pump adequate blood with each heartbeat to working muscles and limits the work you can do in an attempt to protect your body from overheating. The greater your fluid loss, the greater your risk of dehydrating and experiencing physical symptoms (see table 7.1).

In addition to losing water in sweat, we also lose electrolytes. Electrolytes play a crucial role in the body. When our levels are out of balance, it can affect both health and performance.

I Hear a Lot About Electrolytes, but What Are They?

An electrolyte is a substance that conducts an electric current when dissolved in liquid. In the body, sodium, chloride, and potassium are the major electrolytes found in blood and the fluids of body tissues (calcium and magnesium are also electrolytes but have a lesser role in managing fluid balance). Electrolytes are important for fluid balance, conduction of nerve impulses, muscle contraction, and more. With regard to hydration, the differences in electrical charges allow for fluids to move inside, outside, and around cells. Having enough of each electrolyte allows for fluids to be balanced throughout body tissues and blood.

Table 7.1   Symptoms of Fluid Loss at Various Levels

Percentage of body weight lost	Amount of weight for 130 lb (60 kg) athlete	Amount of weight for 200 lb (90 kg) athlete	Physical symptoms
1%	1.3 lb (.6 kg)	2 lb (.9 kg)	Become thirsty and experience lowered ability to regulate body temperature; work capacity begins to decrease
2%	2.6 lb (1.2 kg)	4 lb (1.8 kg)	Stronger thirst; vague discomfort and sense of oppression; loss of appetite
3%	3.9 lb (1.8 kg)	6 lb (2.7 kg)	Dry mouth; more concentrated blood; reduced urine output (in effort to conserve body fluid)
4%	5.2 lb (2.4 kg)	8 lb (3.6 kg)	Loss of 20-30% physical work capacity
5%	6.5 lb (2.9 kg)	10 lb (4.5 kg)	Difficulty concentrating; headache; impatience; sleepiness
6%	7.8 lb (3.5 kg)	12 lb (5.4 kg)	Severe impairment in temperature regulation during exercise; increased respiratory rate, leading to tingling and numbness of extremities
7%	9.1 lb (4.1 kg)	14 lb (6.3 kg)	Likely collapse if combined with heat and exercise

Adapted, with permission, from J.E. Greenleaf and M.H. Harrison, 1986, Water and electrolytes. In *Nutrition and aerobic exercise,* edited by D.K. Layman (Washington, DC: American Chemical Society), 107-124. Copyright 1986 American Chemical Society.

Sweat is more than just water; although there are more than a dozen minerals and electrolytes lost in sweat, sodium, chloride, and potassium make up the largest losses (see table 7.2). These substances need to be replaced every day through diet and, except for sodium, do not necessarily need to be replaced during most training or competitions. One glass of orange juice has more than twice the potassium lost in an average liter of sweat, for example; about a quarter of a cup of milk will replenish the calcium lost in that same amount.

In hot, humid weather your body may produce more sweat in an effort to cool off, so fluid and electrolyte losses may be greater than in cooler temperatures. Although you may not sweat as much in cooler temperatures, it is still important to replace lost fluids. Your hydration strategy may also be different if you train or compete in different climates or even if you train at different altitudes because higher altitudes can cause a greater loss of fluid. Depending on the duration and intensity of the sport, hydrating during training or an event is often important. Dehydration puts a strain on the heart—it's harder for the heart to pump your blood and harder to get rid of the heat you produce during exercise. Losing even 1 percent of body weight through dehydration may subtly affect an athlete's performance. For every 1 percent loss, heart rate increases by five to eight beats per minute, and core body temperature increases by .4 to .5 degrees Fahrenheit (.2 to .3 degrees Celcius). Of course, greater fluid losses can more severely affect not only performance but also health. See table 7.3 for weight changes through fluid loss and the recommended amount of fluid that should be consumed for replenishment.

Table 7.2   Electrolyte Losses in 1 L of Sweat

Electrolyte	Average lost (mg)	Range lost per L (mg)
Sodium	920-1150*	460-1,840
Chloride	1,065	177-2,130
Potassium	195	117-585
Calcium	40	12-80
Magnesium	19	5-36

*sodium concentration is highly varible

Adapted from E.F. Coyle, 2004, "Fluid and fuel intake during exercise," *Journal of Sports Sciences* 22(1): 39-55.

Table 7.3   Fluid Intake and Frequency Based on Amount of Weight Lost During Exercise

Weight loss		Fluid intake		Frequency
(lb/hr)	(kg/hr)	(oz)	(ml)	(min)
1	.45	4	120	15
2	.9	8	225	15
3	1.4	8	240	10
4	1.8	10	300	10
5	2.3	12*	380*	10
6	2.7	16*	450*	10

*It would be an extreme challenge to consume this much at 10-minute intervals; rehydration is key, and monitoring symptoms of dehydration is extremely important.

Why is sodium balance so important and challenging?

Fluids in the body exist both inside cells and outside cells surrounding all body tissues. Sodium, which is found mostly in the extracellular fluids surrounding cells (e.g., blood plasma), is responsible for maintaining the proper fluid balance. It acts like a pump to move fluid, as needed, from the outside to the inside of a cell. Sodium distributes fluid to the appropriate places, in the necessary amounts throughout the body, so that all our organs, muscles, and other tissues will function properly. Under resting conditions, the body works to keep the concentration of sodium in the blood within a certain range. The rise and fall of certain hormones (e.g., vasopressin, an antidiuretic hormone, and aldosterone) tell the kidneys (1) when to release water (urinate) or hold on to it and (2) when to release sodium or reabsorb it. When we are not exercising, the hormones and kidneys work together to make sure our body fluids and electrolytes are at the proper levels through a system similar to a thermostat. When we sweat, we lose some of the fluids from inside and outside cells, along with sodium. Sweating makes the job of fluid balance more challenging.

Athletes sweat at different rates and lose sodium at different rates. You probably know athletes who look as if they walked out of the shower after practice. And then there are those who, when their shirts dry, have a white band of salt across their backs. The salt may even dry on their faces and arms, and certainly they may be able to taste the saltiness of their sweat. These athletes are heavy salt sweaters. However, an athlete may also have a high sodium loss without these telltale signs.

In one liter (about 2 lb/1 kg) of sweat, sodium loss typically ranges from 460 to 1,610 mg (20 to 80 mmol), the average being somewhere around 920 to 1,150 mg (a teaspoon of salt contains 2,300 mg of sodium). Athletes who are acclimated to the heat typically lose less sodium in their sweat. Athletes who are not acclimated or are genetically heavy salt sweaters can lose substantial amounts of sodium. Depending on the brand, one liter of a sports drink may have 230 to 800 mg/L of sodium; so drinking a sports beverage before, during, and after may or may not be sufficient, particularly if athletes are training for long periods of time and are losing much more sodium than they are able to take in. Some athletes need to ingest even more sodium via high-sodium foods, as shown in figure 7.1.

Athletes sometimes develop cramps during training and competition. Heat cramps may be caused by a loss of large amounts of water and sodium. The term *heat cramps* can be misleading because athletes may experience cramps in cooler temperatures if large losses of sodium occur and are not replaced with food and fluids. Because the dangers of excess sodium intake have been publicized in the media, many people refrain from adding salt to foods. Athletes, particularly those experiencing cramps, those who become significantly dehydrated, and those who sweat profusely, may benefit from liberally adding sodium to their diets. To replace sodium losses, some athletes need to use the salt shaker, salt tablets/packets, and/or add more sodium to sports drinks. Some athletes may not have a taste for salt immediately after training. However, if fluids are taken, the desire for salt usually follows. It is important to consume enough salt—a large fluid intake without sufficient sodium can result in hyponatremia (low sodium levels, discussed next) even after exercise is over. Additionally, sodium is required to retain and distribute the water properly. If you crave salt, salt your food! As part of your training diet, include foods such as red or marinara sauce, pickles on a sandwich, and soups. Of course, cramps can result from causes other than dehydration, including fatigue and working above your level of conditioning.

FIGURE 7.1
High-sodium foods

Food	Serving size	Sodium content (mg)
Table salt	1 tsp	2325
McDonald's Premium Grilled Chicken Classic	1 sandwich	1190
Pickle	4 in	1181
Chicken noodle soup	1 cup	1106
Ham	3 oz	1095
Cottage cheese	1 cup	918
Soy sauce	1 tbsp	900
Cheese pizza, 14"	1 slice	740
Tomato juice, canned	8 oz	654
Bagel	4 oz	604
V-8 vegetable juice	8 oz	586
Pretzels, hard	1 oz (10 twists)	560
American cheese	1 oz (1 slice)	417
Saltines	10 crackers	380
Ketchup	2 tbsp	335
Salted peanuts	1 oz (about 30)	231

What is hyponatremia?

As a result of the many years of advice to drink, drink, drink, some athletes overdo it. Yes, it is possible to drink too much. Hyponatremia occurs when blood sodium levels become too low because *too much* water and other fluids are consumed. It can happen with sports drinks, too, because all sports drinks have a sodium concentration that is far less than one's blood. Hyponatremia is generally defined as blood sodium levels of 130 mmol/L or less.

This dangerous condition usually occurs in events lasting four hours or more such as a marathon or ultra-marathon—when the athlete has plenty of time to drink a lot of fluid. In marathon running, hyponatremia occurs more often in smaller, slower, less lean runners who drink heavily. It may even occur in the hours after an event if an athlete drinks a lot of fluid and the pace of drinking is greater than urine production. The lower the blood sodium level drops, the faster it decreases. The longer it remains low, the greater the chance of encephalopathy (brain swelling) and pulmonary edema (fluid around the lungs). One difficult thing about hyponatremia is that the symptoms are very similar to dehydration: nausea, fatigue, and disorientation; however, there is swelling and *weight gain* instead of weight loss throughout an exercise bout or competition. Following are a few ways to prevent hyponatremia. If you have a medical condition that requires sodium restriction, discuss your specific situation with your medical provider.

- Drink if you are thirsty.
- Drink to replace only the amount of fluid lost through sweat, *not* more.
- Do not limit sodium intake. During continuous days of exercise in hot weather, consume extra sodium with meals and snacks.
- Do not drink so much that you gain weight during training or competition.
- Avoid NSAID medications—ibuprofen (Advil), naproxen (Aleve), and acetylsalicylic acid (Aspirin, 325 mg)—unless directed to take them by your doctor. They may interfere with blood flow to the kidneys and the ability to retain sodium during long distance endurance training or competition. Acetaminophen (Tylenol) is fine.

Although hyponatremia seems to be more about overdrinking than under-consuming sodium, you may also wish to consume sports drinks with higher sodium levels (one of the "endurance" formulas); consider adding additional sodium to your sports drink. Or a salt packet can help boost sodium intake during a long race. One packet has 270 mg of sodium. Some athletes take one packet under the tongue early on, along with fluid and another later in a race.

What happens when I dehydrate?

Dehydration causes very real changes to the body. All can be measured, but some you can feel. When you are dehydrated, the volume of fluid in your body is reduced. Since most of this fluid is in the blood, your blood becomes thicker and harder for the heart to pump; with each beat, the heart sends out less blood. Heart rate also increases because the heart has to work harder to circulate blood and get oxygen and nutrients to the working muscles. Exercise seems harder because it is. Since blood flow to muscles slows, the transport of fuel is reduced also, so muscles use up glycogen faster, leading to fatigue more quickly. Blood flow is also decreased to the brain, impairing sharpness and mental functioning.

As your blood volume reduces, your body signals to preserve fluid, and you begin to sweat less, which means you can't cool off as well; your core temperature rises, making the situation worse; exercise becomes harder, and you have an increased risk of injury; your coordination suffers; physical and mental fatigue sets in, and you may experience mood shifts, perception changes, and irritability as well as muscle cramps, nausea, vomiting, or headaches. These symptoms don't occur with a pound or two of fluid loss—you have to

Timing Tip

Some herbal supplements, such as agrimony, artichoke, buchu, burdock, celery, corn silk, guaiac wood, squill, uva ursi, and yarrow, have diuretic properties. It is difficult to estimate their effects on hydration because dosages and potency may vary, so it is best to avoid them. Avoid taking any over-the-counter diuretics because of the possibility of dehydration and electrolyte imbalances. If you are taking prescription diuretic medications, check with your doctor about their impact on hydration and electrolyte status when training, especially if sweating heavily.

be sweating a lot and not drinking to reach these levels. But it can and does happen, so be aware of the symptoms. Also, dehydration can be additive over time if you do not drink enough during and after training and throughout the day. If you start out a training session inadequately hydrated, your performance may suffer, and you can become dehydrated more quickly than if you began well hydrated.

Many studies have looked at runners, cyclists, and other endurance athletes and the role dehydration can play in reducing endurance and stamina. In team sports, effects of dehydration have been documented in studies on skills as well. For example, in soccer, dehydration can cause an inability to sprint late in the game, an impaired ability to challenge for loose balls, and slower dribbling speeds. Dehydration can cause basketball players to make fewer shots, decrease their sprint-

Making Weight

Jockeys, wrestlers, crew members, judo competitors, some football players, and all others whose weight determines whether you compete: We understand that certain practices you employ for making weight often include dehydrating. How you go about making weight can affect your training, performance, and even long-term health. The NCAA (National Collegiate Athletic Association) implemented weight-loss and hydration guidelines for college wrestlers after the death of athletes in 1997 because of severe dehydration.

If you are gaining and losing more than 5 percent of your body weight on a weekly basis, your performance is going to be off. Restricting food and fluids during the week robs your body of the proper fuel to train with. Being chronically dehydrated means your weekly training won't be as effective in readying you for your meet, match, or game.

For a 175 pound (80 kg) athlete, a 3 or 4 pound (1.4 or 1.8 kg) weight change each week is reasonable (2 percent); 10 pounds (4.5 kg) is not (6 percent). Of course we're not promoting dehydrating yourself, but we do understand that a certain amount of fluid is somewhat dispensable. It is better to be well hydrated most of the week and allow for some fluid loss on the day before weigh-in rather than be dehydrated all week long. Be strategic in your weight management plan so that you are not trying to lose 5 percent of your body weight in one day.

Prepare ahead and develop an appropriate weight plan so you're not caught up in this vicious cycle. By mapping out the year, you can determine realistic weights for yourself during the offseason, preseason, and season. A cycle of weight loss and weight gain is detrimental to performance and influences injury risk, mood, and concentration. Training in a chronically dehydrated state could even be harmful to your long-term health and well-being. Even after postseason weight gain and a return to normal eating patterns, some wrestlers remain dehydrated—their bodies adapt to their chronic dehydration.

ing and lateral movement speed, and decrease their depth perception. There is every reason to believe that athletes in all sports, especially those with large sweat losses, might experience similar performance decrements.

Strength and power are negatively affected by loss of body fluids as well. Weightlifters have difficulty completing all repetitions of an exercise when dehydrated (loss of 2.5 percent body weight). If you're not able to complete the prescribed repetitions, you won't realize the gains in strength and size that you would have seen had you been well hydrated and able to do more work. In addition to limiting your capacity for work, dehydration greatly increases the release of cortisol. If you remember, cortisol increases muscle breakdown, which could interfere with muscle building.

How can I tell if I am dehydrated?

Use the first void of the morning to assess hydration status. If your urine looks like apple juice or iced tea and is of a small volume, chances are you need to step up your hydration strategy. When you're not well-hydrated, there isn't enough

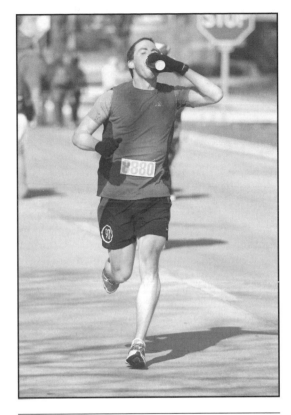

Develop a hydration plan for race day.

extra water available to dilute the waste products that are excreted in urine. That's why it's dark and scant. If your urine looks more like lemonade and you can produce a good volume, then most likely you are well-hydrated. Urine color may be affected by B-vitamins (Riboflavin, B-2) which make the urine bright yellow; betacyanins, a pigment in some dark red vegetables, such as beets, which can tinge urine slightly red; or artificial food colorings which can possibly impart a bluish or greenish color.

If your training is later in the day or evening, be sure to drink adequately throughout the day and check urine before exercise. For students or others who are unable to drink during the day, be sure to get some fluids in whenever possible—between classes, during breaks, and at meals. Get into the habit of grabbing a few sips whenever you pass a water fountain.

Should I force myself to drink, or should I just drink when I'm thirsty?

This is a hot topic of debate among hydration experts. Exercising in a dehydrated state is not ideal and can hurt both performance and, if extreme, health. On the other hand, drinking too much water (without taking in adequate sodium) dilutes the sodium in the blood, which may result in hyponatremia.

Timing Tip

All other variables being equal, athletes who maintain hydration last 33 percent longer than those who don't drink during a workout, so the athlete who is adequately hydrated has a competitive edge over an improperly hydrated athlete.

Which hydration strategy is best?

Some experts suggest that performance begins to suffer at fluid losses greater than 2 percent of body mass. Hydration strategies to prevent losses above this amount include drinking on schedule before, during, and after training lasting more than an hour, and possibly for shorter, intense training. For many athletes, thirst does not match hydration status, and when left to their own devices, they do not intuitively replace adequate fluid to match losses. Others assert that instead of drinking on schedule, athletes should let thirst drive fluid intake; as long as fluid is available and consumed according to thirst, an athlete will not realize decrements in performance. The International Marathon Medical Directors Association (IMMDA) Position Statement explains that thirst is stimulated at levels of 1.7 to 3.5 percent dehydration. The thirst mechanism, according to the IMMDA, should help athletes, in most cases, from drinking too little or too much fluid, preventing the blood plasma from reaching levels that are either too concentrated or too diluted in sodium. However, in an extremely hot environment (greater than 100°F, or 38°C), athletes may need additional fluids until they become acclimated to the temperature; in cooler temperatures (less than 41°F, or 5°C), thirst may be triggered at higher levels of dehydration. An athlete should not gain weight during a race, which would indicate drinking too much, or experience extreme weight loss (more than 4 percent body weight). Both reflect improper hydration. The IMMDA also states that it is fine for athletes to obtain a general understanding of their fluid needs by means of a fluid calculator (see "Determining Your Sweat Rate"), but they should always listen to their bodies' signals—drink if thirsty; don't drink if bloated or weight gain occurs during training or a race.

So who is right? There certainly is validity to paying attention to thirst and drinking accordingly. The problem is that many athletes do not pay attention to their thirst or don't drink adequately to hydrate themselves. Additionally, thirst may not kick in until 3.5 percent dehydration for some athletes, according to the IMMDA, a point at which performance would already be negatively affected. Cardiovascular strain has been shown to occur in hot weather at dehydration rates of 2 percent loss of body weight (3 percent in cooler temperatures), so we think it's a good idea to know how much fluid you lose in conditions you typically train and compete in. Simply be more attentive to your hydration needs. To us, these two positions do not really seem as far apart as they are often made out to be. The take-home message is don't become too dehydrated, and don't over-drink. Since athletes do not know their weight during an event, the best way is to anticipate weight changes by recording changes and practicing hydration during workouts in order to gain a sense of your own sweat rate.

Having a hydration strategy that is based on your typical sweat rate just makes sense. How do you do that? Perform the sweat rate test, and develop a strategy for fluid replacement based on those results. Additionally, a schedule for hydrating can also provide you with a schedule for fueling—particularly if you are using a sports drink. Note that if you train in different temperatures or climatic conditions, you will need to adjust or perform the test under those conditions. Remember that adequate sodium ingestion along with fluid is essential for regulating fluid balance.

Timing Tip

Consuming small amounts of fluid more often is better than a large amount at once (for instance, do not wait to drink until after practice and then down a liter of water). Drinking small amounts more frequently will help you absorb and utilize the fluid better. Be aware that if you drink a lot of fluid at once, gastric emptying is slowed down.

DETERMINING YOUR SWEAT RATE

One of the best ways to understand your fluid needs during exercise is to determine your sweat rate. You may need to do this at different times of the year and in different locations (outdoor versus indoor training, or if you travel for competition) because environmental factors, such as humidity, temperature, and altitude, affect your sweat rate. Try the following for two or three days or even a week to get a sense of your average weight change. You will then use that information to calculate how much fluid you need to ingest to prevent dehydration.

1. Before the measurement, urinate and defecate, if needed.
2. Weigh yourself on a reliable scale, preferably in the nude. If you must wear clothing, be sure to have the same or similar dry clothing available for the postexercise weigh-in.
3. Exercise under the conditions you generally train or are planning to compete.
4. Bring a measured amount of hydration beverage. If you do not drink all of your fluid, make note of the amount of fluid consumed.
5. If you can, avoid using the bathroom until after you weigh in the second time. If you just can't wait, you should try the weigh-in process another day.
6. After exercise, remove wet clothing and dry off. If you need to be clothed, put on clothing that is the same as or similar to what you wore for the first weigh-in. Take body weight.

Record your numbers over several workouts over several days. Now, to assess your fluid losses during exercise, follow these four steps:

1. Starting weight in pounds (_____) – ending weight in pounds (_____) = _____ pounds lost

2. _____ pounds lost x 16 = _____ ounces lost

3. _____ ounces lost + _____ ounces beverage consumed = _____ ounces sweat lost

4. _____ ounces lost ÷ _____ exercise time (in hours) = _____ hourly sweat rate

Or, for a metric measurement of your fluid losses, use this equation:

1. Starting weight in kg (_____) – ending weight in kg (_____) = _____ kg lost

2. _____ kg lost x 1,000 (1 kg = 1,000 ml) = _____ ml lost

3. _____ ml lost + _____ ml beverage consumed = _____ ml hourly sweat rate

4. _____ ml lost ÷ _____ exercise time (in hours) = _____ hourly sweat rate

For example, if an athlete's starting weight is 150 pounds and his ending weight is 149 pounds, and he drank 16 ounces during exercise, this is what the calculation would look like:

1. Starting weight in pounds (___150___) − ending weight in pounds (___149___) = ___1___ pound lost

2. ___1___ pound lost x 16 = ___16___ ounces lost

3. ___16___ ounces lost + ___16___ ounces beverage consumed = ___32___ ounces hourly sweat rate

4. ___32___ ounces ÷ ___1.5___ exercise time (in hours) = ___21___ ounces hourly sweat rate

Or, using the metric system, if an athlete's starting weight is 68 kilograms and his ending weight is 67.5 kilograms, this is what the calculation would look like:

1. Starting weight in kg (___68___) − ending weight in kg (___67.5___) = ___.5___ kg lost

2. ___.5___ kg lost x 1,000 (1 kg = 1,000 ml) = ___500___ ml lost

3. ___500___ ml lost + ___500___ ml beverage consumed = ___1,000___ ml hourly sweat rate

4. ___1,000___ ml lost ÷ ___1.5___ exercise time (in hours) = ___666___ ml hourly sweat rate

To match your fluid loss, divide your hourly sweat rate by 6 or 4, depending on whether it is easiest for you to rehydrate every 10 minutes or 15 minutes each hour. In our example, the athlete would want to drink 3.5 ounces every 10 minutes (21 divided by 6) or 5 ounces every 15 minutes (21 divided by 4). To replace 666 ml, drink 111 ml every 10 minutes or 166 ml every 15 minutes. Essentially, the idea is to divide your training and competition time into manageable segments and to consume fluids throughout.

HYDRATION AND TRAINING

Part of a great hydration strategy is creating a timetable for when to consume fluids. Obviously, drinking milk, juice, or water with each meal will contribute to meeting your daily fluid needs. However, as training gets closer, the type of fluid you select and the amount will become even more specific.

Timing Tip

Drink before and during training lasting 1 hour or more. There is a lag between drinking, fluid leaving the stomach, and delivery to muscle. Having some fluid in the stomach actually speeds the rate of emptying.

Hydration Before Training

You may be tuned into sports nutrition enough to think about *eating* something before you train to fuel the workout, but do you think about drinking to hydrate before exercise? If you answered no, you're not alone. Many athletes, especially early birds, do not think about hydrating before a morning workout, but it's just as important to start an early workout hydrated as one later in the day (Stover et al 2006).

For training or practices lasting more than an hour, pre-hydrate, even if all your body signs are good (light-colored urine, no change in body weight, and lack of thirst). Why? Because it takes time for the pre-exercise beverage to leave your stomach and reach tissues that need the fluid. Also, having some fluid in your stomach helps increase the rate of stomach emptying—so later, when you really need fluid, you'll have access to it. We are not suggesting water loading, just enough to keep fluid levels in balance. General recommendations from the National Athletic Trainers' Association and the International Association of Athletics Federations suggest drinking 17 to 20 ounces (510 to 600 ml) of fluid two to three hours before training and 7 to 10 ounces (210 to 300 ml) of fluid 10 to 20 minutes before training. The American College of Sports Medicine (ACSM) guidelines differ slightly by taking body weight into account. They suggest drinking 5 to 7 ml/kg of body weight at least four hours before training and, if needed, drinking 3 to 5 ml/kg of body weight two hours before training. See table 7.4 to calculate your own prehydration needs.

Hydration During Training

Training and practices lasting an hour or more require you to take in some form of fluid. Water is fine for sessions up to an hour, but for longer sessions or ones of higher intensity, a sports drink (alternated with water, if desired) is beneficial. Replacing sodium, which is a key ingredient in most sports drinks, can help draw fluids into the body and encourage you to drink (see figure 7.2 on page 85 for several acceptable training beverages). Supplying muscles with carbohydrate, another ingredient in sports drinks, is also important during extended training sessions, as we explain in chapter 3. Carbohydrate not only supplies energy to working muscles but also stimulates sodium absorption, which in turn increases water absorption. If you choose to drink water and fuel with a sports gel, check sodium content. Some provide very little sodium, while others provide more.

During training, athletes should avoid juices and other soft drinks, such as soda, because of their high carbohydrate concentration and carbonation, which is best left to nonexercise times.

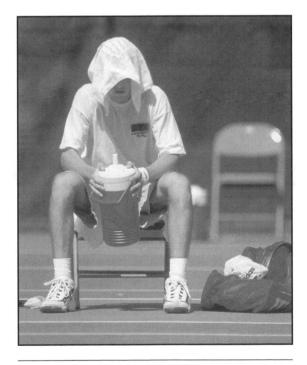

Hydration between play helps to replace lost fluids and rehydrate for the next set.

Table 7.4 Prehydration Needs Based on Body Weight

Body weight kg (lb)	Ounces to drink 4 hours before (5-7 ml/kg)	Ounces to drink 2 hours before (3-5 ml/kg)
41 (90)	7-10	4-7
43 (95)	7-70	4-7
45 (100)	8-11	5-8
48 (105)	8-11	5-8
50 (110)	8-12	5-8
52 (115)	9-12	5-9
55 (120)	9-13	6-9
57 (125)	9-13	6-9
59 (130)	10-14	6-10
61 (135)	10-14	6-10
64 (140)	11-15	6-11
66 (145)	11-16	7-11
68 (150)	11-16	7-11
70 (155)	12-17	7-12
73 (160)	12-17	7-12
75 (165)	13-18	8-13
77 (170)	13-18	8-13
80 (175)	14-19	8-14
82 (180)	14-19	8-14
84 (185)	14-20	9-14
86 (190)	15-20	9-15
91 (200)	15-22	9-15
93 (205)	16-22	9-16
95 (210)	16-22	10-16
98 (215)	17-23	10-17
100 (220)	17-24	10-17
102 (225)	17-24	10-17
105 (230)	18-25	11-18
107 (235)	18-25	11-18
109 (240)	18-26	11-18
114 (250)	19-27	12-19
125 (275)	21-30	13-21
136 (300)	23-32	14-23

FIGURE 7.2
Training beverages

BEVERAGE (8 OZ)	CALORIES	CARBOHY-DRATE (G)	PROTEIN (G)	SODIUM (G)	POTASSIUM (G)
Regular sports drinks					
Accelerade	80	15	4	120	15
All Sport Body Quencher	60	16	0	55	60
Amino Vital	35	7	1,440 mg	10	35
Clif Quench	45	11	0	130	35
Gatorade Endurance Formula	50	14	0	200	90
Gatorade Perform 02	50	14	0	110	30
Gu20 powder mixed with water	50	13	0	120	20
Heed, 1 scoop mixed with water	105	27	0	40	0
Powerade Ion4	50	14	0	100	25
PowerBar Endurance	70	17	0	190	10
Gatorade Prime 01	100	25	0	110	35
Low-calorie sports drinks					
Gatorade Perform 02 (G2)	20	5	0	110	30
Powerade 0 with Ion4	0	0	0	100	25
Propel	20	5	0	75	15

Dense carbohydrates remain in the stomach and intestinal tract longer, causing discomfort. These beverages are fine to drink after exercise, just not during. Because we lose sodium in sweat, an added benefit of sports drinks is that they contain sodium, which helps the body retain water.

If there is no sodium in your fluid, then whatever energy source you consume should provide sodium (crushed pretzels at halftime, for instance, or salt pills along with adequate fluid). The best concentration of a sports drink is 11 to 19 grams of carbohydrate per 8 ounces (5 to 8 percent solution). There isn't firm consensus on the

Timing Tip

Just as you train your muscles to endure more work, practice drinking fluids during training to become more comfortable and to tolerate fluids better. By doing so, and matching your sweat loss within 2 percent of body weight, you will maintain your skills, endurance, power, and body temperature.

Nutrient Timing in Action

Sue, a 16-year-old nationally-ranked female track and field athlete, came to see Heidi after one of the scariest and most uncomfortable experiences in her unfolding career. Being very conscientious, Sue would drink water all day while at school, carrying a water bottle with her everywhere. She would drink before, during, and after training. Sue had a meet a two-hour plane ride away. The team flew down on Friday for Saturday's meet. She had not eaten before getting on the plane because she rushed from school to the airport, but she planned on eating when she arrived at her destination. The plane was late leaving, however, and other than water and a few small bags of pretzels, Sue really did not eat. On Saturday morning, she ate her typical prerace meal (oatmeal). But there were many delays, and instead of running at 9:30, she did not run until 12:30. Sue didn't have any food with her that she felt comfortable eating, and she wanted to run "light" anyway, so all she did was drink water. Her run was three miles, not a distance in which dehydration would even be a great concern. After the race, Sue felt nauseated and uncomfortable. She thought she might be dehydrated. She lay down for a while in the medical tent, then she went back to her hotel, where she started to throw up. Her parents took her to the hospital, where she was finally diagnosed with hyponatremia.

Heidi and Sue worked on a strategy for fueling and drinking more appropriately for the distance she runs. Training and competition may be very different. They worked hard to prevent this from ever happening again. Sue cut back on her water consumption throughout the day and drinks a sports drink around training and competition. Sue now travels with a care package when going on road trips in case delays occur and food is in short supply. Sue weighs herself before and after practice to better match intake with loss, and she has added more sodium-rich foods to her diet.

optimal sodium concentration in sports drinks. A higher sodium concentration will more closely replace losses and increase the desire to drink; however, the beverage has to taste good so that you want to drink it. A high sodium concentration can throw off the flavor. Researchers recommend from 55 mg to more than 200 mg of sodium per 8 ounces (240 ml). Many of the popular sports drinks contain 100 to 130 mg per 8 ounces. Heavy sweaters competing for long periods can either add more sodium or choose beverages containing a higher concentration.

Hydration After Training

Replacing lost fluid takes time and is best achieved by consuming fluids throughout the day after training. For each pound (.5 kg) lost, drink 16-24 ounces of fluid (e.g., water, juice, milk, tea). Be aware that products marketed as recovery shakes or beverages are designed to replace carbohydrate and supply protein but will not provide enough fluid to rehydrate fully. If you sweat heavily, be sure to include ample sodium as well as fluid after training or competing. Since your body absorbs fluid best in small amounts rather than a lot at once, get in the habit of taking in fluid at regular intervals during waking hours to best enhance rehydration. If you are within 1 percent of your body weight from one day to the next, you are doing a good job hydrating. Losses of 3 percent or more of your total body weight indicate that either a "walk-through" at the next day's practice is in order or that you might consider skipping exercises for a day to fully hydrate.

Like so much in sports, you can approach hydration strategically. Although being well hydrated does not *improve* your performance, it allows you to work to your conditioning and skill level. Dehydration will rob you of your potential, lowering your work capacity and impairing your skill. It zaps you of the benefit of all those hours of conditioning, causing early fatigue, depleting glycogen more quickly, increasing your heart rate and even blood pressure at lower workloads. Staying cool requires more than just drinking water, remember to include sodium and monitor weight before and after working out to best create a smart hydration strategy.

Timing Tip

Alcohol is not an adequate hydrator; drinking alcoholic beverages causes fluid losses by increasing urine production. Alcohol acts as a diuretic because it blocks antidiuretic hormone, which helps you hold onto water, and causes you to lose fluid from the body. Instead of replacing fluids, you become more dehydrated. Replace lost fluids with water, juice, milk, sports drinks or even teas in the initial hours post-workout.

8

The Supplement Factor

The supplement industry generates more than $20 billion (US) in annual sales. Supplements range from one-a-day vitamins to hormone mimickers. Many athletes seek a competitive edge in their quest to increase strength, endurance, and performance and to improve body composition. Some surveys report that up to 89 percent of athletes consume supplements, yet there is often no real distinction made between a nutritional supplement like a carbohydrate drink and a stimulant, when clearly the implications for performance and health vary greatly. Two big questions surround supplements: Do they actually work? Is there any danger in taking them? In this chapter, we will discuss important factors to consider before deciding to take a supplement. Have all the facts before taking *anything*, instead of buying the latest item just because your teammate or gym buddy does. There are products on the market that work and those that don't.

WHAT ARE SUPPLEMENTS?

Supplements are substances taken by mouth in addition to one's food. They may be in the form of pills—capsules, tablets, or chewables—or a liquid or powder mixed into a beverage or other food. They are meant to complement one's food intake, not take the place of food. However, there are now so many products on the market, many have little to do with nutrition. Supplements tend to fall into several categories:

- Stimulants that claim to increase energy
- Hormones or hormone mimickers that claim to provide a hormone or act on tissue in a way similar to the hormone they are "copying," which tends to promise a cascade of actions
- Agents that claim to alter energy pathways, such as those claiming to increase fat burning
- Carbohydrate or protein powders and shakes that contain purified sources of one or more amino acids, proteins, or carbohydrates
- Immune boosters that claim to increase production of immune cells or provide immune protection on their own

Clearly, there is a great difference in these categories in terms of need, safety, and risk. There may be times when supplementation is helpful. There may be times when supplementation is hurtful. There are many times when supplementation is filled more with empty promises than substantial benefits. Recognizing the difference is crucial for making wise sports nutrition choices that can further your health and performance goals.

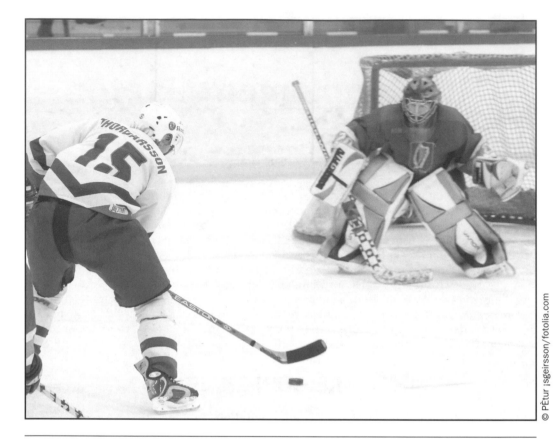

Every governing body agrees: Athletes are ultimately responsible for what they put in their bodies, regardless of what the label says.

Hormone mimickers pose the greatest risk. Stimulants are often abused. Products that promise to alter energy pathways need to be examined on a product-by-product basis. Protein and carbohydrate powders and shakes can definitely be used to an athlete's advantage, although proprietary formulas rarely provide any real advantage over food—it is the convenience that is helpful. Immune boosters can be deceiving; antioxidant supplementation may actually be harmful.

Although there are many excellent supplement manufacturers, there are also some that lack quality controls. If you do decide to take a supplement, purchase it from a reputable and established manufacturer. Tainted and contaminated products are a real threat. Since the laws are not currently stringent in terms of supplement manufacture and labeling, a big challenge is the purity of a supplement. How do you know what is stated on the label is actually what is in the product? If you opened a bag of potato chips and found pretzels you would know the difference, but if you buy a bottle of creatine and it has a steroid derivative in it, how would you know? Some manufacturers skimp on the products included in

Timing Tip

If a product claims to be all natural, it does not necessarily mean safe or effective. There are plenty of poisons found in nature. Some forms of wild mushrooms are all natural but hallucinogenic.

Evaluating Dietary Supplements

Before taking any supplement, really think about why you are doing so. Is there something you are looking for that can be better found through applying the Nutrient Timing Principles (NTP) and adjusting your food intake? Also, play devil's advocate—try to find out the possible negative effects of any supplement you're thinking of taking. Before you purchase or use a supplement, ask yourself these basic questions:

» *What claims are being made about the product?* If a product claims to do many things at the same time, chances are it doesn't do any of them particularly well. Are the product's claims exaggerated and hard to believe? Do the claims match what you really need? For example, if you are an endurance athlete, you don't need a product that claims to improve power.

» *Does the product have a scientific base (published in peer-reviewed scientific journals)?* In peer-reviewed journals such as *Medicine and Science in Sports and Exercise* and *International Journal of Sport Nutrition and Exercise Metabolism,* impartial researchers have examined each study to be sure it followed stringent requirements. Often a supplement will say that clinical trials were done, but these could have been completed in the manufacturer's own lab with no objective person evaluating the work. How do you know the manufacturer's claims are valid? The words clinical findings don't mean anything on their own.

» *What are the ingredients (all the ingredients, not just the headliners)?* All the ingredients must be listed on the label by law. A product that claims to be a proprietary blend isn't necessarily anything special; this is often a marketing ploy. Additionally, you have no idea how much of each ingredient is included in a proprietary blend, as individual quantities are often omitted.

» *Does it work? How do you know? How will you measure its effects?* Do you have a goal and a specific timeframe mapped out so that you will know whether you have succeeded? How will you determine whether you should continue taking the supplement or when to stop?

» *Is it legal? Does It contain substances banned by athletic organizations?* Consult *all* of the governing bodies for sports you participate in to learn which substances are banned.

» *Is it safe?* Can any of the ingredients raise body temperature and cause heat illness? Can it increase blood pressure or heart rate? These are serious side effects that can lead to stroke, heart attack, and even death in otherwise healthy people.

» *What are the possible side effects?* Many supplements do not tell you all the possible side effects, as prescription medications are required to disclose.

» *What is the cost? Is it worth the money?* Because people are eager for a quick fix, many supplements are expensive. You might be able to take in similar nutrients from food for much less (powdered milk versus whey powder, for example). For many athletes, taking that same money and applying it to their food budget would deliver great results.

» *Who and where is the manufacturer?* Is the manufacturer reputable, or is some guy manufacturing the product in his basement (which is possible!)? Research the company to be sure it is a reliable business with a track record of producing safe and effective products.

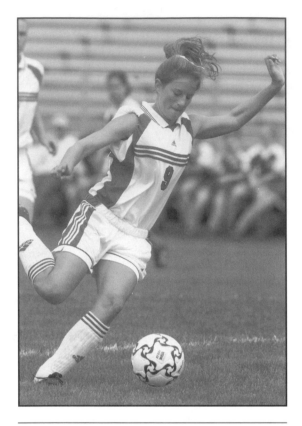

Consider all effects a supplement may have on health and performance.

supplements. For example, ginseng is an expensive ingredient, so it is often adulterated with less expensive products. In a study of 25 different preparations, half of the supplements had less than the label stated, and 6 contained only 1 percent ginseng (Harkey et al 2001). When tested by independent labs, supplements are frequently found to be contaminated or less potent than is claimed on the label.

The policy of schools, colleges, professional teams, and the Olympics state that you are responsible for what you put in your body, regardless of what the label says. You need to educate yourself about the rules of the different governing bodies and decide for yourself the risk versus benefit of taking anything, even over-the-counter products. As you probably know, athletes have been suspended after innocently taking a supplement or cold medication that contained a banned substance. Or sometimes an illegal ingredient is added to a supplement. When tainted supplements are discovered, they are usually recalled, but many consumers don't know about a recall until after they've ingested the product.

THE EFFECTS OF SUPPLEMENTS

Make sure you are fully informed of all effects of a supplement. One good example is the effect of antioxidants on performance. Exercise produces reactive oxygen molecules (free radicals) that may decrease immunity and cause inflammation. Exercise in and of itself also revs up our defense systems, internally producing more immune cells. When exercise becomes very intense and prolonged, our internal systems can't always keep up with the damage being created. It seems to make sense that antioxidant supplementation could help. As it turns out, supplemental antioxidants have been shown in some instances to impair the adaptations to training. How could that be?

Some of the free radical molecules act in ways that cause muscle fatigue, possibly to protect the muscle against further injury. Overriding that natural cautionary signal could cause more damage and increase recovery time. Additionally, some of the cells that enter injured muscle tissue cause inflammation as a result of "cleaning out" metabolic debris, allowing for repair and rebuilding of new, strong muscle tissue. If you stopped this process, would it result in greater harm or older, weaker muscle cells? We actually don't know for sure, but it is a possibility. The point is that there may be repercussions from taking a supplement that go far beyond the hype. Take a good look at any supplement you are

Stay a Step Ahead of the Claims

Even with a science degree, it can be extremely difficult to separate hype from truth when it comes to claims and marketing of supplements. The manufacturers know this, count on this, and use some pretty sophisticated methods to get you to believe what they are saying. Become an educated consumer; be aware of at least the tricks of the trade, and be a bit more savvy on how to separate the sales techniques from real science.

Testimonials

Testimonials are often used to entice you to buy a product. Typically, a famous athlete or coach is touting the benefit of a product. Remember, that athlete was great before he was hired to promote the supplement. Recognize that even though you want to believe the athlete, there may be no real basis of fact. Testimonials are anecdotal evidence, meaning they show one person's experience instead of being based on double-blind scientific studies that look at larger populations for effectiveness, repeatability, and safety. Even if something works for one person, it does not mean it will work for another. This is easier to see with an exaggerated example of a testimonial: "I have an aunt who smoked two packs of cigarettes a day until she died at age 93. Smoking can help you live longer." Because you are now educated about the hazards of smoking, you can see how absurd this testimonial is, even if it is true that the aunt smoked daily and lived to 93 years old.

Extrapolated Data

Extrapolated data are often used to sell products. Science may be behind an ingredient or product, but the product is applied to a different population than the one the research was conducted on, or the conclusion is "stretched" to support a claim. For example, take a look at this claim: "Studies show boron increases testosterone." The studies were done on postmenopausal women, but the product is marketed to adolescent boys and young men. Clearly the compound's effect on young, healthy males with high hormone levels should not be assumed to be the same as its effect on postmenopausal females with low hormone levels. Instead of reading the headlines, you may have to really read the research behind the claim. It helps to talk to people in the know, such as an athletic trainer, exercise physiologist, or sports nutritionist.

Sometimes a process in the body is explained in such detail that it is difficult to follow it all the way through—in order to mask that the claim does not hold or that the reaction in the body is rate limited (e.g., adding more chromium does not necessarily mean more glucose gets into the cells). Additionally, even if there is a physiological effect, this does not necessarily mean there is a performance effect.

Scientific-Sounding Vocabulary

Often the advertisements and brochures accompanying a product will use all sorts of scientific jargon (chemical names, plant extracts, and biochemistry) to sound legitimate and impressive, when really this language is used to intimidate us and falsely escalate the product's credibility. Terms such as *cell mediated*, *thermogenic formula*, *scientific breakthrough*, *miraculous*, and *revolutionary* are all examples that you have probably seen.

considering taking. Be a detective. Are there any downsides to the supplement? Do you actually need it? A supplement may make sense for one athlete but not another. For example, creatine may help some strength athletes but would not help an endurance athlete (more about creatine later).

It may take a little work to find out the possible side effects of some supplements. Any supplement that claims to increase metabolic rate will most likely increase heart rate and could also raise blood pressure, which can be dangerous, especially during exercise, when heart rate and blood pressure are already elevated. Some ingredients such as caffeine, ginseng, and bitter orange have "stacking" or additive effects. Licorice can decrease testosterone levels in the blood; acetyl-L-carnitine, bitter melon, ginkgo, vanadium, and vitamin C have all been implicated in causing gastrointestinal upset.

Before supplementing, ask yourself if you have applied all the NTP. For instance, if you need more energy and are skipping meals, the answer may lie not in a bottle but in adding a meal. Are you eating at regular intervals? Are you consuming your recovery snack to help with both muscle gain and stamina? Are you getting sick often, which can be a result of overtraining or under-eating? Are you making nutrient-poor food selections? Some basic questions will help clarify where your diet and patterns can be improved and where you can better apply the NTP to see gains in energy, performance, recovery, and immunity. Once you have clarified your own goals, wants, and ways to achieve aspirations, you may reconsider if supplementing is the best way to go. Are you already doing everything you can in terms of nutrition, training, and rest?

COMMON SUPPLEMENTS

Now that you have learned the basics and can better discern if supplementing makes sense for you and what to look for when choosing a supplement, let's review some of the more popular supplements out there.

Creatine

What's the claim?

Creatine is supposed to increase muscular strength and power. It also is purported to increase lean body mass.

What exactly is it?

Creatine is made in the body from two amino acids but is not an amino acid itself (technically, it's a nitrogen-containing amine). It is found in meat, so strict vegetarians may be low in creatine.

During weightlifting and other anaerobic activities, the ATP–Cr (adenosine triphosphate–creatine) system is used to produce the energy that helps muscles contract and generate the force to lift weight. The ATP–Cr system is important for rapid energy production inside the muscle. Supplemental creatine provides more of the ingredient used in generating this energy.

How is it taken?

Creatine comes in powder form or mixed in with bars and shakes. The most common and effective method of supplementing creatine is with a powder mixed in with a drink. Taking creatine with a rapidly digested carbohydrate, such as juice, helps deliver more creatine to the muscle than when taken alone because of the insulin release in response to the juice. The recommended does is 3-5 grams a day although some protocols recommend a "loading phase" of 5 days with 20 grams. In addition, one should avoid caffeine during the creatine loading phase because it seems to interfere with a loading mechanism. Studies from Belgium have shown that caffeine inhibits phosphocreatine resynthesis during recovery (Vandenberghe et al 1996). Instead of having a performance-enhancing effect, caffeine eliminates the benefit of creatine, during loading.

Does it work?

Creatine actually does work for most people. Those who have low levels in their muscles respond the most. It's most effective during high-intensity, short-duration activity and has been shown to improve strength, power, and muscle force. Creatine supplementation may also improve sprint performance, particularly in repetitive sprints. Additionally, creatine may contribute to an increase in lean body mass. Note, however, that creatine does not appear to help endurance athletes improve stamina.

Is it safe?

Reported side effects include nausea, vomiting, diarrhea, and muscle cramps, pulls, and strains. When broken down, creatine forms a substance, creatinine, that is excreted by the kidneys. Naturally, it is recommended that people with impaired kidney function not take creatine. Pregnant women are urged to refrain from taking creatine. Also, since there are changes in fluid balance and an impaired sweating and thermoregulatory response (ability to cool off) during the loading period, attention to hydration is recommended.

Creatine is probably one of the most widely studied and used sports supplements. However, many medical teams we have worked with discourage its use due to their observation that it increases the risk of hamstring strains and impairs healing, so sometimes the science and the practical application do not align. If you do use creatine, make sure you use a brand from a reputable manufacturer because tainted creatine has been identified and has resulted in fines for several athletes who thought they were taking a pure supplement.

HMB

What's the claim?

HMB is supposed to help build lean body mass, prevent muscle protein breakdown, and decrease body fat.

What exactly is it?

HMB stands for beta-hydroxy-beta-methylbutyrate and has become a popular supplement for strength training and bodybuilding athletes. It is actually a by-product of leucine (a branched-chain amino acid) metabolism and is naturally found in foods such as grapefruit and catfish. In the body, HMB is thought to help stabilize the sarcolemma, which is the muscle cell membrane. It also is thought to help decrease excessive muscle tissue breakdown—and that's where the claim that it helps with body composition and strength training originates. It's been suggested that HMB may help with a certain type of signaling that is used in muscle building (Rowlands and Thomson 2009; Wilson et al 2008; and Gallagher 2000).

How is it taken?

HMB is available as a tablet, capsule, or powder and as an ingredient in some shakes. It peaks in the bloodstream more quickly when taken by itself, and it enters more slowly when taken with glucose. Since larger doses are excreted, an accepted protocol is to divide the daily dose into three.

Does it work?

The results are conflicting as to whether HMB's claims are true or not. Some studies show that HMB does increase strength and lean body mass, but others also show no effect. A good amount of evidence indicates that it helps reduce markers of muscle tissue breakdown after resistance training. HMB will not be effective unless adequate calories and protein are consumed in addition to a resistance training regimen (Nissen et al 1996; Wilson et al 2008; and Rowlands and Thomson 2009).

Is it safe?

At the moment, there is no mention of adverse effects of HMB taken in doses of 1 gram per day, although that is not a guarantee of safety. Additionally, it seems to have little effect on well-trained individuals and only a very small effect on novice weightlifters. The timing of the supplement in regard to training was not specified in the studies. However, HMB has a short half-life, meaning the body clears it from the blood and reduces its strength in only two to three hours, which could affect the outcome of these studies (Nissen et al 1996; Wilson et al 2008; and Rowlands and Thomson 2009).

Glutamine

What's the claim?

Glutamine is supposed to prevent decreased immunity after prolonged endurance exercise and increase strength and lean body mass after resistance training.

What exactly is it?

Glutamine, a nonessential amino acid, is the most abundant amino acid in both blood plasma and muscle. It can be made in muscle tissue and is needed by many cells in the body. It transports parts of amino acids to the liver and kidneys where they can be reused or excreted. The absorptive cells of the digestive tract take up glutamine, and it is also used to make and provide energy for certain immune cells (lymphocytes, cytokines, neutrophils). It is involved in acid–base regulation and glycogen synthesis and is used to make the building blocks of DNA and RNA. After prolonged exercise, blood and muscle levels are low, and the immune cells that need glutamine can be negatively affected. It has been thought that a shortage of glutamine might be the reason, or part of the reason, that strenuous training increases some athletes' susceptibility to colds and infections.

How is it taken?

Glutamine is available in pills and powders. Pills tend to have much smaller doses than powders and are not likely to have any effect at these levels. Glutamine is also found in all foods that contain protein.

Does it work?

Current evidence indicates that although glutamine levels decrease with exercise, they don't go down far enough to be the causative factor in decreasing the immune cells, so supplementing doesn't have an impact on the number or activity of these cells. It may be that release of cortisol and epinephrine during exercise suppresses the creation of T1 immune cells (certain lymphocytes) during exercise. If decreased glutamine isn't the reason for decreased immune cells, supplemental glutamine won't increase their production.

Research studies using .3 gram and .9 gram of glutamine per kilogram of lean mass have not shown any positive effects on strength improvement, increase of muscle mass, prevention of muscle tissue breakdown, or reduction of muscle soreness (Rohde et al 1998 and Walsh et al 2000). At this point, there appears to be a lack of credible proof for strength athletes to take supplemental glutamine. Glutamine may help in other ways, however. It has an important role in keeping the intestinal tract healthy and may provide protection against infections entering the body via this route. It may also affect immunity through its role in manufacturing the antioxidant glutathione.

Is it safe?

Although negative side effects have not been reported, remember that glutamine is an amino acid. When intake is greater than the body can use, the excess nitrogen must be excreted. Glutamine in particular has been shown to form ammonia when metabolized, although it has not been shown to accumulate in the body. The amount recommended for improved immunity (3 to 7 grams) seems to pose no risk.

Caffeine

What's the claim?

Caffeine's claims include keeping you more alert, "pumping you up," increasing endurance, and possessing powerful antioxidants.

What is it?

Caffeine is a stimulant that acts on the central nervous system, heart muscle, and possibly the mechanism that controls blood pressure. Caffeine may increase the release of neurotransmitters such as dopamine (the "feel good" neurotransmitter). Caffeine is present in coffee, tea, cola and some other soft drinks, and, to a lesser degree, chocolate. It is also present in some herbs and dietary supplements.

How is it taken?

Caffeine can be taken in a pill form and is increasingly added to other supplements (powders, pills, and drinks). In doses up to 3 grams per kilogram, it does have a performance-enhancing effect, particularly for endurance exercise. This would be 164 mg for a 120-pound (54 kg) athlete, 246 mg for a 180-pound (82 kg) athlete, and 342 mg for a 250-pound (114 kg) athlete. For comparison, a 16-ounce (480 ml) coffee from Starbucks has about 330 mg of caffeine, and home-brewed coffee can have 120 to 240 mg of caffeine per 16 ounces.

Does it work?

Positive effects, at appropriate doses, have been established. Caffeine consumption can prevent a decline in cognitive capacity, especially when consumed with glucose (carbohydrate). It is also possible that caffeine consumption is linked to increased physical endurance. It may help with fat burning and carbohydrate absorption, both of which improve endurance. Although one study by Burke (2008) shows that caffeine is helpful in power work, there is little evidence supporting its use in sprint work and weightlifting. Caffeine may also help block pain receptors or alter mood receptors so you don't mind the pain (from exercise) as much. Your perceived exertion will seem less at the same workload.

Many studies show that doses above 3 grams per kilogram yield no additional benefit and may inhibit performance. Performance benefits are usually seen at levels well below 3 grams per kilogram. Caffeine's effects last five hours or more. Note that caffeine is still on the NCAA's list of banned drug classes if the concentration in urine is greater than 15 micrograms/mililiters, which is designed to be above normal dietary intake.

Is it safe?

Doses of 250 to 300 mg have proven effective as a performance enhancer, but doses higher than 300 mg per day have been associated with tachyarrhythmias (irregular heart beats). In addition, excess caffeine intake can cause insomnia, nervousness, restlessness, anxiety, ulcers, abdominal pain, heartburn, and diarrhea (which is often accompanied by dehydration) and can increase gastric acid secretion, sweat rate, and catecholamines. Catecholamines are hormones that affect heart rate and cause vasoconstriction—narrowing of blood vessels—which decreases blood flow to working muscles. Caffeine intoxication can also occur from too much caffeine, and individual tolerance varies. Death from overdose can occur at intakes of 10 grams (10,000 mg) and higher. Caffeine's effect can be very individualized and habitual users build up a tolerance.

Also, some herbs naturally contain caffeine, so if you see the following names on the label, you will be taking in extra caffeine: guarana, yerba mate, kola nut, green tea extract. Labeling laws do not require the amount of caffeine to be listed, so you may not have any idea as to how much the product contains. A "stacking," or magnified effect, of some herbals can occur when taken with caffeine. It is hard to predict how you may feel or perform—they can increase heart rate or blood pressure, which puts extra strain on your cardiovascular system. You may also feel overstimulated and jittery. Some of these herbals to watch out for include ginseng, bitter orange, yohimbine, and ephedra.

Omega-3 Fatty Acids (Fish Oil)

What's the claim?

Fish oil, or omega-3 fatty acids, are supposed to decrease inflammation that occurs as a result of training.

What exactly is it?

Omega-3 fatty acids, which are long-chain fatty acids, also have long names: alpha-linolenic acid (ALA), docosahexaenoic acid (DHA), and eicosapentaenoic acid (EPA). ALA is found mostly in plant sources, such as walnuts, flaxseed, and canola oil, and although healthful, it is not as powerful in terms of anti-inflammatory effects as are EPA and DHA found in higher-fat fish, such as salmon, sardines, mackerel, and herring. All three omega-3 fatty acids compete with omega-6 fatty acids for inclusion in cell membranes. Omega-6 fatty acids are found in soybean, safflower, sunflower, and corn oils. One omega-6 fatty acid in particular, arachidonic acid, produces hormonelike substances, eicosanoids, that cause inflammation. Increasing omega-3 intake can reduce the production of the inflammation-causing eicosanoids by replacing omega-6 in cell membranes.

Exercise causes the release of reactive oxygen molecules (free radicals) and other inflammatory substances called cytokines. Omega-3 fatty acids manufacture antioxidant enzymes that help combat the free radicals. The inflammatory cytokines stimulate cortisol and can inhibit muscle building and amplify muscle tissue breakdown. Reducing excess inflammation may facilitate muscle building and repair and improve overall blood vessel health.

Does it work?

DHA and EPA have been shown to influence the type of eicosanoids produced as a result of exercise. Omega-3s may blunt the inflammatory response to exercise because they manufacture specific eicosanoids—leukotrienes, thrombaxanes, and prostaglandins—that are much less inflammatory than those made by omega-6 fats.

A study by Nieman et al (2009) didn't find that omega-3 supplements had much of an effect on inflammation in athletes. They had trained cyclists take 2.6 grams of EPA and DHA daily for six weeks and complete an intensive three-day ride. Compared to the cyclists taking the placebo, there wasn't a significant difference on performance or inflammation. There is evidence that omega-3 fatty acids benefit unfit subjects (Hill et al 2007). More research in this area is needed to find out if larger doses are needed, or if benefits accrue in athletes engaging in other sports, with consumption over a longer time period, at different ages (will an older athlete see different results?), and in athletes who are not trained as well.

How is it taken?

A couple of servings of fatty fish per week can provide a good amount of omega-3 fatty acids (a 4 oz. serving of wild salmon may have close to 3,000 mg of omega-3). Alternatively, supplements are available. Fish oil supplements can contain anywhere from 30-80 percent EPA and DHA, so be aware of the dose of each that is contained in the oil (you can find this by looking at the ingredient label). For a purified form, 4-5 capsules provide 2-3 grams of EPA and DHA—just as much as the wild salmon. Omega-3 fatty acids are also added to many foods, including eggs, bread, cereal, juice, and margarines.

Is it safe?

In the levels recommended, yes. It is not necessary to take larger doses. As previously mentioned, omega-3 fats prevent platelet aggregation, meaning they cause the blood to thin somewhat. Larger doses may cause too much thinning, which can lead to internal bleeding.

These are just a few of many supplements on the market. We urge you to seek out trustworthy information from medical staff, athletic trainers, or sports nutritionists before investing dollars and hope. Here are a few Web sites you can look at as well for more reliable information on supplements:

National Institutes of Health, Office of Dietary Supplements

http://ods.od.nih.gov

National Center for Complementary and Alternative Medicine

http://nccam.nih.gov

MedlinePlus

www.medlineplus.gov

Some Web sites require a subscription and are continually updated with new findings:

www.ConsumerLab.com

ConsumerLab is an independent laboratory that tests supplements for purity and provides extensive information on each supplement. The laboratory posts complete results of its findings, including supplements that are contaminated or fail testing for any other reason. The Web site contains some free information; access to test results requires subscription.

www.naturaldatabase.com

This research-based site provides a thorough listing of all vitamins, minerals, and supplements and explains all possible uses and dosages. It also covers effectiveness and dangers, including interactions with medications. All references are available.

Athletes may wish to consult the Web site of their governing body for lists of allowed and banned substances and other supplement information.

Collegiate Sports

www.ncaa.org

International Olympic Committee

www.olympic.org

World Anti-Doping Agency

www.wada-ama.org

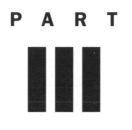

FUELING STRATEGIES, PLANS, AND MENUS

Timing Guidelines for Athletes

By now, Hopefully you understand why timing your intake of certain macronutrients (carbohydrate, protein, fat) and fluids can help maximize your training, conditioning, and competitive goals. Timing your intake before training, conditioning, or competition and taking in the right amount of foods will better prepare your muscles for the work to come. Just as important, some activity requires additional fuel while you're in action to delay fatigue or maximize muscle gains. Finally, all types of sports and conditioning can benefit from recovery nutrition to help build and repair muscle, restore energy, and maintain immune function. Now it is time to apply the Nutrient Timing Principles (NTP), Keep these three smart sports nutrition strategies in mind when creating your own nutrition plan and applying the NTP.

THREE SMART SPORTS NUTRITION STRATEGIES

No matter what sport, no matter how large or small the athlete, how powerful, strong, nimble, or graceful, there are certain tenets that hold true across the board. Although the specifics for each sport and athlete may differ, all athletes will benefit from keeping these three strategies in mind when creating their own plan: aim for consistency, go for quality, and tune in to timing.

Aim for Consistency

Just as consistency in training is important, so is consistency in fueling. Regularly scheduled meals and snacks are a must. Distribute your calories throughout the day. If you eat a lot one day and then skip meals the next or eat unevenly throughout each day, your energy and moods will be inconsistent. Your concentration and stamina will be inconsistent. Your play will be inconsistent. All athletes will benefit from muscles that are ready to perform, meaning they need to be appropriately fueled and hydrated as well as controlled by a brain that is not starved from low blood sugar. If you do not practice well, you won't compete well. Training days are just as important as game days when it comes to reducing the risk of injury and learning and practicing the skills, plays, routines, and strategies needed to win competitions.

A base of adequate calories and nutrients, day in and day out, is essential. Your muscles store and use energy and nutrients throughout the day. A pattern of regular meals and snacks keeps energy levels consistent and keeps muscles and tissues properly fueled from an energy perspective as well as from a repair, growth, healing, immunity, and health perspective. Repair of muscle tissue occurs over many hours—eating strategically provides nutrients the body can use over time. Regular meals help maintain a more even caloric

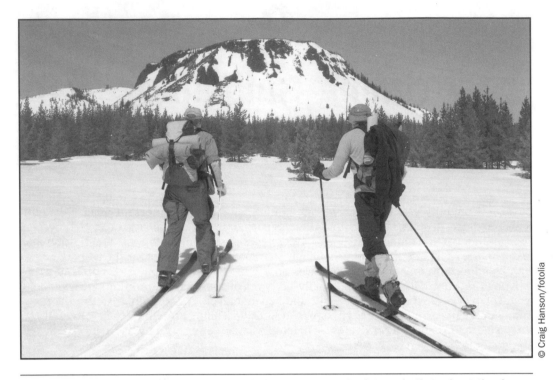

© Craig Hanson/fotolia

Athletes will have more consistent energy if they eat at regular intervals throughout the day.

distribution, which improves body composition even when weight is relatively stable. Distributing calories evenly throughout the day also results in better levels of cholesterol, blood sugar, insulin, and cortisol.

Go for Quality

Choose the quality of food that is right for the timing of intake. Everyone knows there is a significant difference between gummy bears and broccoli, but the gummy bears may be the better choice right before practice. The times around performance are for fueling, meal time is for nutrition. At meal time, choose nutrient-rich foods that will help with long-term resiliency. Before, during, and after training, choose foods and beverages that will help fuel the workout. Although you surely can take in enough calories with any type of food, the quality of the food you eat will ultimately impact health and well-being along with performance. For instance, you may avoid fat right before a workout, but you need healthy fats as part of a healthy training diet. Or, you may avoid fiber right before working out but need fiber as part of your overall diet. Whey and casein proteins may be great as part of a recovery snack, but mealtime proteins ideally provide iron and zinc (lean meats, legumes) or omega-3 fatty acids (tuna steak, sablefish, sardines).

Similarly, tomatoes may not be the food of choice during an event, but the vitamin C they provide is necessary for collagen formation and soft-tissue repair. Vitamins, minerals, and phytochemicals (plant chemicals) in whole foods serve vital functions in your body. Bars, gels, and sports drinks are formulated for consumption around activity, not to replace meals. Carbohydrate eaten throughout the day, further away from training, is best when it is nutrient-rich, such as whole grains, beans, legumes, fruits, and vegetables, including those with more fiber which slow digestion rates. Remember to eat for fuel before, during, and after training and competition, but eat for health and well-being for all other meals and snacks.

Tune in to Timing

Timing is what this book is all about. It matters what you eat, when you eat, and how much you eat. Your training and competition is affected by the nutritional choices you make. Waiting too long between food intake, eating too much or too little, consuming the incorrect types of foods before training or competing, eating or drinking too little or too much during activity, as well as delaying recovery nutrition, all impact every aspect of performance. It can make a big difference, or it can make a small difference that yields a different positive outcome. In the 2008 Summer Olympics, the difference in taking home the Gold was 1.07 seconds in Men's Cycling Mountain Bike; 0.01 seconds in the Men's 100m Butterfly Swim; 0.01 seconds in the Women's 50m Free Swim; .004 seconds in Women's Canoe/Kayak; and 5.19 seconds in the Men's Triathlon! Table 9.1 highlights what is recommended before, during, and after light, moderate, and heavy training. Figure 9.1 explains the different intensities for endurance, strength and power, and stop-and-go athletes.

Table 9.1   Application of Nutrient Timing Principles

TYPE OF TRAINING	TIMING OF NUTRIENTS		
	Before	During	After
Strength and power	**Light and moderate** Snack not needed unless • It's been 4 hours since last meal (15 g carb right before training is suggested) • Training before breakfast (15-25 g carb plus 10-15 g protein or 6 g essential amino acids) **Heavy** Snack is needed: • *2-3 hours before:* 200-400 calories with 35-85 g from carb plus 10-15 g protein or 6 g essential amino acids • *Less than 1 hour before:* up to 200 calories of up to 35 g carb plus 10-15 g protein or 6 g essential amino acids	**Light** Snack not needed unless training before breakfast (8-12 oz [240-360 ml] sports drink suggested) **Moderate** Snack not needed unless training before breakfast (8-16 oz [240-480 ml] sports drink suggested) **Heavy** Snack is needed: • 15-20 g carb/hr for smaller athletes • 20-60 g carb/hr for larger athletes	**Light** Snack not needed **Moderate** Need 7 g/kg carb plus .1-.2 g/kg protein **Heavy** Snack of 1.0-1.2 g/kg carb plus .1-.2 g/kg protein. Repeat intake or have meal within two hours
Endurance	**Light** Snack not needed unless before breakfast (15 g carb right before training is suggested) **Moderate** Snack of 15 g carb right before or 25 g carb 15-30 minutes before **Heavy** Snack is needed, either: • *2-3 hours before:* 300-400 calories from mixed sources • *1-2 hours before:* up to 200 calories with 50 g from carb • *15-30 minutes before:* 25 g carb • *Immediately before:* 15 g carb	**Light** Snack not needed **Moderate** Snack of 30-60 g carb/ hr is needed if training over 60 minutes **Heavy** Snack of 30-60 g carb/ hr is needed and may be increased up to 100 g carb/hr if tolerated	**Light** Snack not needed **Moderate** Snack of .7-1.0 g/kg carb plus .1-.2 g/kg protein is needed **Heavy** Snack of 1.0-1.5 g/kg carb plus .1-.2 g/kg protein. Repeat intake or have meal within 2 hours

(continued)

Table 9.1 *(continued)*

TYPE OF TRAINING	TIMING OF NUTRIENTS		
	Before	**During**	**After**
Stop and go	**Light and moderate** Snack not needed unless • Training before breakfast or 3-4 hours since last meal (15 g carb right before or 25 g carb 15-30 minutes before) **Heavy** Snack is needed: • *1-2 hours before*: 200 calories of up to 50 g carb; protein and fat intake as tolerated • *15-30 minutes before*: 25 g carb • *Immediately before*: 15 g carb	**Light** Snack not needed **Moderate** Snack is needed: • *For activity 60-75 minutes:* 15-30 g carb • *For activity 90 minutes:* 30-45 g carb **Heavy** Snack of 30-60 g carb/hr is needed	**Light** Snack not needed **Moderate** Snack of .7-1.0 g/kg carb plus .1-.2 g/kg protein is needed **Heavy** Snack of 1.0-1.5 g/kg carb plus .1-.2 g/kg protein. Repeat intake or have meal within 2 hours

FIGURE 9.1
Training intensities

STRENGTH AND POWER

Light training	Low volume, low intensity for 30-45 min (<70% HRmax). If weight training, using machines, or doing simple movements with free weights, volume is light with 1-3 sets and reps 10 or more.
Moderate training	Medium volume, medium intensity for 45 minutes or longer at lower intensity (60-90 minutes). 3-5 sets of 8 reps for weight training that utilizes more complex exercises, such as chest presses, squats, cleans; other activities at moderate-effort conditioning training intensity of 6-8 METs for 45 minutes or 4-5 METs for 60-75 minutes (see page 201 in appendix A for an explanation of METs).
Heavy training	Volume of work increased to heavy, intense weightlifting for 60 min or more. More exercises, both complex and isolated, and an increase in sets; may also include conditioning: speed work, agility, lateral speed. Also when volume (time) decreases; intensity increases (sprints; intervals) or volume increases greatly (two-a-days) yet intensity may decrease.

ENDURANCE

Light training	Less than 60 minutes per day; 3-5 days per week; intensity is easy (≤ 70% HRmax).
Moderate training	45 minutes at high intensity (75-80% HRmax) or intervals 60-90 minutes at moderate intensity (≤ 75% HRmax); 5-6 days per week.
Heavy training	60 minutes or more at high intensity (> 75% HRmax) or intervals over 90 minutes at any intensity; 5-6 days per week.

STOP AND GO

Light training	Low volume, lower intensity for 30-60 minutes. May include light conditioning work or sport-specific drills. May also include light endurance at 4-5 METs.
Moderate training	Intensity increases, duration of 60-90 minutes. May include short practices, drill work, or endurance training at 6-8 METs.
Heavy training	1.5-3 hour practices per day or more. May include at least one competition per week with one or two days of shorter practices; multiple competitions per week with light practices between; or tournament participation.

FORMULATING YOUR PLAN

To create your personalized Nutrition Blueprint, your caloric and macronutrient needs (protein, fat, carbohydrate) will first be determined. Then the NTP will be applied by distributing calories and nutrients appropriately and strategically throughout the day and around training. You'll then learn how to translate this Blueprint into food choices. In chapters 10-12, menus specific to your type of sport for both training and competition will be illustrated along with how to deal with the unique challenges that arise for different types of athletes. Be sure to fill in your numbers as we walk you through each step in building your individualized Nutrition Blueprint.

Step 1: Determine Your Caloric Needs

You may be wondering how to figure out what and how much to eat, and if so, the first step is to determine your caloric needs. That's going to depend on your age, height, weight, gender, and activity level (daily activity plus exercise) and whether you are trying to gain, lose, or maintain your weight. Science often uses the metric system for calculations, so your weight in kilograms will be used to determine caloric, carbohydrate, and protein needs. Use table 9.2 to determine your weight in kilograms (your weight in pounds divided by 2.2). Then determine your caloric needs using the steps in appendix A on page 199.

Table 9.2 Weight in Pounds Converted to Kilograms

lb	95	100	105	110	115	120	125	130	135	140	145	150	155	160	165
kg	43	45	48	50	52	55	57	59	61	64	66	68	70	73	75
lb	170	175	180	185	190	195	200	205	210	215	220	225	230	235	240
kg	77	80	82	84	86	89	91	93	95	98	100	102	105	107	109
lb	245	250	255	260	265	270	275	280	285	290	300	305	315	320	350
kg	111	114	116	118	120	123	125	127	130	132	136	139	143	145	159

Your weight in kilograms: _____

Your daily caloric needs: _____

When workouts vary in length, intensity, or even type of activity, calorie needs vary. You might consider creating a table such as the one in table 9.3 which depicts the calories expended for a variety of workouts that Mike, a 200-pound football player, might engage in. Notice how the calones change as time, intensity, and type of conditioning change.

Using this information as a guide, you can create your own chart as a reference to refer to at different stages of training when you have different caloric needs. After you figure out your base number of calories and add your activity calories, you are ready to create your individual Nutrition Blueprint that you will then use to create menus. This will ensure balance and a nutrient-rich diet. The plan will take into account the nutrient timing principles for before, during, and after training to make sure you consume adequate protein and carbohydrate.

Table 9.3   Calories Burned by a 200 lb (91 kg) Athlete

Activity	30 min	45 min	60 min	90 min	120 min
Weightlifting, light workout (3 METs)	137	205	273	410	546
Weightlifting, vigorous effort (6 METs)	273	410	546	819	1092
Circuit training (8 METs)	364	546	728	1092	1456
Calisthenics, light to moderate (4.5 METs)	205	308	410	615	820
Conditioning (push-ups, pull-ups, jumping), vigorous effort (8 METs)	364	546	728	1092	1456

Step 2: Determine Your Protein Needs

Your protein requirement is determined by your weight, level or stage of training, and type of sport. Some athletes think they have to eat large quantities of animal-based foods to provide adequate protein; remember, however, that breads, cereals, nuts, and vegetables also contribute protein (substantially if you eat a lot of them) to your overall intake. See appendix B, Macronutrient Needs by Sport, on page 205 to find out how many grams per kg body weight is needed for your sport and level of training, or consult table 9.4, find your weight, and choose the protein requirement for the total daily amount of protein right for you. If you are unable to find your sport, choose between 1.6-1.8 g/kg if are working on building muscle mass; are an elite endurance athlete or an endurance athlete training long and hard; are a novice athlete of any kind; or are trying to lose body fat. Choose from the lower to middle range (1.2 to 1.6 grams per kilogram) if you are a trained athlete participating in a stop-and-go sport or an endurance athlete training moderately

The number of grams of protein you need daily: _____

Table 9.4 Protein Needs per kg (lb) of Body Weight

Body weight kg (lb)	1.2 g/kg	1.3 g/kg	1.4 g/kg	1.5 g/kg	1.6 g/kg	1.7 g/kg	1.8 g/kg	1.9 g/kg	2.0 g/kg
43 (95)	52	56	60	65	69	73	77	82	86
45 (100)	54	59	63	68	72	77	81	86	90
48 (105)	58	62	67	72	77	82	86	91	96
50 (110)	60	65	70	75	80	85	90	95	100
52 (115)	62	68	73	78	83	88	94	99	104
55 (120)	66	72	77	83	88	94	99	105	110
57 (125)	68	74	80	86	91	97	103	108	114
59 (130)	71	77	83	89	94	100	106	112	118
61 (135)	73	79	85	92	85	104	110	116	122
64 (140)	77	83	90	96	102	109	115	122	128
66 (145)	79	86	92	99	106	112	119	125	132
68 (150)	82	88	95	102	109	116	122	129	136
70 (155)	84	91	98	105	112	119	126	133	140
73 (160)	88	95	102	110	117	124	131	139	146
75 (165)	90	98	105	113	120	128	135	143	150
77 (170)	92	100	108	116	123	131	139	146	154
80 (175)	96	104	112	120	128	136	144	152	160
82 (180)	98	107	115	123	131	139	148	156	164
84 (185)	101	109	118	126	134	143	151	160	168
86 (190)	103	112	120	129	138	146	155	163	172
91 (200)	109	118	127	137	146	155	164	173	182
93 (205)	112	121	130	140	149	158	167	177	186
95 (210)	114	124	133	143	152	162	171	181	190
98 (215)	118	127	137	147	157	167	176	186	196
100 (220)	120	130	140	150	160	170	180	190	200
102 (225)	122	133	143	153	163	173	184	194	204
105 (230)	126	137	147	158	168	179	189	200	210
107 (235)	128	139	150	160	171	182	193	203	214
109 (240)	131	142	153	164	174	185	196	207	218
114 (250)	137	148	160	171	182	194	205	217	228
125 (275)	150	163	175	188	200	213	225	238	250
136 (300)	163	177	190	204	218	231	245	258	272

Step 3: Determine Your Carbohydrate Needs

Next, refer back to appendix B on page 205 to determine your carbohydrate needs based on sport or use table 9.5 to find out the number of daily carbohydrate needed to support your training. Typically, 4 to 6 g/kg body weight is appropriate for strength and power ath-

Table 9.5   Carbohydrate Needs per kg (lb) of Body Weight

Body weight kg (lb)	.7 g/kg	1 g/kg	2 g/kg	3 g/kg	4 g/kg	5 g/kg	6 g/kg	7 g/kg	8 g/kg	9 g/kg	10 g/kg
43 (95)	30	43	86	129	172	215	258	301	344	387	430
45 (100)	32	45	90	135	180	225	270	315	360	405	450
48 (105)	34	48	96	144	192	240	288	336	384	432	480
50 (110)	35	50	100	150	200	250	300	350	400	450	500
52 (115)	36	52	102	156	208	260	312	364	416	468	520
55 (120)	39	55	110	165	220	275	330	385	440	495	550
57 (125)	40	57	114	171	228	285	342	399	456	513	570
59 (130)	41	59	118	177	236	295	354	413	472	531	590
61 (135)	43	61	122	183	244	305	366	427	488	549	610
64 (140)	45	64	128	192	256	320	384	448	512	576	640
66 (145)	46	66	132	198	264	330	396	462	528	594	660
68 (150)	48	68	136	204	272	340	408	476	544	612	680
70 (155)	49	70	140	210	280	350	420	490	560	630	700
73 (160)	51	73	146	219	292	365	436	511	584	652	730
75 (165)	53	75	150	225	300	375	450	525	600	675	750
77 (170)	54	77	154	231	308	385	462	535	616	693	770
80 (175)	56	80	160	240	320	400	480	560	640	720	800
82 (180)	57	82	164	246	328	410	492	574	656	738	820
84 (185)	59	84	168	252	336	420	504	588	672	756	840
86 (190)	60	86	172	258	344	430	516	602	688	774	860
89 (195)	62	89	178	267	356	445	534	623	712	810	890
91 (200)	64	91	182	273	364	455	546	637	728	819	910
93 (205)	65	93	186	279	372	465	558	651	744	837	930
95 (210)	67	95	190	285	380	475	570	665	760	855	950
98 (215)	69	98	196	294	392	490	588	686	784	882	980
100 (220)	70	100	200	300	400	500	600	700	800	900	1,000
102 (225)	71	102	204	306	408	510	612	714	816	918	1,020
105 (230)	74	105	210	315	420	525	630	735	840	945	1,050
107 (240)	75	107	214	321	428	535	642	749	856	963	1,070
114 (250)	80	114	228	342	456	570	684	798	912	1,026	1,140
125 (275)	88	125	250	375	500	625	750	875	1,000	1,125	1,250
136 (300)	95	136	272	408	544	680	816	952	1,088	1,224	1,360

letes and all athletes training less than one hour per day. 6 to 7 g/kg body weight is right for athletes doing one to two hours of cardio training per day. 8 to 10 g/kg is appropriate for athletes training two to four hours per day, and athletes training over four hours need over 10 g/kg body weight.

The number of grams of carbohydrate you need daily: _____

Choosing the appropriate amounts and putting all the macronutrient needs together is a bit of an art as well as a science because you will need to adjust up or down based on how you feel. Sometimes athletes overestimate their energy expenditure; sometimes athletes underestimate the amount of work they are doing. If you are concerned about the difference between training days and rest days, on rest days you could skip the snack before, during, and after exercise, which accounts for a fair amount of carbohydrate and calories. Remember that rest days also help restore energy, so it is not advisable to cut calories too drastically.

Step 4: Determine Your Fat Needs

There are three steps to determining the grams of fat needed to fulfill your nutrition plan.

Step A: Determine Combined Protein and Carbohydrate Calories

Add together the protein and carbohydrate grams from steps 2 and 3. Then, multiply the total number of carbohydrate and protein grams by 4, which is the number of calories each gram contains.

_____ g protein + _____ g carbohydrate = _____ total grams x 4
= _____ total calories

Here's an example: Let's assume our sample athlete, Mike, is 200 pounds (91 kg) and needs the high end of protein (1.8 g/kg), which equals 164 grams, and the lower end of carbohydrate (5 g/kg), which equals 455 grams. Mike would add 164 grams of protein and 455 grams of carbohydrate for a total of 619. Next, he would multiply the total number by 4 to give him 2,476, which is the total number of calories he should consume from carbohydrate and protein combined.

__164__ g protein + __455__ g carbohydrate = __619__ total grams x 4
= __2,476__ total calories

Step B: Determine Calories Needed From Fat

Remember when we asked you to figure out your total calories for the day? Take that number and subtract the number you just calculated (protein and carbohydrate calories) from your total calories. The number you get is the number of calories left for fat in your diet.

_____ total calories − _____ calories from carbohydrate and protein
= _____ calories from fat

Our sample athlete, Mike, needs 3,500 calories per day, so he would take 3,500 and subtract 2,476, leaving him with 1,024 calories from fat, as follows:

__3,500__ total calories − __2,476__ calories from carbohydrate and protein = __1,024__ calories from fat

Step C: Determine Fat Grams Needed

Now that you know the number of fat calories needed per day, you can convert that into grams of fat. To do this, divide the fat calories by 9.

_____ fat calories / 9 = _____ grams of fat needed per day

Our sample athlete, Mike, would divide his 1,024 fat calories by 9 for a total of 114 grams of fat daily, as follows:

_1,024_ fat calories / 9 = _114_ grams of fat needed per day

Step 5: Calculate Macronutrient Percentages

This section is optional. A lot of talk exists about the most desirable distribution of calories. Percentages are not as important as absolute amounts. Athletes require specific amounts of each nutrient in grams per kilogram body weight, not percentages. If you'd like to know the percentage of each nutrient, you may calculate this by dividing the calories provided by each macronutrient by your total calories. The three percentages should equal 100.

_____ g carbohydrate x 4 = _____ calories from carbohydrate /
_____ total calories = _____% carbohydrate

_____ g protein x 4 = _____ calories from protein /
_____ total calories = _____% protein

_____ g fat x 9 = _____ calories from fat /
_____ total calories = _____% fat

For our sample athlete, Mike, it looks like this:

_455_ g carbohydrate x 4 = _1,820_ calories from carbohydrate /
_3,500_ total calories = _52_% carbohydrate

_164_ g protein x 4 = _656_ calories from protein /
_3,500_ total calories = _19_% protein

_114_ g fat x 9 = _1,026_ calories from fat /
_3,500_ total calories = _29_% fat

Typically, training diets for strength and power athletes can be a broad range of 42 to 60 percent carbohydrate, 20 to 35 percent fat (up to 40 percent for adolescents), and 10 to 28 percent protein. Endurance and stop-and-go athletes typically consume 50 to 65 percent carbohydrate, 10 to 20 percent protein, and 20 to 35 percent fat. Be sure that you have selected the right amount for your body weight (grams per kilogram) and training intensity.

Timing Meals for College Athletes

College athletes often claim they sleep in and miss breakfast. In truth, they are really like shift workers; their schedule has them waking later, but they are also going to sleep later. So if a college athlete wakes at 10:00 a.m., but goes to sleep at 2:00 a.m., this is really the same waking hours as someone who wakes at 7:00 a.m. and goes to sleep at 11:00 p.m. It's just the hours that have shifted.

This shift means that for someone who wakes at 10:00 a.m., lunchtime at noon would be breakfast time and dinnertime at 5 or 6 p.m. would be lunchtime. Because of this, a college athlete really needs to plan their nightly snack because it would, in reality, be their dinner! By 10:00 p.m., it is time for a meal and by 12:30 a.m., the athlete may be ready for a smaller snack before he or she goes to bed at 2 a.m. Instead, athletes are often surprised at their own hunger and somehow think they should not be eating a whole meal that "late" at night. Scrambling for food, the fallback is typically pizza or bags of chips, cookies, and candy which are rarely ever satisfying and may lead to an intermittent feeding frenzy that interferes with getting to sleep and staying asleep. A better idea; at lunch (which is dinner for most others) eat a dinner-like meal while it is available. Then, get a sub or hoagie, fruit or juice, side salad, and yogurt to bring back to your room so that you are prepared when hunger hits later in the night. You will certainly feel better and sleep better.

CREATING YOUR NUTRITION BLUEPRINT

Now it's time to determine how often you will eat during the day and how to time your protein, fat, and carbohydrate intake and allot the balance between meals and snacks around training and competition. Never go for long periods without eating; schedule three meals and a snack or two in addition to your training fuel.

Choose one of the templates in figure 9.2 based on when you train during the day. This template will become your Blueprint to help you select the appropriate amounts of food at each meal, snack, and fueling opportunity before, during, and after your training. The Blueprint functions as a guide to help you to map out the right amounts of carbohydrate, protein, and fat to have around training and at all meals and snacks. It will help you to choose the right balance of foods so that you aren't overconsuming one nutrient and underconsuming another.

We will walk you through a blueprint using our sample athlete, Mike. Mike is a strength and power athlete who engages in more strength-building activities than aerobic exercise.

FIGURE 9.2A
Morning workout: Nutrition Blueprint template

Meal/Snack	Carbohydrate (g)	Protein (g)	Fat (g)
Pretraining			
During training			
Recovery			
Breakfast			
Lunch			
Snack			
Dinner			
Snack			

FIGURE 9.2B

Afternoon workout: Nutrition Blueprint template

Meal/Snack	Carbohydrate (g)	Protein (g)	Fat (g)
Breakfast			
Lunch			
Pretraining			
During training			
Recovery			
Dinner			
Snack			

FIGURE 9.2C

Evening workout: Nutrition Blueprint template

Meal/Snack	Carbohydrate (g)	Protein (g)	Fat (g)
Breakfast			
Snack			
Lunch			
Snack			
Pretraining			
During training			
Recovery			
Dinner			

FIGURE 9.2D

Two-a-day workouts: Nutrition Blueprint template

Meal/Snack	Carbohydrate (g)	Protein (g)	Fat (g)
Breakfast			
During training (session 1)			
Recovery			
Preworkout snack			
Lunch			
During training (session 2)			
Recovery			
Dinner			
Snack			

Step 1: Enter Your Training Fuel Into Your Blueprint

In order to understand how to build a Nutrient Blueprint, recognize that some of your total nutrient needs for each day will be reserved for fueling before, during, and after conditioning, practice, or competition. The specific need as it relates to your sport is in table 9.1 on pages 105-106. You need to determine how long before the activity you will be eating based on your schedule, type of sport, and training intensity.

The general guidelines are as follows:

Before: 1 hour to 15 minutes before, consume 30-15 grams of carbohydrate and 10-15 grams of protein

During: 20-60 grams of carbohydrate per hour

After: Recovery is .7-2.5 grams of carbohydrate per kilogram of body weight and .1-2.5 grams of protein per kilogram of body weight. See appendix E on page 214 for more specific guidelines and examples.

For our sample athlete, Mike, here are his training needs based on the information pulled from table 9.1.

Meal/Snack	Carbohydrate (g)	Protein (g)	Fat (g)
Breakfast			
Lunch			
Pretraining	25	15	
During training	15		
Recovery	90	20	
Dinner			
Snack			

Step 2: Enter Your Carbohydrate Needs Into Your Blueprint

The main function for your Nutrition Blueprint is to estimate how you will distribute your "budget" of protein, fat, and carbohydrate throughout the day. After you input your training needs, you can evenly distribute the remainder of your carbohydrate grams between meals and snacks. Around training we like stay close to the numbers we calculate. For meals and snacks, *you don't have to be exact.* You will then use the blueprint to select foods that approximate the amounts you've selected through the rest of the day. For Mike, the remainder of his daily carbohydrate (455 g) would be spread out like this:

Meal/Snack	Carbohydrate (g)	Protein (g)	Fat (g)
Breakfast	110		
Lunch	110		
Pretraining	25		
During training	15		
Recovery	90		
Dinner	75		
Snack	30		

Or, let's say Mike wants to split his carbohydrate between dinner and a bigger snack later on. This is fine, provided he consumes at least two-thirds of his calories in the first two-thirds of the day. For example, Mike could adjust his carbohydrate as follows:

100 grams of carbohydrate at breakfast

115 grams of carbohydrate at lunch

60 grams of carbohydrate at dinner

50 grams of carbohydrate in one evening snack (or split between two evening snacks)

Step 3: Enter Your Protein Needs Into Your Blueprint

Just as we did with carbohydrate, your daily protein requirements need to be distributed through meals and snacks. Here's a blueprint of how Mike may distribute his protein (170 grams) during the day:

Meal/Snack	Carbohydrate (g)	Protein (g)	Fat (g)
Breakfast	110	30	
Lunch	110	45	
Pretraining	25	15	
During training	15		
Recovery	90	20	
Dinner	75	50	
Snack	30	10	

Step 4: Enter Your Fat Needs Into Your Blueprint

Everyone has a fat "budget" to work with that can be organized in several ways. There are added fats, such as using a salad dressing, adding mayonnaise or avocado slices to a sandwich, or using oil to sauté. Then there are "hidden" fats in foods such as cheese, whole milk, ice cream, high-fat cuts of meats, and from the oils and butter used in baking muffins, cakes, cookies, pies or pastries. When it is time to select foods, you might use up the majority of your fat from high-fat food selections, or you might have room to add fat to your diet in selected ways if you choose leaner meats and do not consume high-fat baked goods or sweets often. A general rule of thumb is that if your food item contains fat (cheese, high-fat meats, and fried foods), don't add much more, unless your budget is high. If you've chosen all lean proteins, then add some healthy fats (e.g., olive or canola oil, nuts, nut butter, avocado) to your meal or snack.

Mike, our sample athlete, needs 114 grams of fat per day. Mike's plan contains just a small amount (5 grams) before and after training, leaving him with 105 grams to spread throughout his additional three meals and one snack. This means he can have around 20 to 35 grams per meal or snack. Here's one example of how Mike's fats can be distributed in his blueprint:

Meal/Snack	Carbohydrate (g)	Protein (g)	Fat (g)
Breakfast	110	30	30
Lunch	110	45	25
Pretraining	25	15	5
During training	15		
Recovery	90	20	5
Dinner	75	50	30
Snack	30	10	20

TRANSLATING YOUR BLUEPRINT INTO A FOOD PLAN

So how do you know what foods will equal a certain number of grams of protein, carbohydrate, or fat? The meal and snack ideas in appendix D on page 209 list the grams of macronutrients found in common foods. Macronutrient content of common foods are included in appendix B on page 205, and appendix C on page 206 includes tables of food items and the amount of macronutrients in each.

Even with the charts, it can get tedious counting up every little thing, and we are not necessarily suggesting that you do that all the time. However, it can be helpful to try it, say, for a week, just to get a sense of amounts and proportions, and then return to the "eyeball" method, where you do not have to measure and count every food selection. If you are way off base at first, this kind of exercise in counting can prove to be eye-opening and beneficial. If you are already close to the mark, then rest assured that you are on course. In each of the remaining chapters in part III, we give you examples of meal plans and provide you with a blueprint—a breakdown of grams and percentages of protein, fat, and carbohydrate for a given calorie level—and how it can be translated into foods while keeping the nutrient timing principles in mind.

To get an idea of how our sample athlete's blueprint translates into actual food selections, take a look at figure 9.3 (page 118) for a sample 3,500-calorie meal plan.

Nutrient Timing in Action

A veteran New York Giant lineman, told us he was shocked by how his eating changed after he got married. His wife ensured the refrigerator was stocked and healthy snacks were readily available. Instead of eating a huge lunch before he left the practice facility after off-season training, which often left him feeling groggy, he ate a reasonable portion, knowing he could eat again when he got home. He stopped thinking of eating as *the* way to keep his size and began to think of eating as a way to keep himself fueled as part of his training and conditioning. He began to distribute his calories more evenly throughout the day, more in line with the principles of nutrient timing. His meals and snacks were more balanced. He fueled himself appropriately before and after training. We had talked and worked on this for quite some time, but for this lineman, putting the knowledge into action was a task. He had already experienced much success in his career, doing things the way he was used to. When you are good at what you do, sometimes it is difficult to know how much better or easier things could be. Motivation to try may not be as high as for someone who is struggling.

This newfound way of thinking was clearly in his grasp long before he was married, but, somehow, he never found the motivation to keep food in his fridge. He would join his buddies for dinner out, or he resorted to ordering in when hungry, eating all the food he ordered regardless of whether he was full. He was living in a cycle of eating until stuffed to waiting to eat until he was famished and then starting all over again. For him, it took a lifestyle change, such as getting married, to break the cycle. He can't believe how much better he feels now and that it took him so long. Plan ahead, keep foods around for healthy snacks, and eat reasonable meals that meet your needs rather than exceed them. Any one meal may seem small compared to what you are used to, but when you add all the meals and snacks up, it is just what your body needs. You will feel better and perform better.

FIGURE 9.3
Mike's sample 3,500-calorie menu

Carbohydrate (g)	Protein (g)	Fat (g)	Foods
			BREAKFAST (8:00 A.M.)
45	9	3	1-1/2 cup oatmeal
25	16	4	16 oz. 1% milk
30	0	0	Large banana
4	5	20	1/4 cup chopped walnuts
104	**30**	**27**	*Total for meal: approximately 800 calories*
			LUNCH (12:00 P.M.)
30	6	2	2 slices whole-wheat bread
0	35	8	4 oz (125 g) turkey + 1 oz (30 g) cheese
0	0	5	1 tbsp mayonnaise
0	0	10	1/3 avocado (2 oz)
20	0	0	Apple (5 oz)
50	0	0	12 oz (360 ml) cranberry juice
10	2	0	1 cup baby carrots
110	**43**	**25**	*Total for meal: approximately 800 calories*
			PREWORKOUT SNACK (4:00 P.M.)
26	15	4	Myoplex Lite bar
0	0	0	8 oz (240 ml) water
26	**15**	**4**	*Total for preworkout snack: approximately 215 calories*
			DURING TRAINING (6:00 P.M.)
15	0	0	8 oz (480 ml) sports drink
15	**0**	**0**	*Total for training: approximately 60 calories*
			RECOVERY (7:30 P.M.)
60	23	5	1 scoop EAS Whey protein powder + 16 oz orange juice
34	0	0	Small box of raisins
94	**23**	**5**	*Total for recovery: approximately 450 calories*
			DINNER (8:30 P.M.)
60	9	5	1 cup pasta + 1/2 cup marinara sauce
0	2	4	2 tbsp grated Parmesan cheese
10	4	0	1 cup broccoli
0	28	19	4 oz (175 g) chicken sauteed with 1 tbsp olive oil
5	0	0	Green salad, 2 cups
0	0	5	1 tbsp salad dressing
0	0	0	24 oz (720 ml) water
75	**43**	**33**	*Total for meal: approximately 800 calories*
			SNACK (10:30 P.M.)
4	3	20	1 oz (30 g) pecans
25	8	0	6 oz container non-fat vanilla yogurt
29	**11**	**20**	*Total for snack: approximately 350 calories*
453	**165**	**114**	**Total for day: approximately 3,500 calories**

ADJUST YOUR BLUEPRINT TO MEET INDIVIDUAL GOALS

If you are an athlete who has specific individual and personal needs, such as weight gain or loss, you may need to adjust your Blueprint to better match your goals. Additionally, a vegetarian athlete will also need to modify his or her Blueprint to better reflect this style and philosophy of eating. Other specific needs can be accommodated but are broader than the scope of this book (e.g., gluten-free diets; diets for athletes with diabetes or food allergies). Following are some of the most common individual goals that require adjustments.

Increase in Caloric Needs

At certain times of the year, you may have to revisit your caloric needs if your training time or intensity increases. The off-season, preseason, and season may all require different caloric levels. If you step up training just a notch and need to increase calories, you can do so relatively easily by first increasing fuel around your training. By adding a larger preworkout snack, consuming calories during the workout, and bumping up calories postworkout, you can easily add 300 to 500 extra calories a day. This also makes it much easier to reduce the calories when training pulls back. In each of the remaining chapters, we show you examples of how to boost calories by these amounts.

If your training level increases drastically and you need to do more than just add 300 to 500 calories per day around training, you may need to bump up to a higher calorie plan since carbohydrate needs increase as workout loads increase. Some endurance athletes may need to add a little more fat to their diet if they find they are unintentionally losing weight, and some power athletes may need to add fat if they are consuming such a high intake of calories that it becomes difficult to eat enough food in a day. Generally, protein needs stay relatively consistent because they are based on your weight, whereas carbohydrate requirements are based more on activity levels. We recommend revisiting the caloric calculator in appendix A on page 199 as training changes. Clearly, if you are hungry all the time, losing weight unintentionally, or not seeing gains in strength regardless of time devoted to conditioning, it is worth taking a closer look to see if your caloric intake is matching your output.

Gaining Weight and Keeping Weight On

Some athletes find that gaining weight or keeping weight on is a constant challenge. Many athletes in need of weight gain do not eat as much as they think they do. They may get full easily and so do not eat very much at one sitting, or they may forget to eat and skip meals, not eating as frequently as needed, which deprives them of valuable calories. Following are some strategies for gaining weight or keeping weight on:

- Consistently eat three meals every day.
- Be sure your beverages have calories. Juices, milk, smoothies, or sports drinks are all great choices instead of water.
- Drink beverages at the end of meals and between meals to leave more room for food at mealtime.

Timing Tip

If you are trying to gain weight, add healthy fat and carbohydrates. The general goal is to try to add 1,000 calories more per day than what you are accustomed to eating. The principles of distribution and balance remain the same.

- Choose calorically dense foods such as granola instead of Cheerios; a bean soup instead of a broth-based one; or cornbread rather than a plain roll.
- Eat higher calorie foods first; have soup or salad at the end of your meal.
- Never eat plain bread. Always "dress" your bread with peanut butter, olive oil, jam, honey, apple butter, hummus, occasionally butter or margarine, or any other topping you enjoy.
- Include snacks or mini-meals in between regular meals, especially after practice for recovery and before bedtime.
- Carry snacks with you so that you are prepared to eat when on the run. Peanut butter and crackers, sports bars, granola bars, trail mix, and dried fruit are easy and healthy high-calorie choices that you can keep in your desk or your locker, your briefcase or backpack, and even your car.
- Go for seconds, even if you don't finish them.
- Try to eat just a little more than you are used to—eat a bit past when you think you are full.

Trying to Lose Weight

Although not impossible, trying to lose weight while also gaining muscle can be challenging because weight loss requires a calorie deficit (burning more than you take in). During weight loss, it is common for people to lose some muscle tissue along with body fat; however, you will want to protect against this as much as possible by continuing to strength train while losing weight. Reduce calorie intake but not too much (about 15 percent fewer than your estimated caloric needs to start), while maintaining or slightly increasing protein intake and decreasing carbohydrate and fat. Aim for 2 g/kg protein or slightly more per day. Building muscle tissue requires having sufficient calories and protein available to fuel exercise and promote tissue repair.

It is not unusual for you to lose some strength while losing weight (just one more reason to lose weight during the off-season). Once your goal weight is achieved, slowly add calories so that you can increase your training to increase strength and power. Recalculate your caloric needs based on your new weight and current training regime. Unless training increases substantially, your maintenance calorie needs will most likely be less than before weight loss, as it takes fewer calories to maintain a lower weight. The most important factors to consider when losing weight are supplying enough energy to your muscles to train with and keep hormone levels and immune system functioning and consuming sufficient protein so you do not lose excessive muscle protein (and even bone density) while still reducing carbohydrate sufficiently to actually lose weight.

Typically, there is more than one way to adjust a diet for weight loss. Let's take a look at how you can do this using Mike, our sample strength and power athlete. Let's assume Mike wants to lose weight, so we start by reducing Mike's overall caloric intake by 500 calories, cutting back on fat and carbohydrate and adding some protein to help guard against muscle loss. We will adjust so that he has enough carbohydrate to train with (4 g/kg) and enough protein to preserve lean mass (2 g/kg). The balance of his calories will be fulfilled with fat. Therefore, referring to Mike's 3,500-calorie menu in figure 9.3, we can reduce his intake by around 500 calories by:

- cutting back on oatmeal by 1/2 cup (subtract about 80 calories)
- reducing breakfast nuts by half (subtract about 106 calories)
- replacing juice with water at lunch (subtract about 200 calories)

- adding 2 oz turkey to sandwich (add about 56 calories)
- eliminate 1 tablespoon olive oil by grilling or broiling chicken without added fat (subtract about 135 calories)
- increase portion of chicken at dinner by 2 oz. (add about 74 calories)
- decrease nuts at evening snack by half (subtract about 102 calories)

These changes make Mike's total decrease in calories about 623 and the total addition of calories about 130, equalling a deficit of 493 calories per day. Mike's numbers would now be 380 grams of carbohydrate (51 percent of calories; 4 grams per kilogram), 184 grams of protein (25 percent of calories; 2.0 grams per kilogram), and 81 grams of fat (24 percent of calories; .9 gram per kilogram). At this rate, Mike would lose one pound (.5 kg) per week.

Being a Vegetarian

Vegetarian athletes can meet all their protein needs through food. Since not all sources of protein for vegetarians are of high quality, though, these athletes should plan on consuming a higher percentage of calories from protein, which will help ensure adequate essential amino acids to fill the amino acid pool and support growth and repair. In addition, a greater quantity of nonmeat proteins may be required to deliver the nutrients, particularly iron and zinc, found in animal-based foods. Vegetarian diets are often higher in carbohydrate because many nonmeat proteins contain carbohydrate as well, whereas meats do not. Vegetarians need to plan their meals carefully, since plant forms of these nutrients are absorbed less efficiently. Choosing nutrient-dense foods is important. It's tempting for vegetarian athletes to use protein powders to achieve an adequate protein intake; however, powders do not contain the vast array of vitamins, minerals, and phytochemicals found in food. If dairy foods and eggs are omitted, strict vegetarians (vegans) may need to supplement with B_{12}, which is found only in animal sources.

Figure 9.4 shows how we adapted Mike's diet to a vegetarian menu. This plan meets all his needs in terms of vitamins and minerals without any fortified foods, sports bars, or powders. We wanted to show you that balanced eating can be achieved with all whole foods. Some of the changes to Mike's diet include:

- adding eggs as a source of good-quality protein at breakfast;
- including veggie burgers for protein and sunflower seed butter to provide zinc at lunch;
- replacing the Myoplex Lite bar with a yogurt and berry smoothie to show that a vegetarian athlete's nutrient needs can be achieved without using fortified foods;
- including beans and tofu at dinner (the black beans are especially high in folate, zinc, iron, and thiamine; mushrooms provide niacin; spinach provides iron, folate, and magnesium; tofu is a good source of complete protein); and
- adding pumpkin seeds, which are a rich source of magnesium and zinc.

Mike's protein needs were met with a slight increase, his carbohydrate increased, and his fat decreased while keeping calories very close to his original 3,500. Although healthy vegetarian eating can be achieved without the use of supplements, it is a good idea to consult a sports nutritionist if you are thinking of this style of eating. Achieving a well-balanced intake is not all that easy, even if you include eggs and dairy products. Meeting all vitamin and mineral needs can be tricky because many of the B vitamins are found in greater abundance in animal proteins, as well as iron and zinc as mentioned earlier.

FIGURE 9.4
Mike's sample vegetarian menu

Carbohydrate (g)	Protein (g)	Fat (g)	Foods
			BREAKFAST
45	9	3	1-1/2 cups oatmeal
25	16	6	16 oz low-fat milk
30	0	0	Large banana 8"
0	12	10	2 large eggs
100	**37**	**19**	*Total for meal: approximately 700 calories*
			SNACK
5	10	16	1/4 cup pumpkin seeds
5	**10**	**16**	*Total for snack: approximately 200 calories*
			LUNCH
30	6	0	2 slices whole-wheat bread
12	26	1	2 veggie burgers, 2-1/2 oz each
0	14	16	2 slice cheese
20	0	0	Small apple
8	6	16	2 tbsp sunflower seed butter (on apple)
10	2	0	1 cup baby carrots
80	**54**	**33**	*Total for meal: approximately 825 calories*
			PREWORKOUT SNACK
21	14	0	6 oz Greek Fruited yogurt
5	0	0	1 honey stick
26	**14**	**0**	*Total for preworkout snack: approximately 200 calories*
			DURING TRAINING
15	0	0	8 oz (480 ml) sports drink
15	**0**	**0**	*Total for training: approximately 60 calories*
			RECOVERY
65	20	5	20 oz low-fat chocolate milk
34	5	1	Superpretzel
99	**25**	**6**	*Total for recovery: approximately 450 calories*
			DINNER
10	4	0	1 cup cooked spinach
5	2	0	1/2 cup cooked mushrooms
2	0	0	1/4 cup cooked peppers
0	0	15	1 tbsp olive oil
20	8	0	1 cup black beans
22	7	0	1/2 cup pinto beans
3	13	7	1/4 block tofu
45	5	2	1 cup brown rice
107	**39**	**24**	*Total for meal: approximately 900 calories*
			SNACK
30	10	2	1 cup split-pea soup
30	**10**	**2**	*Total for snack: approximately 180 calories*
462	**189**	**100**	**Total for day: approximately 3,570 calories**

Discretionary Calories

Every athlete has a little room for what are often called discretionary calories—calories that come from empty-nutrient food, or junk food. The idea, though, is to keep these foods to 10 to 15 percent of your total caloric needs per day. So if you need 2,000 calories a day, 200 to 300 calories can come from discretionary calories (say, a candy bar or a soda and a few small cookies). If your caloric requirements are higher, you have more discretionary calories to use each day; a 5,000-calorie daily requirement leaves room for 500 to 750 discretionary calories.

Be flexible in your eating. It's better to include an ice cream cone or a few cookies on a daily basis if you enjoy these foods rather than stuffing yourself silly one day and then eating restrictively to make up for your overindulgence. This can cause performance to suffer, both after the heavy eating and surely during restrictive phases, when the body doesn't get the nutrients or calories to perform and recover optimally. It is just plain healthier to enjoy what you eat and figure out a reasonable way to balance health, performance, taste, and food preferences.

The same way you plan for when to work out, you need to plan for when to eat. Even if your schedule changes daily, you can most likely anticipate each day's timeline Think ahead and be strategic. At the beginning of each day (or the night before), make sure you have a plan for your meals and snacks. Ask yourself the following questions: Do I have the right foods available for my meals? Where and when will I eat? Do I need to buy or bring any foods or beverages today? Two minutes of planning saves lots of time during the day and ensures proper fueling. Make sure you have something healthy and balanced on hand or easily accessible.

Now that you're familiar with all the Nutrient Timing Principles and you've developed your Nutrition Blueprint, let's apply them to your specific sport. In each of the following chapters you will find strategies geared to the particular needs for strength and power athletes, endurance athletes, and stop-and-go athletes, incorporating the NTP with identifiable circumstances you encounter, such as tournament play, back-to-back competitions, game days, or two-a-day training sessions.

10

Strength and Power

Baseball, diving, football, gymnastics, cheerleading, softball, swimming, track and field, volleyball, and wrestling are all considered strength and power sports. Strength and power athletes range from some of the largest athletes to some of the smallest. Practice and competition schedules vary widely. Football is typically played once a week with a mix of heavy and light practices as well as rest days. Professional baseball players can go for more than two weeks of games on back-to-back days—teens and college-age athletes who play for both school and clubs often have similarly grueling schedules. Some sports have all-day tournaments to prepare for (gymnastics, wrestling, volleyball), while others have meets that require many hours of waiting (swimming, diving, cheerleading).

Although strength and power athletes compete in very different sports, an important nutrition point for all these athletes is that they need more fuel during training than for competition. For example, swimmers notoriously spend hours in the pool, yet a race may last less than 30 seconds. Gymnasts and cheerleaders spend hours and hours training, yet competition routines typically are less than three minutes. Clearly, competition does not require the same amount of fuel as training, but muscles need to be prepared with energy nonetheless. Nutrient timing is very important, especially during training and conditioning, for strength development, energy requirements, and weight management.

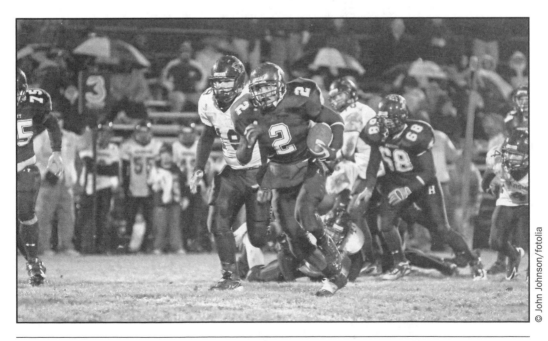

© John Johnson/fotolia

For many strength and power athletes, competition requires less calories and fuel than training.

Nuances of the Different Strength and Power Sports

Nuances of strength and power sports often impose challenges to athletes' fueling and hydration needs that can be overcome with proper planning. The energy requirements throughout the season can change drastically and often differ based on sport and position.

Baseball and Softball Players

Playing softball or baseball does not burn many calories although more calories may actually be needed during off-season training. Players will benefit from beginning games well hydrated. Pitchers and catchers need more fuel and need to replenish during the game. Hectic schedules and travel can pose challenges to eating well, being consistent in patterns, and timing of intake. Planning healthy meals and snacks that contain fruits, vegetables, and adequate carbohydrate without excessive starch or fat is important for proper fueling and avoiding unintended weight gain.

Cheerleaders

Cheerleaders can spend hours at a time practicing, and dehydration can result. Regular meals and snacks during practices and competitions are important for adequate fueling. Cheerleaders may consume too few calories, denying their bodies valuble nutrients. Extreme dieting practices are strongly discouraged. Rather, an intake focusing on adequate calories distributed throughout the day, including healthful selections of fruits, vegetables, whole grains, lean proteins, and adequate fat along with proper hydration, should be encouraged.

Football Players

Football players, particularly larger linemen, may have difficulty regulating body temperature, especially in hot, humid conditions that cause high fluid losses. Because of high body fat, some players have difficulty cooling off. Strict monitoring of weight before and after practice is a must. Replacing 150 percent of lost fluid along with sodium will help prevent the additive effect of dehydration. Some football players are used to eating a lot as opposed to eating well, and therefore may not focus on eating strategically for performance and health. Paying particular attention to caloric distribution, timing, and quality of food selection is of particular benefit.

Gymnasts and Divers

Gymnasts and divers are often conscious of their weight and may eat far fewer calories than their training requires. This practice is not a good solution for weight management and can lead to devastating injuries. Some gymnasts avoid dietary fat in fear that it will cause weight gain. Although fats in food do contribute calories, they are required to keep athletes healthy. Including at least the minimum (1 gram per kilogram) is a must for good health and performance.

Swimmers

Swimming is an all-body exercise, so athletes expend a lot of calories. For athletes training twice a day, getting in adequate calories can be a challenge. Planning for meals and snacks is a must and using the recovery "window" is essential to prevent depletion. Although races are short, swimmers train for hours at a time, crossing into endurance work (see chapter 11). Swimmers work hard, usually in a warm and humid environment, and lose fluids during training. It is helpful to keep fluids poolside and drink throughout practice. Sports drinks can spare glycogen and supply energy during moderate- and high-intensity workouts.

Track and Field Athletes

A big challenge for track and field athletes is adapting to changing energy needs. During heavy training, caloric needs can be high. At other times, athletes may be tapering their training and caloric needs are less, but muscles still need to be fueled for competition. Planning for varying amounts of food and fluid is important during the season and in the off-season. Athletes should not be losing or gaining weight unintentionally.

Volleyball Players

Competitive volleyball players need to monitor hydration carefully because fluid losses may be greater than they realize. Eating properly and taking in sufficient fuel from carbohydrate can be challenging for players who travel frequently. Being prepared with healthy snacks, such as granola bars, dried and fresh fruits, whole-grain crackers, cheese sticks, trail mix, and juice boxes can help players avoid fast food, concession-stand snacks, and other nutrient-void items.

Wrestlers

Wrestlers are notorious for cutting weight by dehydrating. Losing 5 percent or more of body weight in a week to make weight decreases strength and is unhealthy. A smarter strategy is to maintain weight within 5 percent above the weight class then dehydrate slightly and rehydrate slightly, competing in a safe zone of 2 percent dehydration. This allows athletes to train while well hydrated and still make weight. It's impossible to rehydrate enough in the short time between weigh-in and competition if fluid losses are excessive.

PLANNING FOR TRAINING

In chapter 9, we helped you determine your caloric needs and formulate the carbohydrate, protein, and fat needed for training and competition into a Nutrition Blueprint. To illustrate how to apply this information, we will use a sample athlete, Sam, a 154-pound (70 kg) strength athlete who performs heavy conditioning for 60 minutes. We calculated his caloric needs in appendix A on page 199 and determined his macronutrient needs by sport in appendix B on page 205. Sam's estimated caloric needs are 2,800 calories per day: 5 g/kg carbohydrate for a total of 350 grams (50 percent of calories); 1.8 g/kg protein for a total of 126 grams (18 percent of calories); and 99 grams of fat, which come from the balance of calories left (32 percent of calories).

Morning Training

For all morning workouts before breakfast, a small snack 15 to 30 minutes before training is always a good idea. Lighter workouts require less fuel (15 grams of carbohydrate, 10 grams of protein), moderate training slightly more (15 to 25 grams of carbohydrate, 10 to 15 grams of protein). More intense and/or longer-duration training requires more fuel. The type of work (weightlifting versus conditioning drills) may determine what form of fuel is best tolerated. Liquids may sit better before heavy conditioning than solid food. Shakes with 35 or more grams of carbohydrate and 10 to 15 grams of protein are fine. If fuel cannot be taken before, a sports drink during training provides energy to muscles. Moderate and heavy training should be followed by a recovery snack as soon as possible, preferably within 30 minutes, but can be consumed up to 60 minutes after. A regular meal schedule can follow.

Let's take a look at how Sam's daily nutrient needs are spread out if he works out in the morning. First, Sam will need a pretraining snack of 40 grams of carbohydrate and 15 grams of protein before working out in the morning. He will also need 15 grams of carbohydrate during training and between 50-70 grams of carbohydrate and between 7-20 grams of protein for recovery. Here's how Sam's blueprint looks for a day when he trains before breakfast:

Meal/Snack	Carbohydrate (g)	Protein (g)	Fat (g)
Pretraining	40	15	5
During training	15	0	0
Recovery	65	20	0
Breakfast	70	20	25
Lunch	75	25	30
Snack	20	10	10
Dinner	65	40	25
Total	350	130	95

Once Sam's fuel around training is entered into the blueprint, the rest of his nutrient needs can be spread out throughout the rest of the day, as discussed previously. Figure 10.1 shows how Sam's daily nutrient needs translate into real foods when training in the morning for 60 minutes at a high intensity.

FIGURE 10.1

Sam's sample 2,800-calorie menu when training in the morning

Carbohydrate (g)	Protein (g)	Fat (g)	Foods
PREWORKOUT SNACK (6:00 A.M.)			
40	13	4	Carnation Breakfast Essentials
0	0	0	8 oz (240 ml) water
40	13	4	*Total for preworkout snack: approximately 250 calories*
DURING TRAINING (6:30 A.M.)			
15	0	0	8 oz (240 ml) sports drink
15	0	0	*Total for training: approximately 60 calories*
RECOVERY (7:45 A.M.)			
37	2	0	1 1/2 cups Corn flakes to go
12	8	2	8 oz (240 ml) 1% milk
15	10	0	4 oz orange juice + 1/2 scoop whey protein
64	20	2	*Total for recovery: approximately 350 calories*
BREAKFAST (2ND RECOVERY) (9:00 A.M.)			
27	6	1	Whole-wheat English muffin
6	8	16	2 tbsp peanut butter
15	0	0	1 tbsp jam
23	0	0	Small banana
0	6	5	Hard-boiled egg
71	20	22	*Total for meal: approximately 560 calories*
LUNCH (12:30 P.M.)			
30	6	6	10 in (25 cm) wrap
0	21	3	3 oz (90 g) chicken
0	0	10	2 oz (60 g) avocado
2	0	0	Lettuce, tomato, sliced peppers (1 cup)
10	1	0	1 cup baby carrots
0	0	15	2 tbsp ranch dressing (for carrots)
30	0	0	Fruit salad, 1 cup
72	28	34	*Total for meal: approximately 700 calories*
SNACK (4:30 P.M.)			
0	8	5	1 mozzarella stick (1 oz; 30 g)
20	3	5	7 whole-wheat crackers
20	11	10	*Total for snack: approximately 210 calories*
DINNER (7:30 P.M.)			
0	28	15	4 oz (125 g) broiled salmon
3	0	0	1 tbsp teriyaki sauce
35	7	0	1 cup wild rice
12	4	0	1 cup sugar snap peas
0	0	10	2 tsp butter
15	3	0	Small dinner roll
65	42	25	*Total for meal: approximately 650 calories*
347	134	97	Total for day: approximately 2,800 calories

Afternoon or Evening Training

If you've eaten breakfast and lunch and are planning a light workout, no fuel is needed before you train unless it's been more than four hours since you last ate. In that case, a small snack is in order. Drinking a sports beverage during training is just as effective for topping off blood glucose as a pretraining snack, and it can hydrate as well. If you are planning a heavy workout and it has been four hours or more since you last ate, more fuel is needed. Refer to table 9.1 on page 105 of chapter 9 for specific training fuel needs for strength and power athletes.

To help you get a better idea of how a plan is modified for afternoon or evening workouts, let's take another look at our sample athlete and what his blueprint would look like for an afternoon workout:

Meal/Snack	Carbohydrate (g)	Protein (g)	Fat (g)
Breakfast	80	25	20
Snack	35	5	0
Lunch	45	30	35
Pretraining	35	10	5
During training	15	0	0
Recovery	50	15	15
Dinner	90	40	25
Total	350	125	100

Notice how Sam's meals could remain similar by adding to his morning pretraining snack so that it now becomes breakfast. The pretraining snack serves the dual purpose of topping off his energy stores and preventing hunger during his workout. If he were to skip this, chances are he'd be ravenous by dinner. Dinner then fills his needs for the second recovery snack, similar to that when training in the morning. Figure 10.2 shows how Sam's daily nutrient needs translate into real foods when conditioning for 60 minutes at high intensity in the afternoon.

Remember to consume at least two-thirds of your calories in the first two-thirds of your day. Eating frequently is beneficial for muscle repair and optimal body composition. Monitor the time intervals between meals and snacks—more than four hours is generally too long to go without eating. Don't deprive your body of nutrient-rich foods during the day and then overload your system at night, as some athletes do. Skipping meals not only deprives muscles of needed fuel but also puts athletes into hunger overload at night. Additionally, it's difficult to take in enough fruits, vegetables, and dairy servings if you haven't eaten sufficiently all day.

FIGURE 10.2
Sam's sample 2,800-calorie menu when training in the afternoon

Carbohydrate (g)	Protein (g)	Fat (g)	Foods
			BREAKFAST (7:30 A.M.)
			Yogurt parfait:
2	2	10	2 tbsp chopped walnuts
8	17	4	5 oz (150 g) Greek yogurt
15	0	0	1 cup mixed berries
23	0	0	Small banana (6")
35	5	6	1/2 cup granola
83	**24**	**20**	*Total for meal: approximately 600 calories*
			MIDMORNING SNACK (10:30 A.M.)
10	6	0	8 oz latte
27	0	0	1/3 cup dried apricots
37	**6**	**0**	*Total for snack: approximately 172 calories*
			LUNCH (12:30 P.M.)
			Chicken wrap:
30	6	6	10 in (25 cm) wrap
0	21	3	3 oz (90 g) chicken
0	0	10	2 oz (60 g) avocado
2	0	0	Lettuce, tomato, sliced peppers (1 cup)
10	1	15	1 cup baby carrots + 2 tbsp ranch dressing
27	0	0	12 oz (360 ml) iced tea
69	**28**	**34**	*Total for meal: approximately 700 calories*
			PREWORKOUT SNACK (4:30 P.M.)
30	10	5	NuGo dark bar
30	**10**	**5**	*Total for preworkout snack: approximately 200 calories*
			DURING TRAINING (5:30-6:30 P.M.)
15	0	0	8 oz sports drink
15	**0**	**0**	*Total for training: approximately 60 calories*
			RECOVERY (6:45 P.M.)
			Smoothie:
26	11	1	1/2 scoop whey protein + 1 cup orange juice
13	0	0	1/4 cup mango sorbet
11	0	0	1 kiwi
5	6	14	1 oz (30 g) raw almonds
55	**17**	**15**	*Total for recovery: approximately 425 calories*
			DINNER (8:00 P.M.)
0	28	15	4 oz (125 g) broiled salmon
35	7	0	1 cup wild rice
12	4	0	1 cup sugar snap peas
15	3	10	Dinner roll + 2 tsp butter
62	**42**	**25**	*Total for meal: approximately 750 calories*
351	**127**	**99**	**Total for day: approximately 2,800 calories**

Two-a-Day Training

Some strength and power athletes need a lot of energy for two-a-day practices. Be careful in your planning, however—two-a-days for baseball and softball, for example, can require a lot of time but may not expend a huge number of calories. The majority of this energy will come from carbohydrate. When caloric needs do become high, dietary fat may need to be added to ensure caloric needs are met. Although protein is needed for muscle repair, it is not a main source of energy.

When planning, recognize you need to replace muscle glycogen before your next session. Use your total calorie level to adapt to the following recommendations for two-a-days. Although some of the suggestions may seem like a lot of food, or perhaps to others, not that much, realize that your portions should align with your energy expenditure (caloric need).

Before we explain fueling needs around two-a-day sessions, let's first take a look at our sample 154-pound (70 kg) athlete, Sam, and how his daily nutrient needs change for two-a-day practices (see figure 10.3).

FIGURE 10.3
Sam's daily nutrient needs based on two-a-day training

	Daily total (g)	Daily total (calories)	%	g/kg for 70 kg (154 lb)
Fat	167	1,500	26	2.4
Carbohydrate	700	2800	61	10
Protein	175	700	13	2.5
Total		5,000 daily calories	100%	

Now, let's take a look at how Sam's daily nutrient needs are spread out if he participates in two-a-day training:

Meal/Snack	Carbohydrate (g)	Protein (g)	Fat (g)
Breakfast	150	25	25
During training (session 1)	85	0	0
Recovery	70	15	15
Lunch	100	40	50
Preworkout snack	25	0	0
During training (session 2)	45	0	0
Recovery	70	15	10
Dinner	110	70	60
Snack	45	10	10
Total	700	175	170

These daily nutrient needs are based on five hours a day of training, with some of the work being heavy and some more moderate. Note that even though his portions of protein foods are small, his protein ends up being quite high (2.5 grams per kilogram). That's because so many of the high-carbohydrate foods also have some protein. Figure 10.4 shows how Sam's needs translate into real food choices.

FIGURE 10.4
Sam's sample 5,000-calorie menu when participating in two-a-days

Carbohydrate (g)	Protein (g)	Fat (g)	Foods
			BREAKFAST (6:00 A.M.)
60	12	2	4 oz (125 g) plain bagel
9	12	24	3 tbsp peanut butter
26	0	0	2 tbsp jam
60	0	0	16 oz (480 ml) orange juice
155	24	26	*Total for meal: approximately. 950 calories*
			DURING TRAINING (8:15-10:45 A.M.)
60	0	0	32 oz (960 ml) sports drink
25	0	0	Sports gel
85	0	0	*Total for training: approximately 340 calories*
			RECOVERY (11:00 A.M.)
39	12	12	12 oz (360 ml) chocolate milk
34	1	5	Super Pretzel
73	13	17	*Total for recovery : approximately 500 calories*
			LUNCH (11:30 A.M.)
			Turkey sandwich:
45	9	3	6 in (23 cm) sub roll
0	21	3	3 oz (90 g) turkey
2	0	0	Lettuce and tomato
0	7	8	1 slice Swiss cheese
0	0	15	1 tbsp each olive oil and vinegar
28	4	20	2 oz (60 g) potato chips
20	0	0	Orange
0	0	0	Water
95	41	49	*Total for meal: approximately 990 calories*
			PREWORKOUT SNACK (TOP–OFF) (2:30 P.M.)
25	0	0	1 cup grapes
25	0	0	*Total for preworkout snack: approximately 100 calories*
			DURING TRAINING (3:15-5:45 P.M.)
45	0	0	24 oz (960 ml) sports drink
45	0	0	*Total for training: approximately 180 calories*
			RECOVERY (6:00 P.M.)
44	10	3	Stonyfield Farm smoothie
26	6	4	Honey Nut Cheerios cereal bar
70	16	7	*Total for recovery: approximately 400 calories*
			DINNER (6:30 P.M.)
0	62	20	2-4 oz (125 g) pork chops
50	5	0	Large baked potato
0	0	15	3 tsp butter
25	0	0	1/2 cup applesauce
28	2	5	1 piece cornbread
10	4	17	1 cup green beans and almonds in olive oil
0	0	0	24 oz (720 ml) seltzer
113	73	57	*Total for meal: approximately 1,265 calories*
			SNACK (9:00 P.M.)
44	9	8	Frozen burrito (6 oz)
44	9	8	*Total for snack: approximately 285 calories*
705	176	164	**Total for day: approximately 5,000 calories**

Night Before a Two-a-Day

Dinner is a big part of your preworkout fueling. The night before the first workout, and each night for the duration of two-a-days, should focus on carbohydrate with two-thirds of your plate covered by starches along with some vegetables and fruit. The remaining one-third of your plate can be protein. Of course, the fat is interspersed or added to these foods, not really taking up "space" on the plate. Be sure to add healthy fats to your dinner, such as olive or canola oil, nuts, avocados, olives, or high-fat fish, since you may need to limit fat at breakfast or lunch depending on meal and practice times.

High-carbohydrate evening snacks also prepare you for the morning session. Some good ideas are graham crackers with peanut butter; fig bars and milk; pretzels and hummus; a bowl of soup with crackers; cold cereal with milk; a bowl of oatmeal with dried fruit; sorbet, ice cream, or frozen yogurt with berries; or a fruit smoothie. Or, if there is more time between dinner and bedtime, have a mini-meal, such as a pizza bagel; a peanut butter and jelly sandwich; cheese and tomato on an English muffin with a glass of juice; a burrito; or a yogurt parfait. An evening snack helps ensure glycogen levels in the liver are filled. During sleep, liver glycogen helps fuel the brain and central nervous system. Upon waking, liver glycogen is partially depleted. Going to bed with full stores prevents complete depletion by the morning and is especially important if training early before breakfast.

First Two-a-Day Session

During two-a-days, breakfast is one of the three most important meals of the day. You need fuel, and giving yourself time to eat breakfast ensures you get a good start to your day. Without breakfast, it can be difficult to meet caloric needs and easy to create a caloric deficit that will be detrimental to performance, both immediately and certainly within days of two-a-days. Repercussions include increased risk of injury as well as impaired timing, heat intolerance, and reduced power output. What and how much you eat is determined by what time your first practice is scheduled. The more fat and protein you include, the more digestion time you should leave. If time is short, make your breakfast higher carbohydrate.

Also, note that you should not have a high-protein shake for breakfast because you will be burning carbohydrate for energy, not protein. Furthermore, protein takes more energy and more time to digest, so it is not efficient to consume protein as the majority of your intake at this time. A higher carbohydrate smoothie with some protein (30 g or less) is a fine choice.

During the session, consume 30 to 60 grams of carbohydrate per hour to help prevent depleting your glycogen stores. If sports drinks are available, they are a convenient way to fuel and hydrate at the same time. Remember, when you are dehydrated, glycogen depletes faster, so preventing dehydration will also help preserve your energy (see page 81 in chapter 7 to determine your sweat rate, and establish a hydration schedule). Drink at regular intervals, optimally every 10 to 15 minutes. If this is not possible, take advantage of breaks to rehydrate and refuel.

Between Sessions

Since having enough energy for the second session is a top priority, immediately after the first session, focus on consuming sufficient carbohydrate for recovery. Aim for 1.2 g/kg of carbohydrate if you will be able to eat again before the next session, otherwise, you can increase carbohydrate to a greater extent based on your comfort level. Some easy food choices include bagels, bread, corn flakes, grits, farina, pancakes, pasta, pretzels, potatoes, rice, rolls, raisins, bananas, and recovery bars. Right after a hard session, appetites may be suppressed, so going for smoothies, applesauce, ripe bananas, or recovery shakes might be easier and seem most palatable. Be sure to get something in! Protein is of lesser importance at this time. Fluid choices include grape, orange, and pineapple juice; milk or chocolate milk; sports nutrition shakes or recovery beverages; and sports drinks. Hopefully, time will allow for lunch, which should again, contain easily-digested carbohydrate (125 to 175 grams) and a small amount of protein, trying to stay around 4 to 6 ounces. You may include some fat, keeping it on the lower side if you will be returning to practice in the next hour or two. Avoid fried foods, fast food, high-fat meats like salami or sausage, and creamy or cheesy sauces. Better choices are sandwiches with turkey, roast beef, lean ham or grilled chicken; broth-based soups with noodles or rice; pasta salad; pretzels, baked chips, or crackers; fruit; fig bars; or sorbet. If there is time, pasta or rice with chicken or shrimp and cooked vegetables makes for a great lunch. Hydrate at lunch as fluid is absorbed faster with food than on an empty stomach.

Remember, if you begin the second session partially depleted, you will completely deplete your glycogen by the end of the workout. When glycogen is completely depleted, replenishment can take more hours to restore (24 to 48) than you have before the next day's first session. Your training will suffer not only on this day but on the following day as well. So if you have time for both recovery fuel and lunch, then do both. And if you can, rest or nap, which helps the body's restorative power. Before you return for the second session, try to consume another 25-gram carbohydrate snack if possible. It can be consumed just before practice, particularly if it's fast-digesting carbohydrate such as pretzels, raisins, a banana, fig bars, fruit leather, or a sports drink. If practice is in the early evening, make the afternoon snack more substantial. It's important to have multiple eating opportunities during hard training.

Second Two-a-Day Session

The guidelines for the second two-a-day session are the same as for the first session. It may be even more critical to fuel and hydrate properly during the second session because if glycogen becomes depleted by insufficient fueling earlier in the day, you won't have enough time to restock before the following morning. Day after day of insufficient glycogen can impair training and performance and lead to extreme soreness and possibly injury. Additive dehydration can impair performance and lead to heat illness over the course of a week or two in hot weather.

After the second session, another recovery snack is in order, so plan to have something as soon as training is over and before dinner if possible, unless dinner is immediate. Do not purposely wait until dinner—the faster you are able to consume food, the better supplied your muscles will be with glycogen for your workout the following day. Repeated feedings improve muscle glycogen and tissue repair. See pages 216-218 in appendix E for some good recovery ideas. Then for your meal, the same thing as discussed in the Night Before a Two-a-Day section on page 132 applies here. It's fine to include more fat at dinner, particularly for those needing more calories, as you'll have plenty of time to digest.

FUEL FOR COMPETITION

It may be hard to believe but when you think about it, it makes perfect sense; typically, for a game or meet during the regular season, calorie requirements are actually less than they are for a training day. The hours of strength work, conditioning drills, agility work, repetition of routines, and practice require lots of fuel. Strength and power athletes tend to be mesomorphs—with lean mass that needs and burns calories. Whether we're talking about baseball, pole-vaulting, gymnastics, swimming, diving, wrestling, volleyball, or football, the hours devoted to develop the strength needed for competition require much physical work—much more than is expended during a game or a meet. The day of competition, particularly for events lasting only seconds to minutes, your muscles don't need to be loaded, as a marathon runner's should be, but at the same time you shouldn't be hungry or depleted. Often athletes are jazzed up before competition; they may not feel hungry or may actually feel a bit nauseated. Others want to feel "light" or think being hungry will motivate them. Unfortunately, that may help psychologically but not physiologically. Being inadequately fueled can hurt performance.

Night Before the Event

A good meal the evening before competition is important, especially if you are jittery in the morning. Remember that three-fourths of your plate should contain carbohydrate-rich foods. Eating well a full 24 hours before will provide the energy and fluids stored in muscles. Regardless of the timing of the event, meals eaten the day before competition do more to influence stored energy than the meal eaten the morning of an event. The entire day of eating preceding an event influences the body's readiness to perform.

Competition Day

For short events, the goal is to be sure that caloric intake is sufficient to fuel your day, not just your activity. You want adequate fuel available, but there is no need to load. This is particularly true for athletes whose competition is one event lasting less than 10 minutes. Clearly these athletes don't need to eat quite as much on competition day as training days (when activity lasts for hours). You should feel good and not be under-fueled or overloaded. Be sure to include familiar foods that sit well. Avoid spicy and high-fat foods before competition.

For events lasting two hours or more or events with multiple competitions, you will have different fueling requirements based on the timing of your events.

Morning Events

For morning events, a good supply of quick-digesting carbohydrate is in order. If you are able to leave some time for digestion, including protein will help keep you from getting hungry during the game. Keep fat to a minimum, as it will keep food in your stomach longer. Aim to have one-quarter to one-third of your daily calories before the event, so this could mean getting up early to be sure you are properly fueled. Your pre-event meal should be similar in size and style to your normal pretraining meal. For example, if you usually train in the afternoon and eat pasta before training, have pasta for breakfast; otherwise, any carbohydrate-rich breakfast including familiar foods will do.

Afternoon Events

Fueling begins at breakfast, so absolutely no skipping. Your breakfast and lunch should be a meal, not just a bar. Sufficient carbohydrate is the most important thing to focus on here. Include protein and fat at breakfast because, for afternoon events, there is enough time to digest. Depending on the timing of your event and meals, go for a slightly larger carbohydrate-rich breakfast (pancakes or waffles with eggs and juice; add bacon or breakfast potatoes if you like bagel with yogurt and fruit) and smaller carbohydrate-rich lunch (wrap or sandwich with pretzels and an apple). Remember to top off the tank with 15 grams carbohydrate before you begin.

Evening Events

For evening events, be sure you have two-thirds or more of your calories through the day before the event. Think about this: When you need to be fueled to go past 8:00 and possibly until 10:00 p.m., having breakfast, lunch, and *at least* a pregame snack are musts. Imagine, even if you were *not* competing, how hungry you would be by 8:00 p.m. if you had not eaten since lunch. If you don't plan ahead and are under-fueled, you most certainly will not be performing to your potentional toward the end of the event . . . when close competitions are won and lost.

Table 10.1 shows how an athlete who requires 3,000 calories per day may time his or her eating according to competition. Also note that hydration should be included in each: 10-20 oz. fluid 2-3 hours before and 7-10 oz. fluid 10-20 minutes before.

In addition, competing in tournaments or meets that have multiple events at varying time intervals can present a challenge to timing food intake, so having a flexible plan will help. Snacks are a must to have on hand for between-event fueling and hunger management. If your competitions involve a lot of waiting around, be prepared with appropriate snacks instead of winging it and eating whatever you find. You'll be able to fuel yourself properly with carbohydrate for fuel and protein for satiety. If you are not sure about the time interval, graze on small amounts of easily-digested carbohydrate (see appendix E on page 214). If you know you have more time, have some protein to help your satiety and squelch hunger (such as yogurt, turkey, chicken, an egg, or a peanut butter and jelly sandwich). Hydration is important as well. Although short events won't dehydrate you, you still need to remember to stay hydrated while waiting around by drinking periodically throughout the day. Once suited up, athletes don't want to have to run to the bathroom often. Remember, sipping beverages throughout the day rather than gulping a lot at once gives the body time to absorb the fluid into muscles and tissues; the need to urinate will not be as often.

If you are competing in games or matches lasting hours, drink water or sports drinks during the game, such as whenever you're on the sidelines or during a substitution, injury, or timeout, and use your hydration strategy as a guideline. You can then use halftime, changeover, or another break in play as a time to refuel. Research shows that consuming just 25 grams of carbohydrate at halftime, such as a gel, a sports drink, a box of raisins, pretzels, fruit leathers, a banana, or orange slices, can help performance in the last 15 minutes of the game. Think you're doing okay without? Veteran professional players have told us they were just fine and had been for years without consuming anything during halftime. We asked them to experiment just once to see if they felt any different. Time and again, once they tried consuming a small amount of fuel, they couldn't believe the change

Table 10.1 Calorie Distribution Based on Event Time for an Athlete Consuming 3,000 Calories/day

	Total calories prior to event	Meals prior to event	Snacks prior to event
Morning event (10 A.M.)	750-1,000	Breakfast (7 A.M.): 500 to 800 calories	150-200 calories one hour prior (9 A.M.) and 100 calories (25 g carb) immediately before
Afternoon event (1 P.M.)	1,500	Breakfast (8 A.M.): 800 calories Lunch (11:30 A.M.): 500-600 calories	100-200 calories 30 minutes before
Late afternoon event (4 P.M.)	2,000	Breakfast (8 A.M.): 900 calories Lunch (12 P.M.): 600 calories	400 calories two hours prior (2 P.M.) and 100 calories (25 g carb) 15-20 minutes before
Evening event (7 P.M.)	2,200	Breakfast (9 A.M.): 700 calories Lunch (1 P.M.): 900 calories	500 calories two to three hours prior (4-5 P.M.) and 100 calories (25 g carb) 15-30 minutes before

in their energy and performance through the second half, especially the fourth quarter. "I didn't even realize that I wasn't feeling great," one player said. "Now I see the difference, I just had no idea!" Experiment for yourself!

Recovery Fuel

For events lasting less than 10 minutes, a specific recovery snack isn't necessary. For tournaments and meets with multiple events, it is not so much a recovery snack that is needed as a balanced meal since hopefully you have been grazing periodically throughout the day. If you are an athlete who competes for hours, recovery fuel is very important, even if you have a rest day following competition. Your muscles need to repair, and recovery reduces muscle soreness. Be prepared with your own snack since it's not likely to be provided for you (see appendix D on page 209 for recovery snack ideas). If you are traveling and don't have access to refrigeration, a sports bar and sports drink or shakes such as Carnation Instant Breakfast Essentials, Cheribundi/Cherry Pharm Recovery or Boost along with a banana or some fig bars are easy and practical choices. For all competitive events, after the day is over, have a dinner similar to your usual intake.

MENU PLANS FOR STRENGTH
AND POWER ATHLETES

Following are sample menu plans to help illustrate all the facts and put them into practice. Sample meal plans are provided for athletes whose weight ranges from 110 pounds (50 kg) to 300 pounds (136 kg), for light training to heavy training, and for 2,000 calories to 7,500 calories. Use the Blueprint you developed in chapter 9 to plan your meals and use the following sample plans as a guide, adjusting the macronutrients (carbohydrate, protein, fat) based on your training phase (more carbohydrate as training intensity increases, slightly higher protein during initial phases of strength training). Hopefully, these plans offer some great ideas for meals, timing, and distribution of calories. Also illustrated is how to increase or decrease calories depending on training phase. For illustrative purposes, we use exact numbers because we are showing specific calculations. You do not need to be this exact; in real life, few people are when it comes to eating. Rather, use these suggestions and guidelines to build your own meals in order to create a healthy training diet.

Menu Plans for Strength and Power Athletes During Training

Following are menus for athletes of different sizes and energy needs. We'll provide plans for smaller athletes training for shorter and longer sessions; medium-sized athletes training moderately; and larger athletes engaging in two- a-days. Meal and snack times are provided as a guide. Of course these will be adjusted to fit your school, work, or training schedules.

Sample 2,000-Calorie Menu for a 110-Pound (50 kg) Athlete Training Two Hours a Day

For a strength and power athlete who is smaller and lighter, we believe that 2,000 calories per day is the minimum in order to train properly. Many athletes, especially gymnasts, begin their training at a young age, when sufficient calories, protein, fat, and carbohydrate are essential for proper growth and development. Be sure you have estimated your caloric needs as honestly as possible.

In some sports, such as gymnastics, swimming, diving, and some track and field events, appearance and weight can be sensitive topics. When these concerns result in improper fueling, athletes can unintentionally impair their performance. Proper fueling will not result in a gain of body fat. On the other hand, inadequate fueling decreases strength, impairs performance, can slow metabolic rate, and can actually decrease muscle tone. Over the long term, creating a chronic caloric deficit can affect hormonal function, bone health, and immunity; increase risk of injury; and affect daily mood, attitude, concentration, and outlook. During training, most smaller and lighter strength and power athletes need 4 to 8 g/kg carbohydrate, 1.2 to 1.7 g/kg protein, and at least 1 g/kg dietary fat to supply adequate essential fat for cell repair and hormone production. Figure 10.5 shows you a sample menu for a 110 lb athlete.

Sample 2,500-Calorie Menu for a 110-Pound (50 kg) Athlete Training Four Hours a Day

This menu meets the needs for a 110-pound (50 kg) athlete training for four hours: almost 8 g/kg carbohydrate (61% calories); 1.8 g/kg (14% calories); and 1.3 g/kg of fat (24% calories). Figure 10.6 shows you a sample menu for such an athlete.

The additional carbohydrate (from 6 g/kg to almost 8 g/kg) fuels the additional energy expended by this athlete when training increases from two hours to four. Because protein is found in so many foods, it is hard to *not* get enough if including any animal protein sources. You will see, especially for smaller athletes, that the difference in real food when deciding to utilize 1.6 or 1.9 g/kg protein does not amount to much—here the difference is 15 grams of protein, which is about 2 ounces (60 grams) of meat. Fat is increased to help meet caloric needs and keep hormonal systems working: 67 grams. A larger preworkout snack is eaten 1 1/2 hours before training and will help prevent hunger, as dinner is late. Rest assured there are many ways to form this plan. You could have a little less carbohydrate and a little more fat, or a little less protein and more fat if you'd like.

Sample 3,000-Calorie Menu for a 165-Pound (75 kg) Athlete Training Moderately for 90 Minutes a Day

The sample menu in figure 10.7 was developed for a 165-pound (75 kg) athlete training moderately for 90 minutes a day: 5.5 g/kg carbohydrate (55% calories); 1.9 g/kg protein (19% calories); and 1.1 g/kg of fat (26% calories). This menu would also work for any strength athletes weighing between 130 and 187 pounds (59 and 85 kg) who need 3,000 calories per day.

FIGURE 10.5
Sample 2,000-calorie menu for a 110-lb (50 kg) athlete training 2 hr/day

Carbohydrate (g)	Protein (g)	Fat (g)	Foods
BREAKFAST (7:30 A.M.)			
30	3	5	2 toaster waffles
15	0	0	1 tbsp syrup
12	8	0	8 oz (240 ml) nonfat milk
10	0	0	1/2 cup blueberries
67	11	5	Total for meal: approximately 350 calories
MIDMORNING SNACK (10:00-10:30 A.M.)			
17	2	10	1/4 cup nuts and raisins
17	2	10	Total for snack: approximately 165 calories
LUNCH (12:30 P.M.)			
			Turkey sandwich:
30	6	2	2 slices whole-wheat bread
0	14	0	2 oz (60 g) turkey
0	7	8	1 oz (30 g) cheese
10	3	0	2 cups lettuce, carrots, peppers, cucumbers, mushrooms
0	0	10	2 tbsp salad dressing
0	0	0	24 oz (720 ml) water
40	30	20	Total for meal: approximately 450 calories
PREWORKOUT SNACK (3:00 P.M.)			
23	0	0	Small banana (6 in)
0	0	0	Water
23	0	0	Total for preworkout snack: approximately 100 calories
DURING TRAINING (3:30-5:30 P.M.)			
30	0	0	16 oz (480 ml) sports drink + 16 oz (480 ml) water
30	0	0	Total for training: approximately 120 calories
RECOVERY (5:45 P.M.)			
42	11	6	Clif Bar Crunchy Peanut Butter
0	0	0	Water
42	11	6	Total for recovery: approximately 260 calories
DINNER (6:45 P.M.)			
35	3	0	Sweet potato (6 oz)
0	21	0	3 oz (90 g) broiled lemon sole
10	0	0	1 cup sauteed spinach
0	0	10	2 tsp olive oil
0	0	0	16 oz (480 ml) sparkling water
45	24	10	Total for meal: approximately 360 calories
SNACK (9:30 P.M.)			
28	6	1	6 oz (175 g) low-fat yogurt
1	1	5	1 tbsp chopped pecans
29	7	6	Total for snack: approximately 200 calories
293	85	57	Total for day: approximately 2,000 calories

FIGURE 10.6
Sample 2,500-calorie menu for a 110-lb (50 kg) athlete training 4 hr/day

Carbohydrate (g)	Protein (g)	Fat (g)	Foods
			BREAKFAST (7:15 A.M.)
33	10	10	2 slices whole-wheat toast + 1 tbsp peanut butter
2	0	0	1/2 cup cooked spinach
0	6	5	1-egg omelet
12	8	0	8 oz (240 ml) nonfat milk
47	24	15	*Total for meal: approximately 400 calories*
			MIDMORNING SNACK (10:00 A.M.)
20	0	0	Medium orange
15	2	3	Small granola bar
35	2	3	*Total for snack: approximately 175 calories*
			LUNCH (12:00 P.M.)
			Chicken stir-fry:
22	3	1	1/2 cup brown rice
0	0	15	1 tbsp canola oil
10	4	0	1 cup bell peppers and carrots
0	14	2	2 oz (60 g) chicken breast
16	0	0	1/2 cup fresh pineapple
48	21	18	*Total for meal: approximately 440 calories*
			PREWORKOUT SNACK (3:00 P.M.)
26	7	5	6 oz vanilla yogurt + 5 almonds
6	0	0	1/4 cup cereal
23	0	0	Small banana
55	7	5	*Total for preworkout snack: approximately 300 calories*
			DURING TRAINING (4:30-8:30 P.M.)
60	0	0	32 oz (960 ml) sports drink
60	0	0	*Total for training: approximately 240 calories*
			RECOVERY (8:45 P.M.)
39	12	4	12 oz (360 ml) low-fat chocolate milk
11	1	1	1 graham cracker (large rectangle)
50	13	5	*Total for recovery: approximately 300 calories*
			DINNER (9:30 P.M.)
			Tossed salad:
40	18	1	1 cup lentils
2	2	0	2 cups spinach
5	1	0	1/4 cup each bell peppers, shredded carrots, celery, onions
2	2	10	2 tbsp chopped walnuts
0	0	10	2 tbsp salad dressing
23	0	0	6 oz (180 ml) fruit juice + 12 oz (360 ml) seltzer
20	2	0	1/2 cup sweet potato
92	25	21	*Total for meal: approximately 650 calories*
387	92	67	Total for day: approximately 2,500 calories

FIGURE 10.7

Sample 3,000-calorie menu for a 165-lb (75 kg) athlete training moderately for 90 min/day

Carbohydrate (g)	Protein (g)	Fat (g)	Foods
		BREAKFAST (7:30 A.M.)	
45	9	1	3 oz (90 g) bagel
6	8	16	2 tbsp peanut butter
7	0	0	1/2 grapefruit
35	8	2	6 oz low-fat fruit yogurt
93	25	19	*Total for meal: approximately 650 calories*
		MIDMORNING SNACK (10:00 A.M.)	
34	0	0	2 oz box raisins
6	5	14	1 oz almonds (24 nuts)
40	5	14	*Total for snack: approximately 300 calories*
		LUNCH (11:30 A.M.)	
			Roast beef sandwich:
30	6	2	2 slices whole-rye bread
0	35	5	5 oz lean roast beef
0	0	10	2 oz (60 g) avocado
2	0	5	1 cup green salad + 1 tbsp salad dressing
0	0	0	24 oz (720 ml) water
32	41	22	*Total for meal: approximately 500 calories*
		PREWORKOUT SNACK (2:30 P.M.)	
4	10	0	1/2 cup nonfat Greek yogurt
20	2	1	1/4 cup low-fat granola
24	12	1	*Total for preworkout snack: approximately 150 calories*
		DURING TRAINING (3:30-5:00 P.M.)	
30	0	0	16 oz (480 ml) sports drink + 16 oz (480 ml) water
30	0	0	*Total for training: approximately 120 calories*
		RECOVERY (5:15 P.M.)	
50	16	5	16 oz (480 ml) low-fat chocolate milk
30	0	0	Large banana (8 in)
80	16	5	*Total for recovery: approximately 425 calories*
		DINNER (7:15 P.M.)	
			Cashew chicken stir-fry:
67	8	3	1 1/2 cups brown rice
20	4	15	2 cups stir-fried vegetables + 1 tbsp canola oil
0	28	4	4 oz (150 g) chicken
0	0	0	16 oz (480 ml) sparkling water
87	40	22	*Total for meal: approximately 720 calories*
		SNACK (9:45 P.M.)	
33	1	3	3 Fig Newton cookies
0	0	0	1 cup of herbal tea
33	1	3	*Total for snack: approximately 160 calories*
419	140	86	Total for day: approximately 3,000 calories

Menu Plans for Strength and Power Athletes During the Season

Eating can change still from an in-season workout or practice day to the way you'll fuel on the day of an event. Here, you'll see the difference for higher- and lower-calorie need sports and also multiple event days.

Sample 4,500-Calorie Menu for a 200-Pound (91 kg) Athlete Training Moderately During the Season for Three Hours a Day

Figure 10.8 shows you a sample 4,500-calorie menu, for a 200-pound (91 kg) strength and power athlete during the regular season who trains about three hours a day at a moderate level. This plan is appropriate at 6 g/kg carbohydrate (51% calories); 2.3 g/kg protein (18% calories); and 1.7 g/kg fat (30% calories). As you can see, the portions of the chicken and fish are not large, yet protein is high at 2.3 g/kg, showing you that it's easy to meet protein needs through food.

Sample 3,500-Calorie Menu for a 175-Pound (80 kg) Athlete on the Day Before an Event

Pregame fuel isn't just the last meal you have before you compete. The foods eaten a full 24 hours before a competition are used to prepare your body. The day before the game, you must allow for optimal glycogen storage by consuming carbohydrate at each meal. There is plenty of time to digest fat and protein. The challenge for many athletes is that the day before a game may be the least structured day of the week. Creating your own structure by eating on schedule will help ensure adequate and appropriate amounts of carbohydrate are consumed with each meal so that muscles are stocked at game time. Of course, nutrient-rich foods, such as fruits, vegetables, whole grains, and healthy fats, should be included as a matter of routine.

This strength and power athlete's plan includes a good amount of carbohydrate for their sport: 6 g/kg (53% calories) to optimize glycogen stores, particularly the day before a game or competition, which usually includes a light practice if competing once per week. Protein needs are met at 2.0 g/kg (19% of calories), and fat is 1.4 g/kg (28% calories). Figure 10.9 shows a sample 3,500-calorie menu for a 175-pound (80 kg) strength and power athlete the day before an event.

Sample 3,600-Calorie Menu for a 175-Pound (80 kg) Athlete on the Day of an Event

Typically on game day or the day of a competition, caloric needs are equal to or often less than what is needed during training. Remember, you are training many hours for an event that may be much shorter in duration. At the same time, you want to be sure that your muscles are well prepared to perform optimally.

The menu in figure 10.10 would suit the needs of athletes competing in a longer-duration event, possibly a game, who have an opportunity to take in some fuel around midway through. This plan meets the athletes needs: 6 g/kg carbohydrate (55% calories); 1.9 g/kg protein (18% calories); and 1.4 g/kg fat (27% calories).

Sample 2,800-Calorie Menu for a 175-Pound (80 kg) Athlete Competing in a Low-Intensity Sport

The menu shown in figure 10.11 would be appropriate for an athlete on the day of an event, competing in a sport that does not require a large caloric expenditure. Carbohydrate needs are not as great because glycogen levels are not depleted. This plan would provide the right amount of each nutrient for this athlete's needs: 5 g/kg carbohydrate (53% calories); 1.6 g/kg protein (19% calories); and at least 1 g/kg fat (28% calories).

Sample 3,300-Calorie Menu for a 175-Pound (80 kg) Athlete Competing in Two Events in One Day

For athletes competing in two events in one day, such as a doubleheader, calories can be increased from the previous plan of 2,900 calories in figure 10.12 to approximately 3,300 shown in the sample menu in figure 10.12. This plan provides 6 g/kg carbohydrate (58% calories); 1.5 g/kg protein (15% calories); and 1.2 g/kg fat (27% calories).

The increased caloric needs come mostly from carbohydrate, so it is important to be prepared; there may be time for only two formal meals on such a day. Since it can be hard to significantly increase carbohydrate without feeling uncomfortable, we increased the fat slightly to help bring the caloric needs in line. Protein needs are the same, as they are based on body weight.

Few athletes shy away from hard work—hard work is just one of the many characteristics that distinguish the great from the rest. You know that the work you put into your training pays off. This chapter has shown how to tweak your menu plans based on the day's task, be it a morning or afternoon workout, a single competition, or an all-day tournament. Creating a Nutrition Blueprint that takes into account training phase and workload can be somewhat tedious, but the outcome is so beneficial. By creating your own Nutrition Blueprint and incorporating the principles of nutrient timing, you will help ensure a meal plan that keeps all your training efforts going in the same direction: toward a strong, lean, powerful athlete who has energy, resiliency, and a keen ability to concentrate.

FIGURE 10.8

Sample 4,500-calorie menu for a 200-lb (91 kg) athlete training moderately during the season for 3 hr/day

Carbohydrate (g)	Protein (g)	Fat (g)	Foods
BREAKFAST (7:00 A.M.)			
65	6	0	1 cup farina with 1 tbsp syrup
15	0	0	1 cup melon
12	8	5	8 oz (240 ml) 2% milk
0	14	5	2 oz Canadian bacon
92	28	10	*Total for meal: approximately 570 calories*
DURING TRAINING (9:00-12:00 A.M.)			
60	0	0	32 oz (1.5 L) Gatorade + water
60	0	0	*Total for training: approximately 240 calories*
RECOVERY (12:15 P.M.)			
34	0	0	8 oz cranberry juice and water
42	11	6	Clif Bar
76	11	6	*Total for recovery: approximately 400 calories*
LUNCH (1:00 P.M.)			
56	33	26	2 cups bean and beef chili
45	5	2	1 cup brown rice
			Grilled chicken salad:
0	21	3	3 oz (60 g) grilled chicken breast
5	2	0	2 cups salad
4	3	8	2 tbsp sunflower seeds
0	0	10	2 tbsp salad dressing
15	0	0	small papaya, 5 oz
125	64	49	*Total for meal: approximately 1,200 calories*
SNACK (4:30 P.M.)			
11	12	28	2 oz almonds
			Smoothie:
30	9	2	1 cup low-fat vanilla yogurt
15	0	0	1 cup frozen strawberries
11	0	0	1 kiwi
67	21	30	*Total for snack: approximately 620 calories*
DINNER (6:30 P.M.)			
0	42	18	6 oz (180 g) broiled salmon
56	11	16	1 1/2 cups whole-wheat pasta with garlic and 1 tbsp olive oil
0	6	3	3 tbsp grated cheese
20	8	0	1 cup broccoli and 1 cup cooked carrots
76	67	37	*Total for meal: approximately 900 calories*
SNACK (9:30 P.M.)			
50	16	10	16 oz (480 ml) 2% chocolate milk
30	0	8	4 chocolate chip cookies (2.5 in; 6.5 cm)
80	16	18	*Total for snack: approximately 550 calories*
576	207	150	Total for day: approximately 4,500 calories

FIGURE 10.9

Sample 3,500-calorie menu for a 175-lb (80 kg) athlete on the day before an event

Carbohydrate (g)	Protein (g)	Fat (g)	Foods
			BREAKFAST (8:00 A.M.)
			Breakfast burrito:
50	20	16	2 scrambled eggs + 2 tortillas
2	0	10	2 tbsp salsa and 2 oz (250 g) avocado (~1/3 small)
			Fruit smoothie:
23	0	0	Small banana (6 in)
26	7	0	6 oz nonfat vanilla yogurt
15	0	0	1/2 cup juice
116	**27**	**26**	*Total for meal: approximately 800 calories*
			MIDMORNING SNACK (11:00 A.M.)
15	10	0	12 oz latte
18	1	3	Small granola bar
33	**11**	**3**	*Total for snack: approximately 200 calories*
			LUNCH (1:00 P.M.)
30	6	2	2 slices whole-wheat bread
0	21	3	3 oz (90 g) lean roast beef
0	7	13	1 oz (30 g) cheese + 1 tbsp mayonnaise
22	3	0	1 cup vegetable soup
36	3	8	1 oatmeal raisin cookie, 2 oz.
0	0	0	16 oz (480 ml) water
88	**40**	**26**	*Total for meal: approximately 750 calories*
			PREWORKOUT SNACK (2:30 P.M.)
26	6	6	Kashi Pumpkin Spice Flax bar + 8 oz (240 ml) water
26	**6**	**6**	*Total for preworkout snack: approximately 180 calories*
			DURING TRAINING–LIGHT WORKOUT (3:00-5:00 P.M.)
0	0	0	Water
			RECOVERY (5:15 P.M.)
52	16	5	16 oz (480 ml) low fat chocolate milk
52	**16**	**5**	*Total for recovery: approximately 320 calories*
			DINNER (7:00 P.M.)
0	38	13	5 oz (250 g) broiled pork chop
25	0	0	1/2 cup applesauce
13	3	0	1 cup mixed vegetables
34	3	10	1 cup roasted potatoes
19	5	2	1 small dinner roll + 1 tbsp hummus
30	0	0	8 oz (240 ml) lemonade
121	**49**	**26**	*Total for meal: approximately 900 calories*
			SNACK (9:30 P.M.)
31	13	17	Whole-wheat toast + 2 tbsp peanut butter
31	**13**	**17**	*Total for snack: approximately 325 calories*
467	**162**	**109**	**Total for day: approximately 3,500 calories**

FIGURE 10.10

Sample 3,600-calorie menu for a 175-lb (80 kg) athlete on the day of an event

Carbohydrate (g)	Protein (g)	Fat (g)	Foods
BREAKFAST (8:00 A.M.)			
40	6	2	1 cup oatmeal + 1 tbsp brown sugar
4	4	20	1/4 cup chopped walnuts
28	0	0	1/4 cup dried cranberries
24	16	0	16 oz (480 ml) nonfat milk
96	26	22	*Total for meal: approximately 680 calories*
LUNCH (12:00 P.M.)			
			Turkey club sandwich:
45	9	3	3 slices white toast
0	21	0	3 oz turkey
0	6	6	2 slices bacon
3	0	5	1 tbsp mayonnaise
17	6	4	Bowl minestrone soup (1 ½ cups)
28	6	1	6 oz (175 g) low-fat yogurt
15	0	0	Small apple, 4 oz
0	0	0	Water
108	48	19	*Total for meal: approximately 800 calories*
PREGAME MEAL (4:00 P.M.)			
			Roast beef sub sandwich:
45	6	3	Sub roll, 6 in
0	28	4	4 oz roast beef
2	0	0	Tomato, pepper, lettuce (1/2 cup)
0	0	15	1 tbsp oil
35	0	0	20 oz (600 ml) sports drink
82	34	22	*Total for pregame meal: approximately 600 calories*
PREGAME SNACK (TOP-OFF) (6:45 P.M.)			
20	0	0	1 small banana + 8 oz (240 ml) water
20	0	0	*Total for pregame snack: approximately 80 calories*
HALFTIME (8:30 P.M.)			
25	0	0	Sports gel and water
25	0	0	*Total for halftime: approximately 100 calories*
RECOVERY (10:00 P.M.)			
38	20	5	Promax bar
52	0	0	12 oz (360 ml) cranberry juice
90	20	5	*Total for recovery: approximately 485 calories*
DINNER (10:30 P.M.)			
70	30	30	2 slices vegetable and meat pizza
5	2	10	2 cups tossed salad + 2 tbsp salad dressing
0	0	0	16 oz (480 ml) flavored water
75	32	40	*Total for meal: approximately 780 calories*
496	160	108	Total for day: approximately 3,600 calories

FIGURE 10.11

Sample 2,800-calorie menu for a 175-lb (80 kg) athlete competing in a low-intensity sport

Carbohydrate (g)	Protein (g)	Fat (g)	Foods
			BREAKFAST (7:30 A.M.)
25	6	1	1 cup cooked oatmeal
2	2	10	2 tbsp chopped nuts
15	0	0	2 tbsp raisins
15	0	0	1 tbsp brown sugar
24	16	6	16 oz (480 ml) low-fat milk
25	4	1	English muffin
6	8	16	2 tbsp peanut butter
112	36	34	*Total for meal: approximately 900 calories*
			LUNCH (12:00 P.M.)
			Grilled chicken sandwich:
30	6	2	Sandwich roll, 2 oz
0	28	4	4 oz grilled chicken
2	0	0	lettuce and tomato (1/2 cup)
3	0	5	1 tbsp mayonnaise
46	4	3	2 oz (60 g) Baked! Lay's potato chips
8	2	0	2 cups garden salad with tomatoes, carrots, and cucumbers
0	0	10	2 tbsp salad dressing
0	0	0	20 oz (600 ml) water
89	40	24	*Total for meal: approximately 730 calories*
			PREGAME SNACK (3:15 P.M.)
20	0	0	1 orange
0	0	0	8 oz (240 ml) water
20	0	0	*Total for pregame snack: approximately 80 calories*
			DURING COMPETITION (3:30-6:00 P.M.)
30	0	0	16 oz (480 ml) sports drink
30	0	0	*Total for competition: approximately 120 calories*
			POSTGAME SNACK (6:15 P.M.)
52	16	5	16 oz (480 ml) low-fat chocolate milk
52	16	5	*Total for postgame snack: approximately 320 calories*
			DINNER (7:30 P.M.)
			Beef stir-fry:
0	28	8	4 oz (150 g) beef
20	4	0	2 cups vegetables: peppers, broccoli, carrots, celery, onions, mushrooms
45	6	2	1 cup rice
0	0	15	1 tbsp canola oil
0	0	0	12 oz (360 ml) seltzer
65	38	25	*Total for meal: approximately 650 calories*
368	130	88	**Total for day: approximately 2,800 calories**

FIGURE 10.12
Sample 3,300-calorie menu for a 175-lb (80 kg) athlete competing in two events in one day

Carbohydrate (g)	Protein (g)	Fat (g)	Foods
BREAKFAST (10:30 A.M.)			
112	16	8	4 pancakes (6 in; 15 cm)
30	0	0	2 tbsp syrup
0	0	10	2 tsp butter
0	19	18	2 scrambled eggs with 1 oz cheese
11	0	0	1 cup strawberries
153	35	36	*Total for meal: approximately 1,075 calories*
PREGAME SNACK (11:00 A.M.)			
0	14	1	1 oz beef jerky
15	0	0	8 oz (240 ml) sports drink
18	1	3	Granola bar
33	15	4	*Total for pregame snack: approximately 230 calories*
MIDGAME SNACK (1:00-4:00 P.M.)			
15	2	0	Handful of pretzels (12 pretzel nuggets)
15	0	0	8 oz (240 ml) sports drink
30	2	0	*Total for midgame snack: approximately 125 calories*
RECOVERY AND PREGAME SNACK (4:15 P.M.)			
			Peanut butter sandwich:
30	6	2	2 slices white bread
6	8	16	2 tbsp peanut butter
17	0	0	1 tbsp honey
12	8	0	1 cup nonfat milk
30	0	0	16 oz sports drink
23	0	0	Small banana (6 in)
118	22	18	*Total for recovery and pregame snack: approximately 725 calories*
MIDGAME SNACK (6:00-9:00 P.M.)			
29	3	5	Clif Nectar bar
0	0	0	Water
29	3	5	*Total for midgame snack: approximately 175 calories*
RECOVERY AND POSTGAME SNACK (9:15 P.M.)			
			Yogurt smoothie:
26	7	2	6 oz low-fat vanilla yogurt
11	0	0	1 cup strawberries
11	0	0	1 kiwi
15	0	0	1/2 cup orange juice
63	7	2	*Total for recovery and postgame snack: approximately 300 calories*

(continued)

FIGURE 10.12 *(continued)*

Carbohydrate (g)	Protein (g)	Fat (g)	Foods
			DINNER (10:30 P.M.)
			Chicken and vegetable stir-fry
0	28	4	4 oz grilled chicken
5	2	0	1 cup peppers, mushrooms, and tomatoes
0	0	10	2 tsp oil
45	4	10	1 cup rice pilaf
5	2	10	2 cups salad + 2 tbsp dressing
0	0	0	24 oz (720 ml) seltzer
55	36	34	*Total for meal: approximately 670 calories*
481	**120**	**99**	**Total for day: approximately 3,300 calories**

11

Endurance

Endurance athletes participate in distance running, cycling, distance swimming, rowing, race walking, cross-country skiing, triathlon, or any other continuous aerobic activity. Following the NTP is crucial when training on a daily basis. Applying the NTP by consuming fuel before and during longer endurance training is helpful to prevent muscle tissue wasting, promote endurance, and, of crucial importance, can help immune function, which can become suppressed after endurance competition.

Due to the nature of most endurance sports, endurance athletes are sensitive to changes in fueling and relate what they eat to how they perform, especially when going for their personal best. Endurance athletes already recognize the importance of nutrient timing and hopefully will find in this chapter some tools and tips to refine and enhance the efforts they already are making to fuel themselves effectively and efficiently.

PLANNING FOR TRAINING

In chapter 9, you determined your caloric, protein, fat, and carbohydrate needs for training and competition. Now, let's take those requirements and create menu plans for different training times as well as competitions and races. To illustrate how to apply this information, we will use a sample athlete, Sam, a 154-pound (70 kg) endurance athlete who trains at a high intensity for 60 minutes a day. We calculated his caloric needs in appendix A on page 199 and determined his macronutrient needs by sport in appendix B on page 205. Sam requires a total of 3,200 calories per day: 7 g/kg carbohydrate for a total of 490 g (61% calories); 1.6 g/kg protein for a total of 115 g (14% of calories); and 85 grams of fat, which come from the balance of calories left (25% of calories).

Select your template and plug your training level into the Blueprint, so other meals and snacks can be plugged in to match the macronutrient requirement. You don't have to plan every gram or morsel that crosses your lips—few athletes do. It's fine to round off and estimate. The main idea behind the Blueprint is to provide a general guideline as to *about how much* of each nutrient to have around training and at meals and snacks. Developing a template like this helps you create structure, awareness, and goals and can give you a sense of whether you are close to fueling yourself properly or completely off the mark.

Nuances of the Different Endurance Sports

Endurance athletes require hydration and fueling during training and races. It takes practice and ingenuity to learn how to overcome the obstacles and feel comfortable drinking and eating while moving!

Cross-Country Skiing

Fluid losses can be high despite the cold weather. Athletes can use a CamelBak system, perhaps with additional sodium so the sports drink and tubing don't freeze, or an insulated pack with hot fluids or warm sports drink. Beverage temperature may affect the desire to drink.

Rowing

Crew training can be fueled by sports drinks kept in a hands-free hydration system, either a hip belt or CamelBak system. Some rowers keep a water bottle nearby and find they can work in a few sips without losing pace. A sports gel or solid, such as Shot Bloks kept in a pocket or sealable bag, is another fueling option during longer practices or competitions.

Swimming

To maintain hydration during training, water bottles and sports drinks may be kept poolside, but open-water races pose more of a challenge. Feeding stations are usually set up, and some swimmers tuck gels into their swimsuits. This strategy is best practiced in a pool with supervision in the event that blood becomes shunted away from muscles (toward the stomach to aid digestion), causing muscle cramps.

Triathlon

Triathletes may need different fuels for transitions and different legs of their training. Since exercise causes digestion to slow, it is recommended to test liquids, gels, and solid food during training to avoid unexpected reactions to fuel during a race. Many endurance athletes find that liquid nutrition is easier to digest during higher-intensity training when chewing is difficult, especially for runners. During the early stages on the bike, as you are restoring some of the calories and fluids utilized during the swim, liquids may be better tolerated, transitioning to solids midway on the bike and switching back to liquids closer to the run.

Morning Training

Let's take a look at how Sam's daily nutrient needs are spread out if he works out in the morning. First, we determined Sam's fuel needs to be 25 g carbohydrate before training; 30 g carbohydrate during training, and a recovery snack of 70-105 g carbohydrate and 7-14 g protein, depending on his intensity level. Here's how Sam's blueprint looks for a day when he trains at moderate to high intensity aerobic activity before breakfast:

Meal/Snack	Carbohydrate (g)	Protein (g)	Fat (g)
Pretraining	25	0	0
During training	30	0	0
Recovery	75	10	0
Breakfast	90	15	15
Lunch	100	40	25
Snack	20	10	10
Dinner	90	40	30
Snack	60	0	5
Total	490	115	85

Once Sam's training needs are entered into the Blueprint, the rest of his nutrient needs can be spread out throughout the rest of the day. Figure 11.1 shows how Sam's daily nutrient needs translate into real foods when endurance training in the morning for 60 minutes at a high intensity.

As you can see, Sam's daily carbohydrate needs are divided into meals, each with approximately 75-100 grams of carbohydrate. Although it can be challenging to evenly distribute each nutrient, the goal is to not overload any one meal with one nutrient and to distribute your carbohydrate, protein, and fat throughout the day. Crucial Nutrient Timing Principles for morning training are:

- Low-to-moderate activity benefits from a preworkout snack because blood glucose and liver glycogen are low. If it is intolerable to eat before, fuel during exercise with a sports drink. High-intensity sessions require a preworkout snack, and fuel during training (30-60 g/hr carbohydrate).

- Some athletes hesitate to eat before or even during training because they believe exercising on an empty stomach will enhance the loss of body fat. In reality, a lack of carbohydrate will limit the intensity and duration of your workout. Refer to chapter 5 for a discussion on how performance and total calorie expenditure can actually be increased with morning fuel.

- A recovery snack should not be used as breakfast! This practice leads to a calorie deficit, often resulting in increased hunger later in the day. Recovery plus breakfast ideally will equal at least 1/3 of your daily total calories.

FIGURE 11.1

Sam's sample 3,200-calorie menu when training in the morning

Carbohydrate (g)	Protein (g)	Fat (g)	Foods
PREWORKOUT SNACK (6:00 A.M.)			
25	3	1	1 slice white bread and 2 tsp honey
0	0	0	Water
25	3	1	*Total for preworkout snack: approximately 120 calories*
DURING TRAINING (6:30 A.M.)			
30	0	0	16 oz (480 ml) sports drink
30	0	0	*Total for training: approximately 120 calories*
RECOVERY (7:45 A.M.)			
44	10	3	Stonyfield Farms Smoothie drink
34	0	0	Small box of raisins
78	10	3	*Total for recovery: approximately 380 calories*
BREAKFAST (2ND RECOVERY) (9:15 A.M.)			
60	0	0	16 oz (480 ml) orange juice
0	12	10	2 hard-boiled eggs
22	3	3	15 Kashi crackers
82	15	13	*Total for meal: approximately 500 calories*
LUNCH (1:00 P.M.)			
48	18	2	12 oz (350 g) beef and bean chili
0	12	10	2 tbsp shredded cheddar cheese
36	4	0	6 oz (175 g) baked potato
5	2	10	2 cups garden salad + 2 tbsp salad dressing
20	0	0	Medium orange
109	36	22	*Total for meal: approximately 780 calories*
SNACK (4:30 P.M.)			
12	5	8	1/3 cup hummus
6	0	0	baby carrots (1/2 cup)
18	5	8	*Total for snack: approximately 160 calories*
DINNER (7:00 P.M.)			
			Chicken and vegetable stir-fry:
6	0	0	2 tbsp teriyaki sauce
0	28	4	4 oz (125 g) chicken
15	6	0	1 1/2 cup vegetables: carrots, peppers, celery, mushrooms
0	0	21	1 1/2 tbsp peanut oil
68	7	3	1 1/2 cups brown rice
89	41	28	*Total for meal: approximately 780 calories*
SNACK (9:00 P.M.)			
6	3	8	2 tbsp cashews
60	0	0	Banana dipped in 2 tbsp chocolate sauce
66	3	8	*Total for snack: approximately 350 calories*
497	113	83	**Total for day: approximately 3,200 calories**

Afternoon or Evening Training

As long as you eat breakfast and lunch in appropriate portions (trying to divide nutrient needs into thirds for each segment of the day), your afternoon workout will be fueled. Breakfast is key! The fuel from breakfast is important for your late-afternoon energy and the quality of that workout. Refer to table 9.1 on page 105-106 and figure 9.1 on page 106 for specific training fuel needs for endurance athletes.

To help you get a better idea of how a plan is modified for afternoon or evening workouts, let's take another look at our sample athlete and what his Blueprint would look like for an afternoon workout:

Meal/Snack	Carbohydrate (g)	Protein (g)	Fat (g)
Breakfast	100	20	20
Midmorning snack	25	0	0
Lunch	100	35	20
Pretraining	25	0	15
During training	30	0	0
Recovery	75	15	5
Dinner	90	45	25
Snack	70	0	0
Total	515	115	85

Figure 11.2 shows how Sam's daily nutrient needs translate into real foods when conditioning training for 60 minutes at high intensity in the afternoon. Notice Sam has a full breakfast; the lunch changes from beans to a lean turkey burger to avoid gassiness while training. He has a substantial preworkout snack of 300 calories 2 hours before, which both fuels him and prevents ravenous hunger later. If Sam had lunch at noon and were to wait until after his 5:00 p.m. training to eat, he might be going on 6 or 7 hours without eating. Dinner is relatively the same, and his evening snack is smaller at night to meet calorie needs.

If you plan to eat dinner right after your workout, you can use dinner as your recovery. If there will be a delay of more than one hour, though, plan on a recovery snack immediately after. You need not have a big dinner at night. Rather, if you are amply fueled during the day, dinner can be on the small side, such as cereal and milk with fruit; a yogurt parfait; an omelet with toast and mixed fruit; or a small helping of pasta and broccoli with shrimp or chicken. Eating a smaller dinner does not mean that it is okay to skip dinner; it's crucial to restock your muscles and prevent the cycle of becoming energy deficit over time, of overreaching, or feeling dead-legged in the next few training sessions because you haven't eaten properly. Eating a small dinner also will help with sleep as skipping dinner may be counterproductive to getting a good night's rest. On the other extreme, if you have not fueled yourself all day, eating a pint of premium ice cream does not count as the ideal recovery snack.

FIGURE 11.2

Sam's sample 3,200-calorie menu when training in the afternoon

Carbohydrate (g)	Protein (g)	Fat (g)	Foods
			BREAKFAST (7:00 A.M.)
30	0	0	8 oz (240 ml) orange juice
36	12	18	2 slices whole-grain bread + 2 tbsp peanut butter
22	7	2	6 oz (175 g) vanilla low-fat yogurt
20	0	0	1 cup blueberries
0	0	0	Water
108	**19**	**20**	*Total for meal: approximately 690 calories*
			MIDMORNING SNACK (10:00 A.M.)
25	0	0	1/2 cup applesauce
25	**0**	**0**	*Total for snak: approximately 100 calories*
			LUNCH (12:00 P.M.)
30	4	2	Whole-wheat roll
0	28	8	4 oz (125 g) lean turkey burger
4	0	0	1 tbsp ketchup
5	0	5	Sauteed mushrooms (1/2 cup)
23	2	2	1 oz (30 g) Baked! Lay's potato chips
34	0	0	8 oz (240 ml) cranberry juice
96	**34**	**17**	*Total for meal: approximately 675 calories*
			PREWORKOUT SNACK (3:30 P.M.)
29	8	16	1 small banana (6 in) + 2 tbsp peanut butter
0	0	0	Water
29	**8**	**16**	*Total for preworkout snack: approximately 300 calories*
			DURING TRAINING (5:30 P.M.)
30	0	0	16 oz (480 ml) sports drink
30	**0**	**0**	*Total for training: approximately 120 calories*
			RECOVERY (6:45 P.M.)
39	12	4	12 oz (360 ml) low-fat chocolate milk
34	5	1	Super Pretzel
73	**17**	**5**	*Total for recovery: approximately 400 calories*
			DINNER (8:00 P.M.)
			Chicken and vegetable stir-fry:
6	0	0	2 tbsp teriyaki sauce
0	28	4	4 oz (125 g) chicken
15	6	0	1 1/2 cups vegetables: carrots, peppers, celery, mushrooms
0	0	21	1 1/2 tbsp peanut oil
68	7	3	1 1/2 cups brown rice
89	**41**	**28**	*Total for meal: approximately 775 calories*
			SNACK (10:00 P.M.)
41	0	0	1 cup strawberries dipped in 2 tbsp chocolate sauce
41	**0**	**0**	*Total for snack: approximately 165 calories*
491	**119**	**86**	Total for day: approximately 3,200 calories

Extended Training

Some endurance sports are carried out for hours on end. The popularity of century rides (100 miles) for cyclists or extreme races where athletes run anywhere from 50 to 100 miles, are evidence of this. Although we don't address the needs of ultraendurance athletes, many endurance athletes do train for extended periods at least once per week. These sessions can feel much more difficult when athletes are not fueled properly. Although many athletes rely on sports fuels—gels, bars, and the like—for convenience, real food works, also, at a much lower cost.

Let's take a look at our sample 154-pound (70 kg) athlete, Sam's, increased nutrient needs during extended training sessions (see figure 11.3). Then, in figure 11.4, we provide a sample menu for Sam based on training four hours a day at moderate intensity.

FIGURE 11.3
Sam's daily nutrient needs based on extended training

	Daily total (g)	Daily total (calories)	%	g/kg for 70 kg (154 lb)
Fat	131	1,179	25	1.9
Carbohydrate	772	3,088	64	11
Protein	131	524	11	1.9
Total		~4,800 daily calories	100%	

FIGURE 11.4
Sam's sample 4,800-calorie menu when participating in extended training

Carbohydrate (g)	Protein (g)	Fat (g)	Foods
BREAKFAST (6:30 A.M.)			
38	9	3	1 1/2 cups instant oatmeal
14	0	0	1 tbsp brown sugar
37	4	20	1/4 cup raisins + 1/4 cup chopped walnuts
12	8	2	8 oz 1% milk
60	0	0	16 oz orange juice
161	21	25	*Total for meal: approximately 950 calories*
DURING TRAINING (60 G CARBOHYDRATE/HR SPREAD OVER EACH HOUR) (8:30-12:30)			
First hour (beginning ~45 min in):			
60	3	5	2 rectangular fig bars + 4 oz sports drink
Second hour:			
60	10	5	Clif Bar and 8 oz (24 ml) sports drink
0	0	0	24 oz water
Third hour:			
30	2	1	1 slice white bread + 1 tbsp honey
30	0	0	16 oz (480 ml) sports drink, 16 oz. water
Fourth hour:			
30	2	1	1 slice white bread + 1 tbsp honey
30	0	0	16 oz (480 ml) sports drink, 16 oz. water
240	17	12	*Total for training: approximately 1,145 calories*
RECOVERY (12:45 P.M.)			
33	15	0	Isopure Plus
34	5	1	1 Super Pretzel
22	0	0	10 dried apricots
89	20	1	*Total for recovery: approximately 400 calories*
LUNCH (2:30 P.M.)			
54	30	25	Chicken burrito (8 oz)
46	6	27	2 oz (60 g) tortilla chips + 3 oz (90 g) guacamole
34	0	0	8 oz (480 ml) cranberry juice
20	0	0	Medium orange
154	36	52	*Total for meal: approximately 1,225 calories*
DINNER (6:30 P.M.)			
5	2	10	2 cups salad with lettuce, tomato, carrots, peppers, and 2 tbsp Italian dressing
56	11	1	1 1/2 cups whole wheat pasta
17	2	4	1/2 cup meat sauce
4	18	24	4 meatballs (4 oz)
0	4	2	2 tbsp grated Parmesan cheese
27	0	0	12 oz (360 ml) iced tea
25	0	0	Frozen fruit pop
134	37	41	*Total for meal: approximately 1,050 calories*
778	131	131	Total for day: approximately 4,800 calories

Two-a-Day Training

Two-a-day workouts can take their toll if an endurance athlete is not paying attention to the NTP. It is easy to become depleted and dehydrated with two-a-days. You *must* plan your fueling for before, during, and after training.

Breakfast or a snack before your morning workout is a must because if glycogen becomes depleted during the first workout, you won't be able to restock in time for the second workout. In addition, recovery after the first session and fueling before the second workout are vital. Eating frequently helps ensure that glycogen stores are maximized. Take advantage of the time between sessions. For example, have 1g/kg carbohydrate after the first session (you may add .1 to .2 g/kg protein, but enough carbohydrate is essential), and have another 1 g/kg carbohydrate two hours before the second session if time permits; if there are four hours or more, continue to eat at two-hour intervals. If time does not permit for the intake of the second 1g/kg carbohydrate, at least try to have 25 to 30 g in addition to the first recovery snack. Remember, if time is short, liquid carbohydrates may be easier than solids to ingest.

Here are Sam's nutrient needs (our 154-pound (70 kg) athlete), for two-a-day training (see figure 11.5). Following, in figure 11.6, we provide a sample menu for Sam based on three hours a day of combined moderate and heavy training.

FIGURE 11.5
Sam's daily nutrient needs based on two-a-day training

	Daily total (g)	Daily total (calories)	%	g/kg for 70 kg (154 lb)
Fat	122	1,098	26	1.7
Carbohydrate	630	2,520	60	9
Protein	140	560	14	2.0
Total		~4,200 daily calories	100%	

FIGURE 11.6

Sam's sample 4,200-calorie menu when participating in two-a-days

Carbohydrate (g)	Protein (g)	Fat (g)	Foods
			PREWORKOUT SNACK (5:30 A.M.)
24	2	3	Nutri-Grain bar + water
24	2	3	*Total for preworkout snack: approximately 130 calories*
			DURING TRAINING (SESSION 1) (6:00-7:00 A.M.)
45	0	0	24 oz (960 ml) sports drink
45	0	0	*Total for training: approximately 200 calories*
			BREAKFAST (7:30 A.M.)
60	12	2	Bagel
7	5	20	2 tbsp almond butter
39	12	5	12 oz (360 ml) 1% chocolate milk
11	0	0	1 clementine
117	29	27	*Total for meal: approximately 810 calories*
			LUNCH (11:30 A.M.)
30	14	4	Lentil soup (12 oz)
10	4	0	Salad made with 2 cups greens, carrots, peppers, celery, mushrooms
0	14	1	tuna, flaked (2 oz)
0	7	8	1 oz shredded cheese
18	3	8	2 tbsp sunflower seeds + 2 tbsp dried cranberries
0	0	21	1 1/2 tbsp olive oil + vinegar to taste
38	10	7	1 whole-wheat pita (6 in) + 1/4 cup hummus
96	52	49	*Total for lunch: approximately 1,030 calories*
			PREWORKOUT SNACK (3:00 P.M.)
36	3	1	1/2 cup multigrain Cheerios
12	8	0	1 cup nonfat milk
30	0	0	Large banana
78	11	1	*Total for preworkout snack: approximately 365 calories*
			DURING TRAINING (SESSION 2) (5:30-7:30 P.M.)
90	0	0	48 oz (1.5 L) sports drink
90	0	0	*Total for training: approximately 360 calories*
			RECOVERY (7:45 P.M.)
			Shake:
26	10	3	6 oz (175 g) Vanilla low-fat yogurt
30	0	0	8 oz (240 ml) orange juice
25	0	0	1/2 cup sweetened berries
81	10	3	*Total for recovery: approximately 390 calories*
			DINNER (9:00 P.M.)
26	5	5	Bowl minestrone soup
0	21	6	3 oz (125 g) lean sirloin steak
38	4	0	6 oz (175 g) sweet potato (medium)
6	2	15	1 cup sauteed spinach (1 tbsp oil)
30	4	10	2 small dinner rolls + 2 pats butter
100	36	36	*Total for meal: approximately 920 calories*
631	140	119	Total for day: approximately 4,200 calories

Fuel for Competition

Depending on the length of the competition, fueling begins in the days, or even up to a week, in advance of the event. Foods consumed the evening before and day of the event should sit well and, as fuel taken during competition, be tested out during training. New foods or beverages should never be consumed during competition.

One Week to the Days Before an Event

For longer distance events, such as a marathon or triathlon, by three weeks before the race, the taper period begins and weekly mileage begins to decrease. In the week before your event, you are essentially resting, stretching, and putting in a couple of miles or easy laps just to keep blood flowing and your body loose. By three or four days before the event, eliminate all exercise, as even light exercise can interfere with optimizing glycogen storage. The question always arises, "Should I carb-load?" If you do not decrease food intake but rather continue to consume your regular training diet rich in carbohydrate (minus the pre, during, and recovery fuel), this will help stock muscles with energy needed for the event. Essentially, by tapering activity but maintaining intake, you are carb-loading. The rest along with a constant diet will store glycogen. If you have gained a few pounds, do not despair. Each gram of carbohydrate stores water along with it. Weight gain a few days before a race actually means you are doing a good job of storing glycogen. That weight will come off as you use fuel on race day.

Day Before the Event

On the day before an event, a typical strategy is to consume your regular training diet during the day, high in carbohydrate. The night before your event, eat a regular, balanced dinner with foods you are accustomed to. Carbohydrate should cover three-quarters of your plate (grains, fruits, and vegetables), amounting to 150 grams or more of carbohydrate for larger athletes, less for smaller athletes. If you like, have a bedtime snack of 25 to 50 grams of carbohydrate or more based on need and tolerance.

Some athletes prefer to have a larger meal midday and a more moderate dinner and snack in the evening, all of which contain a high proportion of carbohydrate. Other athletes find they are too nervous the day before to eat a larger meal all at once. These athletes take in their larger carbohydrate meals two days before the event (and they are relaxing, so these carbohydrates will be stored). The day before, they take in many high-carbohydrate snacks throughout the day. Any of these strategies will work, as long as sufficient carbohydrate is eaten to stock glycogen stores.

Day of the Event

Foods eaten on event day are to fuel you and, most importantly, should not cause discomfort or impair performance in any way. Be sure breakfast is made up of familiar foods and is low in fiber and fat. Depending on the time before you start, choose mainly carbohydrate with a small amount of protein (30 to 90 grams carbohydrate; 1 to 3 ounces protein) to help the meal "last" and prevent you from getting hungry during competition. Some athletes will eat eggs, turkey, or chicken; milk or yogurt is enough protein for others. Some good choices for breakfast on the day of an event include cereal with nonfat milk and fruit; a bagel with fruit yogurt and water; two eggs, toast with jam, and a glass of juice; instant oatmeal with milk; or a bagel with peanut butter and banana.

For many, race day will be very different in terms of both timing and energy (the jitters or jazzed up). Often, you need to wake and eat breakfast much earlier than for a typical training day, and the time before the race starts is usually much greater than the time between when you usually wake and train. In fact, you may need to eat breakfast and then bring a snack to consume while waiting for the race to begin. If you typically train at night but have a morning race, practice getting up, eating, and training around the same time you will be racing. If you always train in the morning but have an afternoon competition, then practice consuming one or two meals plus a snack before several afternoon training sessions. If the race is later in the day and there is time for another meal, go bigger for breakfast and heavier on protein and fat if you want to (add some nuts or nut butters, for instance), and eat a moderate but high-carbohydrate lunch (e.g., yogurt parfait, a small turkey sandwich or wrap with applesauce or raisins). The bottom line is to practice what you will eat ahead of time and not wait until the day of the event to figure out what works best for you.

Hydrate before the event: Drink 10 to 20 ounces (300 to 600 ml) of water, juice, or milk with breakfast and then another 7 to 10 ounces (210 to 300 ml) of water or sports drink 10 to 20 minutes from the start. If you usually drink coffee or tea in the morning, you've adapted to it, so go ahead and have it. Don't skip it on event day as you may feel tired or out of sorts without it. If you typically do not consume tea, coffee, or any caffeine, event day is not the time to add it.

If your event is after lunch, consume another 17 to 20 ounces (510 to 600 ml) of fluid (juice, water, sports drink, milk) two to three hours before the event and then 7 to 10 ounces (210 to 300 ml) 10 to 20 minutes from the start. Be sure to consume adequate amounts of sodium (see chapter 7), which is needed for proper fluid balance. Sodium-containing foods and beverages should be part of your regular training diet and are also needed on the day of the event. Mild dehydration will hurt performance; heat exhaustion and hyponatremia will hurt health.

During the Event

Figure out your fueling strategy well in advance of your event so that you can practice it during training. Begin fueling before you are depleted because your body will maintain pace and function better. This means you need to begin before you *feel* as if you need it.

To establish your schedule, as long as you have prefueled (with breakfast or other meals), you can begin hydrating at the 10- to 15-minute mark with water according to your sweat rate, typically somewhere between 5 and 10 ounces (150 and 300 ml) every 10 to 15 minutes. At the 45-minute mark, introduce a sports drink as your fuel, or if you continue with water, consume another source of carbohydrate and sodium. If you're aiming for 60 grams per hour, the amount of carbohydrate consumed within every 15 minutes should equal approximately 15 grams.

Make yourself stick to your predetermined plan. You will greatly benefit from having a strategy you've practiced so that during competition there's no need to think about that aspect of competing—you can focus on other elements of the race instead. The plan is not as different as you may think for longer or shorter distances—just the cutoff time is different. If your endurance event is three hours, you will keep on fueling until about 15 to 30 minutes before the finish line. If your event is six hours, you will keep on fueling and hydrating until 30 to 45 minutes from the finish (you may not consume as much carbohydrate per hour, especially if slower).

Recovery After the Event

Right after the event, your body is really in need of some top nutrition. Especially after longer events, the body's defenses are down, and this is where the strategies you've learned during training will help. Eating and hydrating as soon as possible will help muscles recover, even though you are not planning on training the next day. Take advantage of the glycogen-storing enzymes by consuming quickly digested carbohydrate within 30 minutes—at least 1 g/kg. It is very important to take in sodium, so choose sports drinks as part of recovery or eat salty foods because hyponatremia can still set in if you hydrate with plain water. A good recovery suggestion is a 4-ounce (125 gram) bagel, which provides 60 g carbohydrate and 450 to 500 mg of sodium, paired with a pint of orange juice, for a total of 110 grams of fast-digesting carbohydrate, 350 percent of the daily value for vitamin C, and more than

Runners and Gastrointestinal Distress

Gastrointestinal distress is never fun but even less so when it hits in the middle of a run, swim, or ride. 20 to 50 percent of endurance athletes can experience cramping, nausea, flatulence, diarrhea during or after exercise, and even bleeding. Complete reasons are not known for sure, and multiple reasons may be at the root of the problem. Plus each athlete may be affected differently. Possible causes include:

» the up and down motion of running stirring the bowels (running may increase an enzyme that increases peristalsis, or contractions of the intestines)

» the flow of blood to the intestines is diverted

» the underlying possibility of irritable bowel disease

» dehydration on long training runs causing diarrhea

» lactose intolerance effects enhanced by the exercise

» anxiety about the event

There are some strategies you can try to figure how much of your problems are just a timing issue. First, be aware of your bowel habits and try to time your workouts for after such times. Also, keep yourself well hydrated by consuming five to eight ounces of water every 15-20 minutes and avoid drinks that contain more that 10 percent (25 g carb/8 oz) carbohydrate (sugar) content. Some athletes, for fear of creating distress, avoid eating or drinking, but dehydration actually can make this worse because when they do eat or drink, a pooling of water occurs that may cause cramping. Start early, in small amounts, and fuel often to help prevent gastrointestinal distress. In addition, prior to an event or workout, try to avoid:

» fructose, fruit products or juice, especially apple and grape juice which are high in fructose. Also, look for a sports drink that doesn't contain fructose;

» sorbitol and other sugar substitutes (gum, breath mints, and low-calorie or low-sugar products);

» caffeine (including some energy bars and gels that contain caffeine) unless you are sure it does not have this type of a stimulant effect on you;

» high doses of Vitamin C, such as tablets; and

» high-fiber foods, such as many common breakfast items (instead, choose easy-to-digest foods, such as Corn flakes or white bread or a bagel).

As mentioned, you should first experiment with quantity and timing and selection of pretraining fuel and allow adequate time, preferably about two hours if possible, after eating before you engage in activity. If necessary, you can also try an over-the-counter anti-diarrheal product, such as Imodium, but be warned: Some contain substances like phenobarbital, so you'd flunk any drug test. And, they all dehydrate you, so they're not the best choice in long, hot-weather races. A nonsteroidal anti-inflammatory (Advil, Motrin, Aleve, ibuprofen, etc.) the night before an event might alleviate the problem, but increases the risk for hyponatremia and, for some, increases stomach agitation. Also, be sure to rule out lactose intolerance, a parasite, Irritable Bowel Syndrome, allergies, or any other underlying medical condition.

900 mg of potassium. Or, to include protein, try a pint (600 ml) of chocolate milk with a 2-ounce (60 g) bag of pretzels, which together provide 96 g carbohydrate and more than 1,000 mg of sodium; add an orange for 100 percent of your vitamin C.

For major events like marathons and triathalons, recognize that recovery goes on for days or weeks. Remember the Three R's: rest, refuel, and rehydrate. Continue to eat regular meals and snacks choosing nutrient-rich foods; there is a tendency when not training to not want to eat or to feel like you can eat whatever you want because there is no race coming up. Begin to taper your caloric intake toward the end of the first week after you race once your body has had some time to restore and repair some from the stress of competition.

MENU PLANS FOR ENDURANCE ATHLETES

Use the blueprint you developed in chapter 9 to plan your meals and the following sample plans as a guide, adjusting the macronutrients (carbohydrate, protein, fat) based on your training phase (more carbohydrate as training intensity increases, slightly higher protein during initial phases of strength training). Hopefully, these plans offer some great ideas for meals, timing, and distribution of calories. Also illustrated is how to increase or decrease calories depending on training phase. For illustrative purposes, we use exact numbers because we are showing specific calculations. You do not need to be this exact; in real life, few people are when it comes to eating. Rather, use these suggestions and guidelines to build meals in order to create a healthy training diet and apply the NTP.

Menu Plans for Endurance Athletes During Training

Following are two meal plans for each caloric level illustrated: 2,000 calories and 3,500 calories. One is for a morning workout, the other for an afternoon workout. There are add-on calories in case you need more. Remember to go back and calculate your own caloric needs. These sample menus are just illustrations of how to integrate the Nutrient Timing Principles. You can adjust to the time of day you train and your food preferences. The important thing to remember when building your own plan is to account for fuel and hydration before, during, and after training; build out your meals from there, paying attention to distribution of calories and quality of nutrients in each meal.

Sample 2,000-Calorie Menu Plans

For most athletes, 2,000 calories is truly not enough. A 2,000-calorie menu plan is only for smaller athletes who are training for shorter events or in the light to moderate training category. The plans shown here are developed for a 110-pound (50 kg) athlete who trains 60 minutes per day. Figure 11.7 shows this athlete's macronutrient needs, and the following two menus reflect these amounts.

FIGURE 11.7

A 110 lb (50 kg) athlete's daily nutrient needs when training 60 min/day

	Daily total (g)	Daily total (calories)	%	g/kg for 50 kg (110 lb)
Fat	51	459	23	1
Carbohydrate	300	1,200	60	6
Protein	85	340	17	1.7
Total		2,000	100%	

Sample 2,000-Calorie Menu for a 110-pound (50 kg) Athlete Training for 60 Minutes in the Morning

The plan provided in figure 11.8 is for a 110-pound (50 kg) athlete training in the morning who requires 2,000 calories per day. Notice the pretraining snack, the fluid schedule beginning first thing in the morning, the fuel during training, and the full breakfast as a recovery. There is mainly quickly digested carbohydrate consumed around training; foods higher in fiber—such as whole grains, apples, and berries—are included in meals further away. Notice, too, that the calories are well distributed throughout the day. The small yet balanced dinner can still satisfy because the athlete has eaten sufficiently during the day.

A smaller athlete training longer or an athlete who includes interval, hill, or speed work may want to add 300 to 400 calories to the plan. With these additional calories, the plan would also be appropriate for an athlete who weighs about 15 pounds (7 kg) more—a 125-pound (57 kg) athlete training lightly to moderately for 60 minutes. In these cases, the additional calories could come from carbohydrate and fat to burn for energy; protein needs won't change much. Here are some suggestions for adding more fuel around the workout and recovery:

- Add 1 tablespoon of jam to the preworkout snack (13 g carbohydrate) for an additional 50 calories.
- Have a full bagel instead of half (30 g carbohydrate, 6 g protein, and 1 g fat) and add another tablespoon of almond butter (3 g carbohydrate, 2 g protein, and 10 g fat) for an additional 260 calories.
- Add 4 ounces of sports drink to increase carbohydrate by 7 grams and calories by 30.

Together all of these changes would result in an additional 52 grams of carbohydrate, 9 grams of protein, and 11 grams of fat. The total increase by making these changes is approximately 340 calories, and the daily macronutrient percentages are similar: 60 percent carbohydrate; 16 percent protein; and 24 percent fat. Note that the additions would meet the needs of both a 110-pound (50 kg) athlete (1.9 g/kg protein; 7 g/kg carbohydrate) and a 125-pound (57 kg) athlete (1.7 g/kg protein; 6 g/kg of carbohydrate).

Sample 2,000-Calorie Menu for a 110-Pound (50 kg) Athlete Training for 60 Minutes in the Early Evening

The plan provided in figure 11.9 is for a 110-pound (50 kg) athlete who works out in the early evening instead of the morning. The midmorning snack is moved to become pretraining fuel. The hydration strategy remains moderate but present, as this athlete's fluid loss is minimal. Because the calories are relatively low, most hydration comes from water and other food.

You may want to add about 400 calories to the afternoon plan if you're planning to incorporate some sprints or hill work; if you're a larger athlete, needing a little more of each macronutrient; or if you are a "high burner" and struggle to keep weight on. In these cases, since the plan is already fairly high in fruits and vegetables, we can add a little to all the other groups. Here's what we'd suggest:

- Add half a cup of juice at breakfast (15 g carbohydrate) and one more tablespoon of nuts (1 g carbohydrate, 1 g protein, and 5 g fat) for an additional 120 calories.
- Add 3 tablespoons hummus plus 1/2 cup raw carrots and water as a midmorning snack (14 g carbohydrate, 5 g protein, and 3 g fat) for an additional 100 calories.
- Replace the rye bread at lunch with a roll (15 g carbohydrate, 3 g protein, and 1 g fat) for an additional 80 calories.
- Add a granola bar to the recovery snack (15 g carbohydrate, 3 g protein, and 2 g fat) for an additional 90 calories.

The total increase by making these changes is approximately 400 calories. Percentages are now 60 percent carbohydrate; 17 percent protein; and 23 percent fat. Also, the additions would meet the needs of both a 110-pound (50 kg) athlete at the high end (7 g/kg carbohydrate and 2 g/kg protein) and a 125-pound (57 kg) athlete (6 g/kg carbohydrate and 1.7 g/kg protein).

FIGURE 11.8
Sample 2,000-calorie menu for a 110 lb (50 kg) athlete training 60 min in the morning

Carbohydrate (g)	Protein (g)	Fat (g)	Foods
			PREWORKOUT SNACK (5:45 A.M.)
15	3	1	1 slice white bread and water
15	3	1	*Total for preworkout snack: approximately 80 calories*
			DURING TRAINING (5:55 A.M.)
15	0	0	8 oz (240 ml) sports drink
0	0	0	Water
15	0	0	*Total for training: approximately 60 calories*
			RECOVERY/BREAKFAST (7:30 A.M.)
30	6	1	1/2 large bagel
3	2	10	1 tbsp almond butter
30	0	0	8 oz (240 ml) Cheribundi/CherryPharm Tart Cherry Juice
27	8	0	1 cup hot cocoa made with nonfat milk
90	16	11	*Total for recovery/meal: approximately 525 calories*
			SNACK (10:30 A.M.)
0	7	8	Cheese stick
20	0	0	Medium orange
20	7	8	*Total for snack: approximately 180 calories*
			LUNCH (12:00 P.M.)
30	6	2	2 slices whole-wheat bread
0	14	0	2 oz (60 g) turkey breast
10	2	0	2 cups tossed salad
0	0	5	1 oz (30 g) avocado
0	0	5	1 tbsp salad dressing
20	0	0	Small apple
0	0	0	12 oz (360 ml) flavored water
60	22	12	*Total for meal: approximately 440 calories*
			SNACK (3:30 P.M.)
13	10	3	6 oz (175 g) plain low-fat yogurt
15	0	0	3/4 cup mixed berries
28	10	3	*Total for snack: approximately 165 calories*
			DINNER (7:00 P.M.)
30	6	1	2/3 cup brown rice
0	21	0	3 oz (90 g) shrimp
10	4	0	1 cup grilled vegetables
0	0	15	1 tbsp olive oil for cooking
15	0	0	1/2 cup sliced pineapple
18	0	0	8 oz (240 ml) sweetened iced tea
73	31	16	*Total for meal: approximately 560 calories*
301	89	51	Total for day: approximately 2,000 calories

FIGURE 11.9
Sample 2,000-calorie menu for a 110 lb (50 kg) athlete training 60 min in the early evening

Carbohydrate (g)	Protein (g)	Fat (g)	Foods
BREAKFAST (8:00 A.M.)			
30	6	2	1 cup cooked oatmeal
12	8	2	1 cup 1% milk
2	2	10	2 tbsp chopped walnuts
30	0	0	1/4 cup dried cherries and apricots
74	16	14	*Total for meal: approximately 485 calories*
LUNCH (12:00 P.M.)			
			Tuna sandwich:
30	6	2	2 slices rye bread
0	14	2	2 oz (60 g) tuna
0	0	5	1 tbsp canola mayonnaise
5	2	0	Lettuce, tomato, and onion on sandwich; 1/2 cup of red pepper slices to eat on the side
11	1	0	4 oz carrot juice
23	2	2	1 oz (60 g) Baked! Lay's potato chips
69	25	11	*Total for meal: approximately 475 calories*
PREWORKOUT SNACK (3:00 P.M.)			
20	0	0	Medium orange
27	8	2	Hot cocoa made with 1% milk
47	8	2	*Total for preworkout snack: approximately 240 calories*
DURING TRAINING (5:30-6:30 P.M.)			
15	0	0	8 oz (240 ml) sports drink
15	0	0	*Total for training: approximately 60 calories*
RECOVERY			
46	7	3	Smoothie made with 1/2 cup plain low-fat yogurt 1 cup frozen berries, 1 tbsp honey, and 1 tbsp ground flaxseed
46	7	3	*Total for recovery: approximately 240 calories*
DINNER (8:30 P.M.)			
15	20	17	2 oz (60 g) lean ground turkey, 1-1/2 cups mushrooms, tomatoes, spinach, and zucchini, sauteed with 1 tbsp canola oil
34	7	0	3/4 cup whole-wheat pasta
0	4	2	2 tbsp grated Parmesan cheese
49	31	19	*Total for meal: approximately 500 calories*
300	87	49	**Total for day: approximately 2,000 calories**

Sample 3,500-Calorie Menu Plans

The following 3,500-calorie menu plans were developed for an athlete who weighs 145 pounds (66 kg) to 160 pounds (73 kg) and who trains 90 to 120 minutes. Figure 11.10 shows the daily carbohydrate, protein, and fat needs of this athlete, which are then used to determine when, what, and how much to eat in the two sample menu plans—one for a morning training session and one for an afternoon training session

FIGURE 11.10
A 145 lb athlete's daily nutrient needs when training 90 to 120 min/day

	Daily total (g)	Daily total (calories)	%	g/kg for 66 kg (145 lb)
Fat	95	855	25	1.4
Carbohydrate	525	2,100	60	8
Protein	135	540	15	2
Total		Approximately 3,500 daily calories	100%	

Sample 3,500-Calorie Menu for a 145-Pound (66 kg) Athlete Training for 90 to 120 Minutes in the Morning

For the 3,500-calorie meal plan provided in figure 11.11, the athlete works out in the morning. The 60 grams of carbohydrate during the workout is sufficient because the preworkout snack helps in fueling. Meals throughout the day include many different fruits, vegetables, and whole grains, providing an array of beneficial nutrients. Notice also that the protein is well allocated—there isn't a large intake at any one snack or meal. Athletes utilize protein more efficiently in this manner.

Cutting back on calories may be necessary for shorter training or lighter workouts. These changes are not about weight loss; they are for athletes who need to cut back to match caloric needs. To do this, an athlete should cut back on fat and cut back on some added sugars since they do not provide valuable vitamins or minerals. Here's what we suggest:

- Swap the sweetened iced tea for water or seltzer (less 18 g carbohydrate) for a total of 70 calories.
- Have half a cup of regular cereal instead of the granola at the afternoon snack (less 15 g carbohydrate, 4 g protein, and 6 g fat) for a total of 130 calories.
- Eliminate the cashews from the stir-fry (less 10 g fat) for a total of 90 calories.

The distribution of protein, fat, and carbohydrate stay the same; however, the calorie difference is about 300 less when taking these changes into account.

Sample 3,500-Calorie Menu for a 145-Pound (66 kg) Athlete Training for 90 to 120 Minutes in the Afternoon

For the 3,500-calorie meal plan provided in figure 11.12, the same 145-lb (66 kg) athlete works out in the afternoon, shifting his intake to include a larger breakfast, including fiber-rich foods that wouldn't interfere with training since they were eaten many hours before. Foods at lunch should settle well and not cause any discomfort while training, such as pasta with cooked vegetables and chicken.

FIGURE 11.11

Sample 3,500-calorie menu for a 145 lb (66 kg) athlete training 90 to 120 min in the morning

Carbohydrate (g)	Protein (g)	Fat (g)	Foods
PREWORKOUT SNACK (6:30 A.M.)			
45	6	2	2 slices white toast + 1 tbsp jam
45	6	2	*Total for preworkout snack: approximately 220 calories*
DURING TRAINING (7:30-9:30 A.M.)			
60	0	0	Water + 32 oz (900 ml) sports drink
60	0	0	*Total for training: approximately 240 calories*
RECOVERY (9:45 A.M.)			
30	8	0	8 oz (240 ml) Cheribundi/CherryPharm Natural Recovery
34	0	0	Small box of raisins
64	8	0	*Total for recovery: approximately 290 calories*
BREAKFAST (11:15 A.M.)			
30	6	2	1 cup cooked oatmeal
2	2	10	2 tbsp chopped walnuts
12	8	2	8 oz low-fat milk
11	0	0	1 kiwi
0	6	5	1 hard-boiled egg
30	0	0	1 cup orange juice
85	22	19	*Total for meal: approximately 600 calories*
LUNCH (2:30 P.M.)			
30	6	2	2 slices whole-wheat bread
0	21	0	3 oz (90 g) turkey breast
0	0	10	2 oz (30 g) avocado on sandwich
0	0	10	2 tbsp Italian salad dressing
17	4	5	2 cups salad with 2 tbsp dried cranberries and 8 olives
18	0	0	8 oz (240 ml) sweetened iced tea
15	0	0	1 peach
80	31	27	*Total for meal: approximately 690 calories*
SNACK (5:00 P.M.)			
35	5	6	1/2 cup granola
13	10	3	6 oz (175 g) plain low-fat yogurt
15	0	0	3/4 cup blueberries
63	15	9	*Total for snack: approximately 400 calories*
DINNER (8:00 P.M.)			
27	36	23	4 oz (125 g) yellowfin tuna; 1 1/2 cups mushrooms, broccoli, red peppers, and onions; and 2 tbsp cashews, sauteed in 1 tbsp canola oil with soy sauce and garlic
45	6	2	1 cup brown rice
15	0	0	1/8 honeydew melon
87	42	25	*Total for meal: approximately 740 calories*
SNACK (10:00 P.M.)			
12	8	2	8 oz 1% milk
29	3	11	4 chocolate chip cookies
41	11	13	*Total for snack: approximately 325 calories*
525	135	95	**Total for day: approximately 3,500 calories**

FIGURE 11.12

Sample 3,500-calorie menu for a 145 lb (66 kg) athlete training 90 to 120 min in the afternoon

Carbohydrate (g)	Protein (g)	Fat (g)	Foods
BREAKFAST (9:00 A.M.)			
37	9	3	1 cup vanilla low-fat yogurt
7	0	0	1/2 cup raspberries
2	2	10	2 tbsp walnuts
41	6	6	Oat bran muffin, medium (3 oz)
0	0	0	Water
87	17	19	*Total for meal: approximately 590 calories*
MIDMORNING SNACK (10:30 A.M.)			
16	5	11	Kind bar
40	10	0	Sweetened latte
56	15	11	*Total for snack: approximately 385 calories*
LUNCH (12:30 P.M.)			
			Chicken and vegetable pasta:
0	28	4	4 oz (125 g) chicken breast
65	12	2	1 1/2 cups pasta
10	4	15	1 cup carrots and zucchini + 1 tbsp olive oil
0	2	1	1 tbsp grated Parmesan cheese
20	0	0	Medium orange
30	0	0	8 oz (360 ml) lemonade
125	46	22	*Total for meal: approximately 880 calories*
PREWORKOUT SNACK (2:30 P.M.)			
22	1	2	2 fig cookies
0	0	0	Water
22	1	2	*Total preworkout snack: approximately 110 calories*
DURING TRAINING (3:00-5:00 P.M.)			
60	0	0	32 oz (960 ml) sports drink
60	0	0	*Total for training: approximately 240 calories*
RECOVERY (5:15 P.M.)			
52	12	6	16 oz (480 ml) low-fat chocolate milk
25	2	0	10 pretzel twists
77	14	6	*Total for recovery: approximately 415 calories*
DINNER (7:15 P.M.)			
0	35	15	5 oz (150 g) lean steak
45	4	10	1 1/2 cups roasted red potatoes
5	2	0	1/2 cup carrots
30	4	11	Medium dinner roll + 2 tsp butter
80	45	36	*Total for meal: approximately 825 calories*
SNACK (9:30 P.M.)			
20	0	0	Small baked apple with cinnamon
20	0	0	*Total for snack: approximately 80 calories*
527	138	96	Total for day: approximately 3,500 calories

Menu Plans for Endurance Athletes During the Season

Following are two meal plans for an athlete running a marathon that illustrate the NTP. The first is a 3,400-calorie menu for a 110-pound (50 kg) marathoner, and the second is a 5,000-calorie menu for a 160-pound (73 kg) runner We'll walk you through how to calculate your energy needs, which can be applied whether you are participating in a triathlon, cross-country ski race, riding a century, or competing in any other distance event. Depending on the sport, your fueling choices may vary, but the steps we show you are helpful in developing a fueling strategy around the Nutrient Timing Principles.

Sample 3,400-Calorie Menu for a 110-Pound (50 kg) Athlete Running a Marathon

Although this plan is designed with a marathoner in mind, endurance athletes such as cyclists and cross-country skiers need to fuel and hydrate often just as runners do. The choice of race-day foods may be very different for a runner, a cyclist, and a skier. That's because food tolerance differs depending on mode of exercise as well as preferences and even the culture of the sport. For illustrative purposes, figure 11.13 shows you an example of how a 110-pound (50 kg) athlete might eat for a marathon.

First, let's calculate this athlete's daily caloric needs for both daily living and activity, including the marathon. A 110-pound (50 kg) athlete who runs a 10-minute mile burns approximately 83 calories per mile. We figure this by taking the athlete's weight in kilograms (50) and multiplying it by 10 (a 10-minute mile is 10 METs) to get a total of 500 calories that the athlete burns per hour while participating in the marathon (see page 201 for a list of METs). We then divide this by 6 miles per hour for a total of 83 calories burned per mile, which when multiplied by 26.2 miles (the number of miles in a marathon), gives a total of approximately 2,200 calories that the athlete will burn when running the marathon. So as not to overestimate, we now deduct her resting metabolic rate for the approximate four and a half hours she'll be running. Since 1 MET represents resting metabolic rate, we subtract 50 (her weight in kilograms multiplied by 1 MET) multiplied by the amount of time spent in the race for a total of 225 resting calories. Based on this, here's how we figure out the athlete's total caloric needs for marathon day (see appendix A on page 199 for detailed instructions on how to figure your daily caloric needs):

Calories needed for daily living	1,400
Add calories needed for marathon	+2,200
Subtract calories needed for daily living for the duration of the marathon (4 1/2 hr)	−225
Total caloric needs for the day of the marathon	3,375

Although this athlete will burn approximately 3,400 calories on race day, it's *not required* that she eat that exact amount. She should eat what is comfortable and tolerable with an eye to her needs. For athletes accustomed to less food, the preexercise meals we show may be larger than they are used to, and it may prove uncomfortable. Too much food before a race can impair performance just as much as being underfueled.

During the event, the sweat rate for this athlete is 1 pound (.5 kg) per hour, so she will need to drink 4 ounces (120 ml) every 15 minutes. In addition, to have adequate fuel during the event, she should consume 30 grams of carbohydrate per hour, which can be divided further into 7- to 8-gram increments every 15 minutes. Some good suggestions to meet this need are 4 ounces (250 ml) sports drink, 1 Shot Blok with 4 ounces water, or 7 to 8 pretzel nuggets with 4 ounces water. For recovery, the runner should consume nutrient-rich carbohydrate with adequate fluid after the race; protein can be added to the first or second recovery snack. Then follow up with a balanced, nutrient-rich meal.

FIGURE 11.13
Sample 3,400-calorie menu for a 110 lb (50 kg) athlete running a marathon

Carbohydrate (g)	Protein (g)	Fat (g)	Foods
BREAKFAST (5:00 A.M.)			
24	3	0	1 cup Cheerios
12	8	3	8 oz low-fat milk
15	5	10	1 slice toast with 1 tbsp peanut butter
30	0	0	8 oz (240 ml) orange juice
81	16	13	*Total for meal: approximately 500 calories*
PRERACE SNACK (7:00 A.M.)			
45	9	2	3 oz (90 g) bagel
15	0	0	8 oz (240 ml) sports drink
60	9	2	*Total for prerace snack: approximately 300 calories*
DURING RACE (9:00 A.M.)			
Beginning 15 min after start of race, begin consuming 2 oz (60 ml) of water every 15 min until ~45 min after start of race, when you will consume the following up to ~15 minutes before the end of the race:			
7-8 (4x/hr)	0	0	4 oz (120 ml) sports drink or 4 oz (120 ml) water every 15 min and either 1 Clif Shot Blok or 6-7 pretzel nuggets every 15 min (3 1/2 hours of fueling)
105	0	0	*Total for race: approximately 420 calories*
FIRST RECOVERY (IMMEDIATELY POST-1:30 P.M.)			
24	10	5	Luna bar
23	0	0	Small banana (6 in)
35	0	0	20 oz (600 ml) sports drink
82	10	5	*Total for first recovery: approximately 400 calories*
SECOND RECOVERY (3:30 P.M.)			
60	12	2	4 oz (125 g) bagel
52	16	16	16 oz (480 ml) chocolate milk
112	28	18	*Total for second recovery: approximately 725 calories*
DINNER (6:00 P.M.)			
0	42	30	6 oz (150 g) steak
30	3	0	6 oz (175 g) baked sweet potato
0	0	10	2 pats butter
10	4	5	1 cup broccoli sauteed with 1 tsp olive oil
51	0	0	12 oz cranberry-grape juice
91	49	45	*Total for meal: approximately 965 calories*
SNACK (9:00 P.M.)			
33	0	0	1/2 cup sorbet
33	0	0	*Total for snack: approximately 120 calories*
564	112	83	Total for day: approximately 3,400 calories

Sample 5,000-Calorie Menu for a 160-Pound (73 kg) Athlete Running a Marathon

In the menu provided in figure 11.14, we show you how a 160-pound (73 kg) athlete may eat on the day of a marathon. First, let's calculate this athlete's daily caloric needs for both daily living and activity, including the marathon: A 160-pound (73 kg) athlete who runs an 8 minute mile burns approximately 122 calories per mile. We figure this by taking the athlete's weight in kilograms (73) and multiplying it by 12.5 (an 8-minute mile is 12.5 METs) to get a total of 912 calories that the athlete burns per hour while participating in the marathon. We then divide this by 7.5 miles per hour for a total of 122 calories burned per mile, which when multiplied by 26.2 miles (the number of miles in a marathon), gives a total of approximately 3,200 calories that the athlete will burn when running the marathon. So as not to overestimate, we now deduct his resting metabolic rate for the approximate three and a half hours he'll be running. Since 1 MET represents resting metabolic rate, we subtract 73 (his weight in kilograms multiplied by 1 MET) multiplied by the amount of time spent in the race for a total of 255 resting calories. Based on this, here's how we figure out the athlete's total caloric needs for marathon day (see appendix A on page 199 for detailed instructions on how to figure your daily caloric needs):

Calories needed for daily living	2,100
Add calories needed for marathon	+3,200
Subtract calories needed for daily living for the duration of the marathon (3 1/2 hr)	−255
Total caloric needs for the day of the marathon	**5,045**

FIGURE 11.14

Sample 5,000-calorie menu for a 160 lb (73 kg) athlete running a marathon

Carbohydrate (g)	Protein (g)	Fat (g)	Foods
			BREAKFAST (5:00 A.M.)
30	6	2	2 slices white toast
6	8	16	2 tbsp peanut butter
26	0	0	2 tbsp jelly
33	4	5	1 cup farina + 2 tsp sugar + 1 tsp butter
34	0	0	8 oz (240 ml) cranberry juice + 8 oz (240 ml) water
129	**18**	**23**	*Total for meal: approximately 800 calories*
			PRERACE SNACK (7:00 A.M.)
30	0	0	Large banana (8 in)
33	2	3	3 fig cookies
15	0	0	8 oz (240 ml) sports drink
78	**2**	**3**	*Total for prerace snack: approximately 350 calories*
			DURING RACE (9:00 A.M.)
Beginning 15 min after start of race, begin consuming 2 oz (60 ml) of water every 15 min until ~45 min after start of race, when you will consume the following up to ~15 minutes before the end of the race:			
7 (6x/hr)	0	0	4 oz (120 ml) sports drink every 10 min
8-10 (2x/hr)	0	0	1 shot blok or 3-4 jelly beans every half hour
~150	**0**	**0**	*Total for race: approximately 600 calories*
			FIRST RECOVERY (IMMEDIATLY POST-12:45 P.M.)
60	12	2	Large bagel
39	12	4	12 oz low-fat chocolate milk
99	**24**	**6**	*Total for first recovery: approximately 530 calories*
			SECOND RECOVERY (2:45 P.M.)
46	10	4	Clif Bar Carrot Cake
28	6	1	6 oz (175 g) fruit on bottom yogurt
60	0	0	16 oz (480 ml) orange juice
134	**16**	**5**	*Total for second recovery: approximately 640 calories*
			DINNER (6:00 P.M.)
0	42	18	6 oz (250 g) salmon steak
45	10	14	1 cup pasta with 1/4 cup pesto sauce
30	6	10	2 pieces Italian bread with 2 tsp olive oil
10	4	0	1 cup grilled peppers and mushrooms
75	0	0	20 oz apple cider
160	**62**	**42**	*Total for meal: approximately 1,260 calories*
			SNACK (9:00 P.M.)
39	12	12	12 oz (360 ml) low-fat chocolate milk
72	4	24	4 Toll House Chocolate Chip cookies
111	**16**	**36**	*Total for snack: approximately 830 calories*
861	**138**	**115**	**Total for day: approximately 5,000 calories**

The large caloric needs for this plan are met by two morning fuelings with adequate carbohydrate and a small amount of fat added to the early meal. To maximize glycogen stores this athlete has been tapering and fueling the entire week prior to the day of the event. Since this athlete's sweat rate is 1.5 pounds (.7 kg) per hour, he will drink 4 ounces (120 ml) every 10 minutes (7 grams of carbohydrate per 10 minutes) (a sports drink supplies 42 grams per hour) and he can then add 18 grams of carbohydrate per hour (for a total of 60/hr) by consuming one shot blok or 3-4 jelly beans every 30 minutes (see table 11.1 for some ideas for carbohydrate during activity; also see appendix C on page 206 for a list of the grams of carbohydrate in certain foods or even appendix E on page 214 for some great preexercise and recovery foods that would also work well during an event). For recovery, the runner should consume nutrient-rich foods and adequate fluid containing sodium and potassium as well as sufficient carbohydrate and protein for muscle repair and immunity.

Table 11.1 Carbohydrate food ideas during activity

Food	Quantity	Carbohydrate (g)
Jelly beans	10 large	26
Jelly Belly jelly beans	35 small	37
Sport beans	1 package	25
Pretzel nuggets	20 pieces	25
Twizzlers	1 piece	9
Gummy bears or Swedish fish	1 piece	2
Clif Shot Bloks	3 pieces	24
Powerbar gel	1 packet	27
Powerbar Performance bar	1 bar	46
Powerbar Fruit Smoothie bar	1 bar	27
Boiled potato	1, 2 1/2" diameter	27
Fig Newtons	2 cookies	22
Raisins	Small box	34

Applying the principles of nutrient timing to endurance training and competition will result in better-fueled training and recovery, diminishing muscle tissue breakdown, inflammation, and soreness and promote immunity. Determining your caloric needs based on your training and establishing your carbohydrate, protein, and fat requirements are the basis for creating an individualized Nutrition Blueprint. The timing principles are incorporated into the blueprint, helping to ensure your fuel is accounted for before, during, and after training. From this point, you can formulate training or competition-day meal plans, adjusted for time of day. It takes some work to create your own Nutrition Blueprint and meal plan, but it also takes work to train as hard as you do. Make it count. Create a plan incorporating the principles of nutrient timing to get the most out of your efforts.

CHAPTER

12

Stop and Go

Basketball, field hockey, figure skating, ice hockey, lacrosse, rugby, soccer, and tennis are all considered stop-and-go sports. As diverse as these sports are, athletes participating in them must develop both strength and power as well as endurance to compete. Even more specifically, honing skills in agility, speed, power, precision, stamina, mental sharpness, and in some cases, grace, will mean the difference between excellence or mediocrity. Developing and fine-tuning your skills during training requires the right fuel at the right times.

One commonality of athletes in all stop-and-go sports is the use of fast-twitch muscle fibers for power. These fibers use carbohydrate only to fuel muscle contraction. When the carbohydrate is used up, the muscles fatigue quickly. Since fast-twitch fibers don't use oxygen well, they can't rely on fat as fuel, so it's vital that athletes replace the carbohydrate if they want to remain strong and energized. When matches or games go into tiebreakers, sudden death, or overtime, the better-fueled athlete has the advantage—a lack of proper fueling can lead to fatigue, inattention, slowness, cramping, missed opportunities, injuries, and defeat. The faster, more powerful, more precise athlete who maintains physical and mental stamina often wins or helps his or her team win. Inadequate fueling day in and day out can lead to staleness and decreased performance as the season goes on.

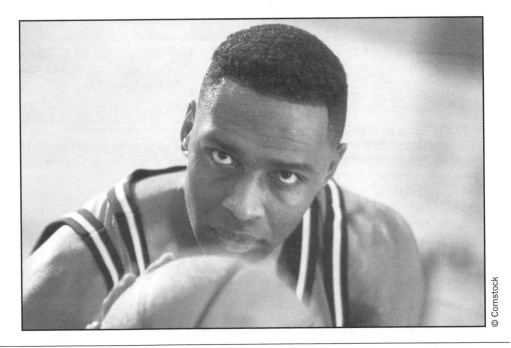

© Comstock

Maintaining intensity of play up through the end of a game is related to how well-fueled you start the game.

Nuances of the Different Stop-and-Go Sports

Stop-and-go athletes may be competing a few times per week during the season. Complicated by their heavy travel schedules, remaining well-hydrated and well-fueled can pose challenges. Applying the NTP before, during, and after practices and especially during competition can make the difference between winning and losing.

Basketball

Basketball players require a substantial amount of carbohydrate and fluids to prevent physical and mental fatigue. Because games are scheduled frequently and at varying times of day, players may go for long periods without eating. Inconsistency in fueling can result in inconsistency in energy and play on the court. Eating on the road often, players may choose high-fat foods, and although calorically many players can handle this, they just have to be sure high-fat does not crowd out carbohydrate-rich foods, which will serve to replace glycogen and prevent staleness over the course of the season. Weight should remain stable or within 1 to 2 percent from day to day. Prehydration is a must, as is drinking at intervals of 10 to 20 minutes during play in order to replace some of the fluids lost in sweat.

Field Hockey

During a game, players can cover more than 5 miles (8 km), which means legs can become depleted of glycogen. Starting out with adequate carbohydrate stores is vital so that energy doesn't wane in the last 15 minutes of play, when 30 percent of all goals are scored. Consuming fuel and fluid during play can ensure that players perform up to their skill level.

Figure Skating

Skaters often burn more calories than they realize and may undereat and underhydrate. Appropriate caloric intake and nutrient timing satisfies hunger, fuels training, improves body composition, and minimizes muscle tissue breakdown. Skaters need to take in sufficient protein, fat, calcium, and vitamin D, as some athletes may be at risk for stress fractures. Because figure skating is performed in a cool environment, hydration is not always a top priority, but regular water breaks are a must.

Ice Hockey

Fueling strategies must be adapted from morning practices to afternoon or evening games. Because rinks are cool, players may not feel the need to drink during play. Additionally, hockey players may not realize how much fluid they lose in sweat. If losses aren't replaced, it's easy to accumulate dehydration. When an athlete is dehydrated, both solid foods and liquids remain in the stomach, causing sloshing of liquids in the stomach which is bothersome to some players. When sloshing occurs, some players refrain from taking in enough fluid, causing further dehydration! This can lead to glycogen depletion because a delay in stomach emptying delays fuel reaching working muscles. The muscles may use up stored glycogen before ingested fuel is able to supply additional energy, even from fluids, when an athlete is in a dehydrated state.

Soccer, Rugby, and Lacrosse

Research done on soccer players is believed to apply to rugby and lacrosse players as well. A soccer player can cover between 4.5 and 7 miles (7 and 11 km) in a game. There is a heavy demand in these athletes for carbohydrate and fluids, which should be ingested before, during, and after games. Beginning games with high glycogen stores is essential for second half energy. Carbohydrate intake during play is glycogen sparing and has been shown to facilitate greater running distances and more goals scored with less conceded. High carbohydrate intake on a daily basis is imperative to replace glycogen for subsequent matches. Athletes should drink 17 to 20 ounces (510 to 600 ml) two hours before the game; another 7 to 10 ounces (210 to 300 ml) 10 to 20 minutes before taking the field; and 20 to 40 ounces (600 to 1,200 ml) per hour depending on outside temperature, intensity of play, and whether substitutions are allowed. If drinking during play is prohibited, athletes must drink and fuel up (30 grams of carbohydrate) during halftime.

Tennis

Players need to take in sufficient carbohydrate, fluid, and sodium throughout the day. Even with a prematch snack, muscular fatigue can set in after 60 to 90 minutes of intense play. Taking in 30 to 60 grams of carbohydrate per hour can help prevent this. Players should begin matches hydrated by taking in 17 to 20 ounces (510 to 600 ml) two hours before the match and 7 to 10 ounces (210 to 300 ml) 20 minutes before. During the match, players should have 4 to 8 ounces (120 to 240 ml) at each changeover and consume 20 ounces (600 ml) for each pound lost, including extra sodium if sweating is excessive. Between sets and matches, higher carbohydrate intake, such as gels or honey sandwiches, provide quick energy to glycogen depleted muscles. See recovery ideas in appendix E on page 214.

PLANNING FOR TRAINING

In chapter 9, we help you determine your caloric needs and formulate the amounts of carbohydrate, protein, and fat needed for training and competition. To illustrate how to apply this information, we will use a sample athlete, Sam, a 154-pound (70 kg) stop-and-go athlete who trains for two hours at a moderate to high intensity. We calculated his caloric needs in appendix A on page 199 and determined his macronutrient needs by sport in appendix B on page 205. Sam requires a total of 3,200 calories per day: 7 g/kg carbohydrate for a total of 490 g (61 percent calories); 1.7 g/kg protein for a total of 119 g (15 percent calories); and 84 g fat, which come from the balance of calories left (24 percent calories).

First, we will plug Sam's training fuel into his Nutrition Blueprint, as described in chapter 9. To do this, it helps to first answer the following questions. Let's assume Sam works out in the morning; here's what his answers would be:

- Do you need a pretraining snack? Yes
- Based on the time between your snack, when you will train, and the type of work you will do, what are your pretraining fueling needs? 30 grams of carbohydrate and 0 grams of protein
- Do you need fuel during training? If so, how much? Yes, 60 grams of carbohydrate
- What are your recovery needs? 70 grams of carbohydrate (1 gram per kilogram × 70) and 7 to 14 grams of protein (.1 to .2 gram per kilogram × 70)

Now that the Blueprint is created for training, the remaining macronutrients can be distributed for meals and snacks. You don't have to plan every gram or morsel that crosses your lips—few athletes do. It's fine to round off and estimate. The main idea behind the Blueprint is to provide a general guideline as to *about how much* of each nutrient to have around training and at meals and snacks. Developing a template like this helps you create structure, awareness, and goals and can give you a sense of whether you are close to fueling yourself properly or completely off the mark.

Morning Training

Let's take a look at how Sam's daily nutrient needs are spread out if he works out in the morning. Since Sam is training before breakfast he needs a preworkout snack and fuel during training will help fuel muscles and keep his coordination sharp. His two recovery snacks can serve as breakfast and frequent feedings work well to begin restoring glycogen. Here's how Sam's blueprint looks for a day when he trains at a high intensity before breakfast:

Meal/Snack	Carbohydrate (g)	Protein (g)	Fat (g)
Pretraining	30	0	0
During training	60	0	0
Recovery	70	15	10
Breakfast/2nd recovery	70	15	5
Lunch	75	40	30
Snack	30	5	15
Dinner	105	45	20
Snack	50	0	5
Total	490	120	85

Figure 12.1 shows how Sam's daily nutrient needs translate into real foods when training in the morning for two hours at a high intensity.

For shorter or lower-intensity workouts in the morning, a snack before training is always a good idea. Blood sugar and liver glycogen are lowered after an overnight fast, so without food, your coordination, timing, and mental sharpness suffer. Just 15 grams—as simple as 8 ounces (240 ml) of sports drink, a slice of bread, or a handful of dry cereal—is all it takes. For longer or higher-intensity workouts, have at least 25 grams of carbohydrate or more before if time permits. Also, be ready with a recovery plan, and have foods available to begin repairing and restocking muscles for the next practice. Training fuel plus breakfast should make up at least one-third of total daily calories so that calorie distribution will be equitable throughout the rest of the day.

FIGURE 12.1

Sam's sample 3,200-calorie menu when training at high intensity for 2 hr in the morning

Carbohydrate (g)	Protein (g)	Fat (g)	Foods
PREWORKOUT SNACK (5:30 A.M.)			
15	2	1	1 slice white bread
15	0	0	1 tbsp jam
0	0	0	Water
30	2	1	Total for preworkout snack: approximately 125 calories
DURING TRAINING (6:00-8.00 A.M.)			
60	0	0	32 oz (960 ml) sports drink
60	0	0	Total for training: approximately 140 calories
FIRST RECOVERY (8:15 A.M.)			
60	15	10	12 oz (360 ml) 2% chocolate milk
11	1	1	Graham cracker
71	16	11	Total for first recovery: approximately 450 calories
SECOND RECOVERY (9:30 A.M.)			
47	13	0	Smoothie made with 1/2 cup frozen sweetened berries and 1 cup plain nonfat yogurt
22	1	3	2 graham crackers
69	14	3	Total for second recovery: approximately 360 calories
LUNCH (1:00 P.M.)			
38	7	1	1 cup whole-wheat pasta
6	4	19	1/4 cup pesto sauce
0	24	1	4 oz (125 g) shrimp
4	2	0	1 cup steamed broccoli
24	3	7	1 slice garlic bread
0	0	0	Sparkling water
72	40	28	Total for meal: approximately 700 calories
MIDAFTERNOON SNACK (4:30 P.M.)			
5	6	14	1 oz almonds
23	0	0	Banana
28	6	14	Total for snack: approximately 260 calories
DINNER (7:00 P.M.)			
10	32	12	Kebabs made with 4 oz (125 g) lean beef and 2 cups vegetables (mushrooms, peppers, zucchini, cherry tomatoes)
45	5	2	1 cup brown rice
20	0	0	3 tbsp grilling sauce
31	5	11	2 slices rosemary olive bread dipped in 2 tsp oil
106	42	25	Total for meal: approximately 805 calories
SNACK (9:30 P.M.)			
18	0	6	3 butter cookies
33	0	0	1/2 cup sorbet
51	0	6	Total for snack: approximately 260 calories
487	120	88	Total for day: approximately 3,200 calories

Afternoon or Evening Training

One more reason to eat breakfast: Breakfast and lunch provide the energy needed for workouts later in the day. Having these two meals is an absolute must. Try to consume two-thirds of daily calories before a late-afternoon practice. Since food and fluids at meals also contribute to hydration needs, do not skip meals, and remember to drink according to your hydration plan. Add a snack, and consume fuel around training. Recovery, dinner, and a snack will all help restore you before your next workout. Here's how to determine when and how much to eat before training:

	2 hrs or less since last meal	4 hrs or less since last meal
Light workout	Nothing needed	15 g carbohydrate
Moderate workout	Nothing needed	15 g carbohydrate
Heavy workout	*< 1 hr before*: 25 g carbohydrate or 15 g carbohydrate right before	*2-3 hrs before*: 300-400 calories, protein and carbohydrate ok; low in fat *< 1 hr before*: 200 calories, 25-50 g carbohydrate

To help you get a better idea of how a plan is modified for afternoon or evening workouts, let's take another look at our sample athlete and what his Blueprint would look like for an afternoon workout:

Meal/Snack	Carbohydrate (g)	Protein (g)	Fat (g)
Breakfast	100	20	25
Snack	20	0	5
Lunch	100	45	20
Pretraining	25	0	0
During training	60	0	0
Recovery	70	10	10
Dinner	100	45	20
Snack	15	0	5
Total	490	120	85

Figure 12.2 shows how Sam's daily nutrient needs translate into real foods when training heavily for two hours in the afternoon. Breakfast and lunch will help fuel Sam later in the day during his high-intensity practice and ensure he is getting better-quality foods during meals. Since it's been four hours or more since his last meal, he takes 25 grams of quick-digesting carbohydrate before practice. As you'll notice, dinner isn't all that large because he's well fueled all day long. A small bedtime snack helps provide glycogen to the liver.

FIGURE 12.2

Sam's sample 3,200-calorie menu when training at high intensity for 2 hr in the afternoon

Carbohydrate (g)	Protein (g)	Fat (g)	Foods
BREAKFAST (7:00 A.M.)			
0	12	10	2 eggs, scrambled
45	6	2	2 slices whole-wheat toast + 1 tbsp jam
0	0	5	1 tbsp cream cheese
27	2	10	1/2 cup hash-brown potatoes
11	0	0	1 kiwi
17	0	0	Green tea with 1 tbsp honey
100	20	27	*Total for meal: approximately 725 calories*
MIDMORNING SNACK (10:30 A.M.)			
18	1	3	Granola bar
18	1	3	*Total for meal: approximately 100 calories*
LUNCH (12:30 P.M.)			
45	8	0	1 cup pasta
10	4	0	1 cup cooked carrots, broccoli, and zucchini
0	0	15	1 tbsp olive oil
0	28	4	4 oz (90 g) chicken
0	2	1	1 tbsp grated Parmesan cheese
45	0	0	12 oz (360 ml) orange juice
100	42	20	*Total for meal: approximately 750 calories*
PREWORKOUT SNACK (3:00 P.M.)			
25	0	0	1/2 cup applesauce
25	0	0	*Total for preworkout snack: approximately 100 calories*
DURING TRAINING (4:00-6:00 P.M.)			
60	0	0	32 oz (960 ml) sports drink
60	0	0	*Total for training: approximately 240 calories*
RECOVERY (6:15 P.M.)			
45	11	7	12 oz (360 ml) 2% chocolate milk
25	0	0	1 oz packet Craisins
70	11	7	*Total for recovery: approximately 390 calories*
DINNER (7:30 P.M.)			
10	32	10	Kebabs made with 4 oz (125 g) lean beef and 2 cups vegetables (mushrooms, peppers, zucchini, cherry tomatoes)
36	6	0	1 cup whole-wheat couscous
20	3	0	3 tbsp grilling sauce
31	5	11	2 slices rosemary olive bread dipped in 2 tsp oil
10	0	8	8 oz tomato juice
107	46	29	*Total for meal: approximately 800 calories*
SNACK (9:30 P.M.)			
12	1	6	3 pieces dark chocolate
12	1	6	*Total for snack: approximately 100 calories*
492	121	92	Total for day: approximately 3,200 calories

Fuel for Competition

Eating for competition is about fuel and timing, not quality per se, so it may differ from eating for training. Remember, the precompetition meal begins *the day before* a game or match.

Day Before an Event

Beginning at lunch on the day before an event, you should think *pregame fuel*. Each meal will ideally be balanced with two-thirds of the calories coming from grains, fruits, vegetables, and milk or yogurt and one-third from protein. At this point there is no need to restrict fat as there is still plenty of time to digest it. Try something as simple as a bowl of pasta with shrimp and vegetables with some Parmesan cheese and a glass of cranberry juice; or a piece of barbecued chicken with mashed potatoes and carrots, a roll, and a glass of iced tea. Dinner should be something comparable. By adding a bedtime snack such as fig bars and hot cocoa; sorbet and a few vanilla wafers; low-fat frozen yogurt with fruit; cookies and milk; or a peanut butter and jelly sandwich, you are helping to ensure stocked muscles by game time.

Day of the Event

On the day of the event, the distribution of calories, carbohydrate, and fluid is based on what time the competition is and target intakes can be created by counting backward from game time. Table 12.1 shows several example competition times and intake distribution for an athlete requiring 600 to 900 g carbohydrate per day. If your intake is less, you can adjust using this as a guide: for a 1:00 p.m. game, at least 1/3 of your carbs should be taken in before; for a 4:00 p.m. game, 1/2 to 2/3 of your daily carbs should be taken in before; and for a 7:00 p.m. game, 2/3 or more of your carbs should be taken in before.

Remember, the goals for competition fueling are to fuel you and keep you hydrated, ward off hunger, and keep blood sugar levels stable. Preevent fueling should not interfere with play: No spicy or gas-producing foods such as beans, broccoli, cauliflower, or other foods you find disagreeable.

Breakfast on the Day of the Event

Precompetition meals are typically consumed 3-4 hours prior to the event start time. For morning or early afternoon, breakfast is the precompetition meal. For afternoon games or matches, many athletes may think extra sleep is helpful. However, consuming breakfast in addition to your precompetition meal ensures that you'll get *more* energy into your system.

Table 12.1   Carbohydrate intake distribution based on competition times

Competition time	Total carbohydrate intake prior to the competition	Timing of precompetition fuel
1:00 p.m.	200-300 g (at least 1/3 of day's total)	Breakfast/pregame meal: 100-150 g; just before start of game: 25 g; and halftime or break in play: 25 g
4:00 p.m.	400-500 g (1/2 to 2/3 of day's total)	Breakfast: 200 g; brunch/pregame meal: 150 g; just before start of game: 25 g; and halftime or break in play: 25 g
7:00 p.m.	500 g or more (at least 2/3 of day's total)	Breakfast: 100 g; brunch/lunch: 200 g; pregame meal: 150 g; just before start of game: 25 g; and halftime or break in play: 25 g

Precompetition Meal

Although all the meals you've consumed in the 24 to 36 hours before your event help fuel your muscles, the foods you eat 3 to 4 hours before are frequently referred to as the precompetition meal. You may have this meal with your team or on your own. Choose smaller portions of lean protein and foods that are high in carbohydrate, low in fat, and low in fiber and that you are accustomed to eating. Include fluids to hydrate during and between meals on competition day so you start the event fully hydrated. In addition, it is wise to top off your tank after your warm up with a small snack, especially if your meal was 3 to 4 hours earlier.

During the Event

Take advantage of a break in play to hydrate and fuel. For some, halftime is the only opportunity; try to use substitutions and timeouts if possible. Here are a few suggestions for some 25-30 g carbohydrate foods to keep on hand during competition: 1 slice white bread with 1 tbsp jam or honey, a 2-inch mini-bagel, a small box of raisins, a medium banana, 4 orange wedges and 3-5 pretzels, 2-3 Fig Newtons, a handful of crushed pretzels, or 1 cup of grapes.

Also, sports drinks hydrate and refuel and are vital for athletes who are unable to drink during play. Sports gels, gus, and bars may also be a convenient way to refuel, but water needs to be consumed along with them, and check the label to make sure you are taking in adequate sodium. Also, many contain caffeine and caffeine-like stimulants, so check levels and be aware of the "stacking effect" of taking in more than one product. Remember, the longer a game or match goes (extra sets, overtime), the closer it is—any edge that you have in terms of energy and hydration is in your favor. Players who hydrate and are well fueled are better able to play up to their skill level.

Recovery After the Event

Be prepared with a recovery snack after games and matches, even if you are planning to have a meal soon after. Stop-and-go sports use fast-twitch muscles that deplete quickly, so getting a jump start on restocking will benefit athletes who compete day after day. It may help prevent soreness and the feeling of "staleness" a few weeks into the season. Adding more carbohydrate (pretzels, fig bars, raisins) to a recovery drink—Met-Rx, Surgex, Accelerade, Isopure, Boost, Carnation Instant Breakfast Essentials—speeds muscle readiness for your next event. You may add nonfat dried milk to any recovery drink or even to regular milk to boost carbohydrate and protein. It's a much less expensive alternative to protein powder, and it includes both whey and casein—milk proteins known for muscle repair. See page 214 in appendix E for more recovery food ideas.

Fuel for Tournament Play

Pregame eating for tournaments is the same as fueling for a typical competition. What's most crucial in tournament play is what you eat in between matches or games. You need to begin restocking your muscles immediately after the first event. And, since the availability of food is unreliable, you must be sure to bring appropriate fueling snacks with you.

An Hour or Less Between Competition

For athletes who have an hour or less between matches, recovery really means restocking fuel, so go with easily-digested carbohydrate only. Try honey and white-bread sandwiches, jelly beans, applesauce, sports gels or gus, or soft pretzels—these will restock your muscles and are quick digesting. Hydrate with water or sports drinks, and you'll be ready to go for your next competition.

Two to Three Hours Between Competition

For athletes with more time between matches, such as two to three hours, snacks can include some *protein* to prevent hunger and can be slightly larger, such as a peanut butter and honey or jelly sandwich with a banana and sports drink or water; a bagel or bread with two or three slices of turkey, baked chips or pretzels, and sports drink; a high-carbohydrate bar (Clif, NuGo, Kashi Roll!) and a carton (16 ounces; 480 ml) of juice or low-fat chocolate milk; yogurt, fruit, and cereal; or Carnation Breakfast Essentials or Boost with pretzels and a piece of fresh fruit or a couple of fruit leathers. Note that although sports foods are convenient and fine as part of your food arsenal, relying solely on them may leave you unsatisfied. You'll have to eat quite a few bars or gels if your event goes for extended hours or there are delays. Whole foods will make you feel more nourished and satisfy your hunger.

In the case that it's hard to predict when your next competition will begin, be prepared with small, quick-digesting carbohydrate snacks that will last, such as mini-bagels, fresh fruits, low-fat granola bars, fruit cups, fruit leathers, low-fat muffins, cold sweet potatoes, graham crackers, fig bars, rice cakes and pretzels, juices, or instant oatmeal. Then, if it is determined that you have time between events, you can add some protein and fat to these carbs, such as cheese sticks; peanut or almond butter; small cans or vacuum-sealed packs of tuna or chicken. Just be sure to experiment ahead of time to see what works for you and be sure you get a good supply of carb with the protein.

Also, for tournaments, remember that bringing a cooler can greatly expand your food choices. Even reusable freezer packs in an insulated bag are a convenient way to keep foods cold. Some additional food options in this case might be low-fat yogurt (mix in cereal to boost carbs); fruit and cottage cheese with crackers; fruit smoothies; cold pasta salad; edamame and rice bowl; hummus; low-fat cheeses; or lean meats, such as chicken, turkey, roast beef, or ham.

Nutrient Timing While Traveling

Some sports require out-of-state travel or even travel outside of the country. Athletes sometimes seek out fast-food restaurants because they are familiar and inexpensive. Most food items, though, are high-fat and not necessarily the best in terms of pregame fare.

When fast-food is your only option, some good breakfast ideas could be an English muffin or other breakfast bread with jam; fruit; hot or cold cereal; yogurt with low-fat granola; low-fat muffins; or pancakes or French toast. Egg McMuffins from McDonald's, for example, really are a good choice (11 g fat); just skip the croissants, sausage, and other high-fat meats.

For lunch and dinner, also seek lower fat options, such as grilled chicken or roast beef, or choose a regular hamburger instead of one with cheese and bacon. Other options may include deep-dish pizza; noodle or pasta dishes; broth- or tomato-based soups; salads; or grilled, roasted or broiled meat, fish, or poultry with ample vegetables, potatoes, and bread. In addition, yogurt parfaits, milk, and juices are on many menus.

Another great idea when traveling is to pack your own snacks! Many food items travel well and are great to have on hand. You can travel with a jar of peanut butter, powdered milk, bags or cans of tuna, cups of soup, dried fruits, cold or hot cereals, and sport bars. Also, it is important to remind you that if you are flying, drink 1-2 cups of water per hour on the flight. The decompartmenatlized air can have a dehydrating effect, and jet lag is associated with dehydration.

MENU PLANS FOR STOP-AND-GO ATHLETES

Following are sample menu plans to help illustrate the Nutrient Timing Principles and put them into practice. Use the Blueprint that you developed in chapter 9 to plan your meals, and use the following sample plans as a guide. Hopefully, these plans offer some great ideas for meals, timing, and distribution of calories. You don't need to be as precise as these menus are; being in the general vicinity of the numbers will work.

Menu Plans for Stop-and-Go Athletes When Training Needs Are Greater Than Competition Needs

Following are two meal plans for stop-and-go athletes; the first is a 4,000-calorie training menu for a 165-pound (75 kg) stop-and-go athlete who trains about three hours per day. The second is a competition menu for the same athlete, reduced to 3,800 calories because the length of competition is less than the time this athlete spends training. Remember to go back and calculate your own caloric needs. These sample menus are just illustrations of how to integrate all we have recommended with the principles of nutrient timing. You can adjust to the time of day you train and your food preferences. The important thing to remember when building your own plan is to account for fuel and hydration before, during, and after training; build out your meals from there, paying attention to distribution of calories and quality of nutrients in each meal.

4,000-Calorie Training Menu

Figure 12.3 shows the training needs for a 165-pound (75 kg) stop-and-go athlete who practices for three hours a day; the menu plan in figure 12.4 shows how these needs are translated into real food choices. Note that this menu could also be suitable for a larger athlete training for a shorter time.

3,400-Calorie Competition Menus

Practice sessions may be longer than competition for some stop-and-go athletes. In this case, we cut back on the fat to accommodate a decreased energy need. Competition may be at any time of day, so athletes need to adjust intake to provide adequate fueling. Figures 12.5 and 12.6 provide sample 3,400-calorie menus for a 165-pound (75 kg) athlete participating in a two-hour competition. The first menu shows how a 165-pound athlete's needs translate into real food choices for a two-hour competition at 7:00 p.m. In this menu, since competition ends rather late, a bedtime snack is not needed. As you see in figure 12.6, which shows how this athlete's menu would be adjusted for a 4:00 p.m. competition, a snack is needed.

FIGURE 12.3

A 165 lb (75 kg) athlete's daily nutrient needs when training 3 hr/day

	Daily total (g)	Daily total (calories)	%	g/kg for 75 kg (165 lb)
Fat	120	1,080	27	1.6
Carbohydrate	600	2,400	60	8.0
Protein	130	520	13	1.7
Total		4,000 daily calories	100%	

FIGURE 12.4
Sample 4,000-calorie menu for a 165 lb (75 kg) athlete training 3 hr/day

Carbohydrate (g)	Protein (g)	Fat (g)	Foods
BREAKFAST (7:45 A.M.)			
27	6	3	1 cup cooked oatmeal
12	8	5	8 oz 2% milk
9	0	0	2 tsp brown sugar
4	4	18	1/4 cup walnut halves
60	0	0	16 oz (480 ml) orange juice
112	**18**	**26**	*Total for meal: approximately 750 calories*
SNACK (10:20 A.M.)			
14	4	14	Kind bar
33	0	0	1 1/2 cup cherries
47	**4**	**14**	*Total for snack: approximately 330 calories*
LUNCH (12:40 P.M.)			
15	6	2	8 oz cup chicken noodle soup
22	2	2	8 saltine crackers
0	21	7	3 oz (90 g) ham
0	8	8	1 oz (30 g) Swiss cheese
30	6	0	2 slices rye bread
5	1	2	1 cup cucumber and tomato salad
50	0	0	12 oz (360 ml) fruit slush drink
122	**44**	**21**	*Total for meal: approximately 850 calories*
PREWORKOUT SNACK (3:00 P.M.)			
15	1	0	Handful of pretzel nuggets (about 12)
15	0	0	8 oz (240 ml) sports drink
30	**1**	**0**	*Total for preworkout snack: approximately 125 calories*
DURING TRAINING (3:30-6:30 P.M.)			
90	0	0	2 sports gels and water, 16 oz sports drink
90	**0**	**0**	*Total for training: approximately 240 calories*
RECOVERY (6:45 P.M.)			
39	12	4	12 oz (360 ml) low-fat chocolate milk
34	0	0	Box of raisins
73	**12**	**4**	*Total for recovery: approximately 360 calories*
DINNER (8:15 P.M.)			
37	7	1	1 cup whole-wheat pasta
0	28	4	4 oz (125 g) grilled chicken
15	0	3	1/2 cup tomato sauce
10	4	15	1 cup sauteed spinach with 1 tbsp olive oil
0	12	10	2 tbsp Parmesan cheese
30	4	20	2 slices Italian bread dipped in olive oil
34	0	0	8 oz (240 ml) cranberry juice mixed with seltzer
126	**55**	**53**	*Total for meal: approximately 1,190 calories*
600	**134**	**118**	**Total for day: approximately 4,000 calories**

FIGURE 12.5

Sample 3,400-calorie menu for a 165 lb (75 kg) athlete competing for 2 hr beginning at 7:00 p.m.

Carbohydrate (g)	Protein (g)	Fat (g)	Foods
BREAKFAST (7:30-8:00 A.M.)			
30	6	3	1 cup cooked oatmeal
12	8	0	1 cup nonfat milk
33	3	15	1/4 cup raisins + 3 tbsp walnut halves
30	0	0	8 oz (240 ml) orange juice
105	**17**	**18**	*Total for meal: approximately 650 calories*
LUNCH (11:30 A.M.)			
0	28	8	4 oz (125 g) grilled chicken breast
4	0	1	2 tbsp barbeque sauce
32	5	10	6 in (15 cm) corn on the cob + 2 tsp butter
5	2	1	Tomato and cucumber salad, 1/2 cup
35	4	9	1 cup mashed potatoes
20	3	2	1/2 cup frozen yogurt
96	**42**	**31**	*Total for meal: approximately 800 calories*
PREGAME MEAL (3:30 P.M.)			
15	6	2	8 oz cup of chicken noodle soup
30	4	2	Hamburger roll
4	21	8	3 oz (90 g) lean turkey burger + 1 tbsp ketchup
23	2	2	1 oz (30 g) Baked! Lay's potato chips
72	**33**	**14**	*Total for meal: approximately 550 calories*
SNACK (5:30 P.M.)			
20	0	0	1 apple
0	7	6	1 cheesestick
20	**7**	**6**	*Total for snack: approximately 160 calories*
PREGAME TIPOFF (6:30 P.M.)			
15	0	0	8 pretzel nuggets or 8 oz (240 ml) sports drink
15	**0**	**0**	*Total for pregame snack: approximately 60 calories*
DURING GAME (7:00 P.M.)			
55	0	0	Sports gel + 16 oz sports drink
55	**0**	**0**	*Total during game: approximately 200 calories*
RECOVERY (9:00 P.M., WITHIN 15 MINS OF COMING OFF FIELD)			
43	10	6	Clif Bar
34	0	0	8 oz cranberry juice
77	**10**	**6**	*Total for recovery: approximately 400 calories*
DINNER (10:00 P.M.)			
73	30	1	1 1/2 cups rice with 3 oz (90 g) shrimp and vegetables
5	0	10	2 cups green salad and 2 tbsp dressing
27	0	0	1/2 cup mango sorbet
0	0	0	Sparkling water
105	**30**	**11**	*Total for meal: approximately 745 calories*
545	**139**	**86**	**Total for day: approximately 3,400 calories**

FIGURE 12.6

Sample 3,400-calorie menu for a 165 lb (75 kg) athlete competing for 2 hr beginning at 4:00 p.m.

Carbohydrate (g)	Protein (g)	Fat (g)	Foods
BREAKFAST (8:30-9:00 A.M.)			
48	6	9	3 4-inch waffles
30	0	0	2 tbsp maple syrup
10	0	0	1/2 cup berries
0	19	18	2 scrambled eggs and 1 oz cheese
88	25	27	Total for meal: approximately 700 calories
SNACK (10:00 A.M.)			
20	3	2	1 cup Cheerios
12	8	2	1 cup 1% milk
32	11	4	Total for snack: approximately 200 calories
LUNCH (12:30 P.M.)			
65	40	20	4 oz (125 g) ham on a sub roll with lettuce, tomato, "light on the oil," and vinegar
48	6	0	2 oz (60 g) bag pretzels
27	2	4	4 oz (125 g) chocolate pudding
140	48	24	Total for meal: approximately 970 calories
PREGAME SNACK (3:30 P.M.)			
25	0	0	1/2 cup applesauce
0	0	0	Water
25	0	0	Total for pregame snack: approximately 100 calories
DURING GAME (4:00 P.M.)			
55	0	0	Sports gel and water + 16 oz sports drink
55	0	0	Total during game: approximately 220 calories
RECOVERY (6:00 P.M.)			
28	12	5	Kashi Go Lean Roll Bar
52	0	0	Tropical juice blend, 12 oz.
80	12	5	Total for recovery: approximately 415 calories
DINNER (7:00 P.M.)			
10	25	1	Kebabs made with 3 oz (90 g) lean beef and 2 cups vegetables (mushrooms, peppers, zucchini, cherry tomatoes)
54	9	0	1 1/2 cups couscous
20	0	3	3 tbsp grilling sauce
84	34	4	Total for meal: approximately 500 calories
SNACK (9:30 P.M.)			
25	1	14	2 small brownies
12	8	2	8 oz 1% milk
37	9	16	Total for snack: approximately 330 calories
541	139	80	Total for day: approximately 3,400 calories

Menu Plans for Stop-and-Go Athletes When Competition Needs Are Greater Than Training Needs

Some athletes, such as tennis players, may require more calories for competition because play is unpredictable and could go longer than scheduled. Following are two meal plans for stop-and-go athletes; the first is a 2,400-calorie training menu for a 125-pound (57 kg) stop-and-go athlete who trains about two hours per day. The second is a competition menu for the same athlete, increased to 2,900 calories because the time spent participating in competition is more than the time this athlete spends training. When building your own plan, take fuel and hydration before, during, and after training into account; pay attention to distribution of calories and quality of nutrients in meals and snacks throughout the day.

2,400-Calorie Training Menu

Figure 12.7 shows the training needs for a 125-pound (57 kg) stop-and-go athlete who practices for two hours in the afternoon; the menu plan in figure 12.9 shows how these needs are translated into real food choices.

FIGURE 12.7
A 125 lb (57 kg) athlete's daily nutrient needs when training for 2 hr in the afternoon

	Daily total (g)	Daily total (calories)	%	g/kg for 57 kg (125 lb)
Fat	72	648	27	1.3
Carbohydrate	337	1,348	56	6
Protein	99	396	17	1.7
Total		2,400 daily calories	100%	

2,900-Calorie Competition Menu

For this athlete, competition is longer than the time spent in practice sessions, so in order to accommodate the increased caloric need, we added more carbohydrate to fuel extended play and added fat to increase overall calories (figure 12.8).

FIGURE 12.8
A 125 lb (57 kg) athlete's daily nutrient needs when participating in a 3 hr competition

	Daily total (g)	Daily total (calories)	%	g/kg for 75 kg (165 lb)
Fat	81	729	25	1.4
Carbohydrate	440	1,760	60	8
Protein	106	424	15	1.8
Total		2,900 daily calories	100%	

For competition, this athlete needs 8 g/kg carbohydrate (63% calories); 1.7 g/kg protein (13% calories); and 1.4 g/kg fat (24% calories). Although the athlete's protein needs don't change, it's almost impossible to increase carbohydrate intake without increasing protein, so we will account for that. The menu plan in figure 12.10 shows how these needs are translated into real food choices. Here's how we adjusted the 2,400-calorie training menu so that it became a 2,900-calorie menu appropriate for a three-hour competition:

- Increased soup at lunch by 4 oz and added 1/3 cup of rice (32 g carbohydrate, 2 g protein, and 1 g fat) for approximately 145 calories
- Added more sports drink during play (30 g carbohydrate) for a total of 120 calories
- Increased recovery snack by trading fruit leather for large banana (+ 8 g carbohydrate) for about 32 calories
- Added 1 tbsp sunflower seeds at dinner (2 g carbohydrate, 2 g protein, and 4 g fat) for about 45 calories
- Added evening snack of 1/2 cup frozen yogurt (30 g carbohydrate, 2 g protein, 2 g fat) for an addition of 150 calories

FIGURE 12.9

Sample 2,400-calorie menu for a 125 lb (57 kg) athlete training 2 hr in the afternoon

Carbohydrate (g)	Protein (g)	Fat (g)	Foods
BREAKFAST (7:00 A.M.)			
30	4	2	1 cup oatmeal
12	8	3	1 cup 1% milk
3	3	15	3 tbsp chopped walnuts
15	0	0	2 tbsp dried cherries
5	0	0	Green tea + 1 tsp honey
65	15	20	*Total for meal: approximately 500 calories*
MIDMORNING SNACK (10:00 A.M.)			
11	0	0	1 kiwi
0	7	6	1 cheesestick
11	7	6	*Total for snack: approximately 125 calories*
LUNCH (12:30 P.M.)			
30	4	2	Whole–wheat sandwich roll
0	21	3	3 oz (90 g) grilled chicken
2	0	0	Lettuce and tomato
0	0	10	2 oz (60 g) avocado
33	4	2	1 cup tomato soup
0	0	0	Water
65	29	17	*Total for meal: approximately 525 calories*
PREWORKOUT SNACK (3:30 P.M.)			
16	2	1	2 cheddar rice cakes
0	0	0	Water
16	2	1	*Total for preworkout snack: approximately 80 calories*
DURING TRAINING (4:00-6:00 P.M.)			
60	0	0	32 oz (960 ml) sports drink
60	0	0	*Total for training: approximately 240 calories*
RECOVERY (6:15 P.M.)			
39	12	8	12 oz reduced-fat chocolate milk
22	0	0	2 fruit leathers
61	12	8	*Total for recovery: approximately 365 calories*
DINNER (7:30 P.M.)			
0	28	15	4 oz (125 g) broiled salmon
36	6	0	1 cup couscous
2	0	0	2 cups leafy greens
0	0	5	1 tbsp Italian dressing
22	0	0	2 clementines
60	34	20	*Total for meal: approximately 560 calories*
338	99	72	Total for day: approximately 2,400 calories

FIGURE 12.10

Sample 2,900-calorie menu for a 125 lb (57 kg) athlete participating in a 3 hr competition

Carbohydrate (g)	Protein (g)	Fat (g)	Foods
BREAKFAST (8:00 A.M.)			
30	4	2	1 cup oatmeal
12	8	3	1 cup 1% milk
3	3	15	3 tbsp chopped walnuts
15	0	0	2 tbsp dried cherries
5	0	0	Green tea + 1 tsp honey
65	15	20	*Total for meal: approximately 500 calories*
MIDMORNIING SNACK (10:00 A.M.)			
11	0	0	1 kiwi
0	7	6	1 cheesestick
11	7	6	*Total for meal: approximately 125 calories*
LUNCH (11:30 A.M.)			
30	4	2	Whole–wheat sandwich roll
0	21	3	3 oz (90 g) grilled chicken
2	0	0	Lettuce and tomato
0	0	10	2 oz (60 g) avocado
65	6	3	8 oz tomato soup with 1/3 cup rice
0	0	0	Water
97	31	18	*Total for meal: approximately 675 calories*
PREWORKOUT SNACK (2:30 P.M.)			
16	2	1	2 cheddar rice cakes
0	0	0	Water
16	2	1	*Total for preworkout snack: approximately 80 calories*
DURING COMPETITION (3:00-6:00 P.M.)			
90	0	0	48 oz sports drink
90	0	0	*Total for training: approximately 360 calories*
RECOVERY (6:15 P.M.)			
39	12	8	12 oz reduced fat chocolate milk
30	0	0	Large banana
69	12	8	*Total for recovery: approximately 400 calories*
DINNER (7:30 P.M.)			
0	28	15	4 oz (125 g) broiled salmon
36	6	0	1 cup couscous
2	0	5	2 cups leafy greens + 1 tbsp Italian dressing
2	2	4	1 tbsp sunflower seeds
22	0	0	2 clementines
62	36	24	*Total for meal: approximately 600 calories*
SNACK (10:00 P.M.)			
30	2	2	1/2 cup low-fat frozen yogurt
30	2	2	*Total for snack: approximately 150 calories*
440	105	79	Total for day: approximately 2,900 calories

Menu Plan for Stop-and-Go Athletes When Participating in Tournaments

High-carbohydrate recovery and fueling during the event are of utmost importance for stop-and-go athletes who need to compete in more than one game or match per day, such as when participating in tournaments. Beginning the day with well-stocked glycogen is crucial. Assuming a 165-pound (75 kg) stop-and-go athlete competes in two events, one in the afternoon and one in the early evening, lasting about 90 minutes to two hours each, with only a short time between events, here is a look at the Blueprint showing his nutrient needs:

	Daily total (g)	Daily total (calories)	%	g/kg for 75 kg (165 lb)
Fat	120	1,080	22	1.6
Carbohydrate	820	3,280	66	11
Protein	155	620	12	2.0
Total		5,000 daily calories	100%	

Figure 12.11 shows how a 165-pound (75 kg) athlete's daily nutrient needs translate into real foods when participating in such a tournament. This menu reflects how athletes on the road may still make wise choices and take in sufficient carbohydrate. If the tournament continues with a game the next morning and there is very little time between waking and playing, we recommend that players take in a pure carbohydrate breakfast, which can be packed ahead of time, such as a bagel with two tablespoons of jelly (90 grams) and 16 ounces (480 ml) of sports drink (30 grams). If there is more time, a peanut butter and jelly, egg, or turkey sandwich and a banana will provide longer-lasting fuel; athletes should also have a snack just before the game, such as a small box of raisins and water or sports drink.

By applying the principles of nutrient timing during training, you'll be giving your body the fuel needed to become more powerful, agile, and precise while staying mentally focused. Once the season hits, fueling properly with these principles will play a major role in your being able to perform to the best of your ability, day after day, especially during long seasons with many days of back-to-back competition.

As you've learned, achieving stamina is much more than eating a pregame meal. The timing and composition of your workout fuel along with the quality of your food at mealtimes will affect your resiliency during the season. Postexercise intake of protein influences muscle repair, but only a small amount is needed right after your activity. Taking in smaller amounts through the day makes better use of your protein allowance than having a large dose all at once. Hydration, an important and vital aspect of being properly fueled, is something you must always pay attention to. The quality of the foods you consume contributes to immunity, protection against inflammation, and overall well-being. Putting all these principles together will ensure that you are ready to work to the very best of your ability.

FIGURE 12.11

Sample 5,000-calorie menu for a 165 lb (75 kg) athlete participating in a tournament with 2 competitions in one day

Carbohydrate (g)	Protein (g)	Fat (g)	Foods
BREAKFAST (8:00 A.M.)			
29	18	12	Egg and cheese sandwich made with 1 egg, 1 slice cheese, and English muffin
105	9	18	Pancakes (one order at fast food restaurant) with 3 tbsp syrup and 2 pats margarine
60	0	0	16 oz (480 ml) orange juice
12	8	2	8 oz (240 ml) 1% low-fat milk
206	**35**	**32**	*Total for meal: approximately 1,250 calories*
LUNCH (11:30 A.M.)			
			Turkey sub sandwich:
45	9	2	6-in sandwich roll
0	21	0	3 oz turkey
2	0	0	Shredded lettuce and 3 slices tomato
0	0	15	1 tbsp oil and vinegar to taste
23	2	2	1 oz (60 g) Baked! Lay's potato chips
26	0	0	12 oz (480 ml) iced tea
30	3	8	Oatmeal cookie (1.5 oz; 45 g)
126	**35**	**27**	*Total for meal: approximately 900 calories*
PRECOMPETITION SNACK (2:30 P.M.)			
15	0	0	8 oz (240 ml) sports drink
15	2	0	handful of pretzels (about 8)
30	**2**	**0**	*Total for precompetition snack: approximately 130 calories*
DURING FIRST COMPETITION (HALFTIME, 3:00-5:00 P.M.)			
30	0	0	16 oz (480 ml) sports drink
30	**0**	**0**	*Total for competition: approximately 120 calories*
RECOVERY (BETWEEN COMPETITION) (5:15 P.M.)			
			Peanut butter and honey sandwich:
30	4	2	2 slices white bread
6	8	16	2 tbsp peanut butter
17	0	0	1 tbsp honey
30	0	0	Large banana 8"
35	0	0	8 oz cran-apple and water as needed
118	**12**	**18**	*Total for recovery: approximately 680 calories*
DURING SECOND COMPETITION (7:00-9:00 P.M.)			
30	0	0	16 oz (480 ml) sports drink and water
30	**0**	**0**	*Total for competition: approximately 120 calories*

Carbohydrate (g)	Protein (g)	Fat (g)	Foods
	**RECOVERY (AFTER SECOND COMPETITION) (9:00 P.M.)**
30	15	0	Isopure Plus recovery drink
46	3	0	Small bag pretzels, 2 oz
76	**18**	**0**	*Total for recovery: approximately 375 calories*
	**DINNER (10:00 P.M.)**
82	35	1	Pasta with roasted vegetables, 1 1/2 cups + shrimp
21	3	4	3/4 cup pasta sauce
0	6	5	1 tbsp grated cheese
5	0	10	2 cups salad with 2 tbsp Italian dressing
30	6	17	2 slices Italian bread + 1 tbsp olive oil for dipping
44	4	8	4 fig cookies
21	0	0	4 oz (240 ml) grape juice
203	54	45	*Total for meal: approximately 1,425 calories*
819	**156**	**122**	**Total for day: approximately 5,000 calories**

A

Calculating Your Caloric Needs

As exercise intensity and duration change, so do caloric needs. Calculating your total daily caloric needs is a helpful step in putting together your Nutrition Blueprint. It provides a framework for understanding how much fuel is required by the body on a daily basis. The first step estimates the calories required while the body is resting: Your heart, lungs, kidneys, and liver need a minimum of calories to function. Next, the energy used to support daily activity apart from training (e.g., walking to and from the car, doing housework, pacing the corridor) is accounted for. Lastly, the calories expended to support training are calculated. This section may be referred to at different points in the season to recalculate caloric requirements as training becomes more or less intense.

STEP 1: CALCULATE YOUR BASAL METABOLIC RATE

Basal metabolic rate (BMR) is the amount of calories required to carry out all of your body's vital functions in the waking state without any physical activity (i.e., as if you were lying in bed all day). BMR reflects the energy your body needs for respiration; nerve transmission; and function of the brain, liver, and all other organs. A number of formulas have been created to estimate BMR. We show three different formulas here: the Harris-Benedict equation, the Cunningham equation, and a simplified method—you can select one or try all three. If you know your lean body mass, the Cunningham equation may be more accurate if you are very muscular.

Harris-Benedict Equation

This equation uses height, weight, gender, and age to estimate one's needs. It can be used by most athletes. However, it does not include lean body mass, so it will underestimate BMR in muscular people and overestimate BMR in people with high levels of body fat.

Men

> BMR = 66 + (6.23 x weight in pounds) + (12.7 x height in inches) − (6.8 x age in years)
>
> or
>
> BMR = 66 + (13.7 x weight in kg) + (5 x height in cm) − (6.8 x age in years)

Women

> BMR = 655 + (4.35 x weight in pounds) + (4.7 x height in inches) − (4.7 x age in years)
>
> or
>
> BMR = 655 + (9.6 x weight in kg) + (1.8 x height in cm) − (4.7 x age in years)

Cunningham Equation

This equation uses lean body mass but does not consider age or height, and the same equation applies to both men and women. Highly muscular athletes may use this method if they know their lean body mass. Weight in kilograms equals weight in pounds divided by 2.2.

BMR = 370 + (21.6 x kg of lean body mass)

Simplified Method

The simplified method is possibly less accurate because the information is not as specific. However, for those who prefer less math, it provides a reasonable estimate.

Men

BMR = weight in pounds x 11

BMR = weight in kg x 24

Women

BMR = weight in pounds x 10

BMR = weight in kg x 22

Now, after you have figured out your estimated BMR using one of the three methods, write it down: _____

STEP 2: INCLUDE PURPOSEFUL ACTIVITY AND EXERCISE

For this step, you have two choices: You can either get a general estimate based on time spent training, or you can use METs, a more specific multiplier, to estimate the calories spent on training.

General Estimate

For a general estimate of the calories you burn during daily activity and exercise, use one of the following (BMR is the number you got in step 1):

BMR x 1.375 for light activity (1 to 3 days per week)

BMR x 1.55 for moderate activity (3 to 5 days per week)

BMR x 1.75 for heavy activity (6 to 7 days per week)

BMR x 1.9 for exceedingly heavy exertion or very physical exertion throughout the day (e.g., heavy-duty construction worker or lumberjack) or two-a-day hard workouts

Specific Calculation

In this step, you will first estimate your daily calorie requirement without exercise. Then, you will calculate the calories burned during training using METs. Added together, they provide your total daily calorie needs.

METs stands for metabolic equivalents, which are multiples of the resting metabolic rate. It is a more sport-specific estimation of caloric expenditure. It assumes that at rest, you use 1 calorie per kilogram of body weight per hour, and as intensity of physical work increases, so too does the MET level (or calories burned). The MET value for each sport or activity is based on intensity (see table A1). If a sport or activity has a MET value of 5, it means you are burning five times the number of calories you would at rest while you are exercising. But, before you factor in your daily activity, you need to first determine how many calories you burn without additional exercise. Based on the MET values, you can assume that daily activity factors are as follows: sitting all day has a MET value of 1.2; walking a lot and not sitting much has a MET value of 1.3; and for physically demanding daily activity, such as a job as a construction worker, the MET value would be higher, around 1.5. For you, fill in the following based on this example:

_____ BMR x _____ (daily activity factor) = ___ ___ total calorie needs without exercise

Next, you need to find MET value for additional activity by multiplying your weight (in kg) by the MET value of an activity and estimate the number of calories burned. For example, a 154-pound athlete weighs 70 kg (154 divided by 2.2). If this athlete participates in a sport that has a MET value of 5, he would burn 350 calories in one hour (70 kg × 5 METs × 1 hr = 350 calories). For you, fill in the following based on this example:

_____ (weight in lb) / 2.2 = ___ __ (weight in kg) x _____ (MET value of your activity) x _____ (number of hours of activity) = _____ (number of calories burned)

Table A1   MET Values for Common Sports and Activities

Activity	MET value
Baseball	
Fielding	5
Pitching and catching	6
Basketball	
Shooting baskets	4.5
Basketball game	8
Boxing	
Punching bag	6
In ring	12
Conditioning	
Pull-ups, push-ups, vigorous effort	8
General, light to moderate effort	4.5
Circuit training	8
Free weights or universal weights, light to moderate effort	3
Free weights or universal weights, vigorous effort	6

(continued)

(continued)

Activity	MET value
Cycling	
10-11.9 mph (16-19.2 km/hr)	6
12-13.9 mph (19.3-22.4 km/hr)	8
14-15.9 mph (22.5-25.6 km/hr)	10
16-19 mph (25.7-31 km/hr)	12
20+ mph (32+ km/hr)	16
Dancing, ballet or modern	6
Diving	3
Football, competitive	9
Golf	
Using power cart	3.5
Carrying clubs	5.5
Gymnastics	4
Hockey, field or ice	8
Judo, jujitsu, karate, kickboxing, or taekwondo	10
Race walking	6.5
Lacrosse	8
Rope jumping, general	10
Rowing	
2-3.9 mph (3.2-6.3 km/hr)	3
4-5.9 mph (6.4-9.5 km/hr)	7
6+ mph (9.6+ km/hr)	12
Competition or crew, or sculling	12
Rugby	10
Running	
5 mph (8 km/h) (12 min mile)	8
6 mph (9.7 km/hr) (10 min mile)	10
6.7 mph (10.8 km/hr) (9 min mile)	11
7.5 mph (12.1 km/hr) (8 min mile)	12.5
8.6 mph (13.8 km/hr) (7 min mile)	14
10 mph (16 km/hr) (6 min mile)	16
Skating	
9 mph (14.5 km/hr) or less	5.5
9+ mph (14.6+ km/hr)	9
Skiing, cross-country	
2.5 mph (4 km/hr), light	7
4-4.9 mph (6.4-7.9 km/hr), moderate	8
5-7.9 mph (8-12.7 km/hr), vigorous	9
8+ mph (12.8+ km/hr)	14

Activity	MET value
Skiing, downhill	
Light effort	5
Moderate effort	6
Vigorous effort, racing	8
Soccer	
Casual	7
Competitive	10
Softball	
General	5
Pitching	6
Stretching, hatha yoga	4
Swimming	
Crawl, slow (50 yd/min; 50 m/min)	8
Crawl, fast (75 yd/min; 75 m/min)	11
Butterfly, general	11
Breaststroke, general	10
Tennis	
Doubles	6
Singles	8
Volleyball	
Noncompetitive	3
Competitive	4
Beach	8
Wrestling	6

Source: B.E. Ainsworth, W.L. Haskell, A.S. Leon, et al., 1993, "Compendium of physical activities: Classification of energy costs of human physical activities," *Medicine & Science in Sports & Exercise* 25(1): 71-80.

STEP 3: DETERMINE NET CALORIES BURNED DURING TRAINING

To get the most accurate estimation of caloric needs, the time you calculated into your 24-hour resting metabolic rate (BMR) should be deducted from your total exercise time. Because you are not resting when you are training, you have to deduct that resting rate, otherwise you will be counting your body at rest *and* exercising, which will overstate your caloric needs. For example, if you exercise for two hours a day, and you were to add the calories burned in those two hours, you'd be accounting for 26 hours worth of metabolism. To do this, for every hour you train, deduct 1 MET (your weight in kilograms). This basically represents your resting metabolic rate.

For example, to determine how many calories you would have burned if you had just rested instead of trained, take your weight in kilograms and multiply it by the number of hours spent training. If the 154-pound (70 kg) athlete spent two hours exercising, we would multiply 70 kg by 2, which equals 140 calories. Then, once we figure in step 3 that his exercise expenditure was 700 calories for the two hours spent training, we subtract the 140 calories from this, for a total of 560. Therefore, two hours of training increases this athlete's daily caloric needs by 560, not 700 calories. For you, fill in the following based on this example:

_____ (total caloric expenditure from step 3) − _____ resting calories (weight in kg x hours spent training) = _____ NET calories burned while training

STEP 4: CALCULATE YOUR TOTAL DAILY CALORIC NEEDS

Now you will use all your calculations from steps 1 to 4 to determine your total caloric needs for a day. To do this, take your calories for daily living (BMR × 1.2 or 1.3) and add additional calories burned through exercise to get the number of calories needed to maintain your weight and support your training.

For example, using the quick method, a 154-pound (70 kg) athlete's caloric needs would be figured like this:

154 lb x 11 calories per pound (for a male) = 1,694 calories for basal metabolic rate

Next, multiply this by his activity factor to get his calories for daily living (activity without exercise):

1,694 calories x 1.3 = 2,202 calories

Then, assuming the athlete trains two hours at a MET level of 5 METs, you figure out the number of calories expended during training and subtract resting calories to determine the number of training calories the athlete needs in addition to his calories for daily living:

70 x 5 METs = 350 x 2 hr = 700 calories expended during training

700 − 140 resting calories (1 MET [wt. in kg] x 2 hr) = 560 calories for daily living

And, finally, you add the number of calories for daily living to the number of calories for training to get the total number of calories the athlete needs per day:

2,202 + 560 = 2,762 total calories per day

Macronutrient Needs by Sport

SPORT	MACRONUTRIENTS		
	Carbohydrate	Protein	Fat
Baseball and softball	Pitchers and catchers: 6-8 g/kg; fielders: 5-7 g/kg (50-60% total calories)	1.2-1.7 g/kg (12-20% total calories)	1.0 g/kg (<30% total calories)
Basketball	Low intensity: 5-7 g/kg; high intensity: 8-10 g/kg	1.4-1.7 g/kg	Balance to fill caloric needs (25-35% total calories)
Cross-country skiing	Light workout: 5-7 g/kg; moderate: 7-10 g/kg; high intensity or 2 sessions/day: 10-12+ g/kg	Low and moderate intensity: 1.2-1.6 g/kg; high intensity: 1.2-2.0 g/kg	Low intensity: 1.0 g/kg; moderate intensity: 1.4 g/kg; high intensity: 1.5-2.0 g/kg
Cycling	Moderate intensity: 6-8 g/kg; high intensity or long endurance: 8-10+ g/kg (65% total calories)	1.2-1.7 g/kg	Balance to fill caloric needs
Figure skating	5-8 g/kg (50-55% total calories)	1.2-1.8 g/kg	At least 1.0 g/kg (20-30% total calories)
Football	Training camp: 8-10 g/kg (lower end for linemen); in-season: 5-8 g/kg (lower end linemen); off-season/light training: 4-6 g/kg	1.4-1.8 g/kg	<35% total calories
Gymnastics	5-8 g/kg (60-65% total calories)	1.2-1.8 g/kg	At least .8-1.0 g/kg (20-25% total calories)
Ice hockey	8-10 g/kg (60-65% total calories)	1.4-1.7 g/kg	Balance to fill caloric needs (20-35% total calories)
Martial arts	5-8 g/kg	1.2-1.7 g/kg	20-30% total calories
Rowing (crew)	5-7 g/kg	1.2-1.7 g/kg	1.0 g/kg; more if necessary to meet caloric needs
Running	Low intensity under 60 min: 5-6 g/kg; low to moderate intensity over 60 min: 6-10 g/kg; high intensity: 7-10 g/kg, 10 g/kg or more long distance	1.2-1.8 g/kg	.8-2.0 g/kg (depends on calorie needs)
Soccer	8-10 g/kg (60-65% total calories)	1.4-1.7 g/kg	<30% total calories
Swimming	Racing: 5-8 g/kg; endurance: 8-10+ g/kg	1.2-1.7 g/kg	Balance to meet caloric needs
Tennis	Training: 5-8 g/kg; tournament play and frequent matches: 8-10 g/kg	1.2-1.7 g/kg	At least 1.0 g/kg; more if necessary to meet caloric needs
Track and field	Jumpers and throwers: 5-8 g/kg; sprinters: 100-400 m: 6-8 g/kg; 800+ m: 5-7 g/kg; multiple events: 7-10 g/kg	1.2-1.7 g/kg	1.0 g/kg; more if necessary to meet caloric needs
Volleyball	7-10 g/kg (60-65% total calories)	1.2-1.7 g/kg	20-30% total calories
Wrestling	5-8 g/kg	1.2-1.8 g/kg, higher end when cutting weight	Balance to meet caloric needs

Note: kg = weight in pounds / 2.2; also note that protein intake may be higher to meet larger athlete's calorie needs.

Adapted from C.A. Rosenbloom, 2000; American Dietetic Association, 2006, and N.L. Meyer, S. Parker-Simmons, and J.M. Erbacher, n.d.

C

Carbohydrate, Protein, and Fat Grams of Selected Foods

CARBOHYDRATE

The following table lists the carbohydrates in specific foods by category.

FOOD	SERVING SIZE	GRAMS	FOOD	SERVING SIZE	GRAMS
Breakfast cereals			**Grains, Pasta, Starch (cont'd)**		
Granola	1/4 cup	18	English muffin	One muffin	25
Raisin Bran	1 cup	45	Pancakes (4")	2 cakes	30
Shredded Wheat	1 cup	40	Pita bread (8")	1 piece	44
Cheerios	1 cup	20	Bran muffin	1 medium (4oz)	60
Grapenuts	1/4 cup	23	Bagel	4 oz	60
Cornflakes	1 cup	24	**Beverages**		
Oatmeal	1 cup cooked	30	Sports drink	8 oz	14-15
Fruits			Milk	8 oz	12
Apple	1 medium	20	Beer	12-oz can	13
Orange	1 medium	20	Chocolate milk	8 oz	25
Banana	6"	23	Orange juice	8 oz	30
Pear	1 medium	25	Apple juice	8 oz	30
Raisins	(1.5-oz box)	34	Cranberry juice	8 oz	34
Dried apricots	8 halves	18	Cola	12-oz can	40
Vegetables			**Entrees, Convenience foods**		
Zucchini	1/2 cup	4	Sushi (California roll)	6 pieces	45
Broccoli	1 stalk (1 cup)	10	Split-pea soup	1 bowl, 12 oz	42
Green beans	1/2 cup	5	Cheese pizza, NY-style slice		65
Carrot	1 medium 7"	7	Chili	1 cup	30
Peas	1/2 cup	10	Bean burrito		50
Tomato sauce	1/2 cup	14	**Sweets**		
Corn	1/2 cup	18	Fig Newton	1 cookie	11
Grains, Pasta, Starch			Chocolate chip cookie	1 cookie	10
Submarine sandwich roll	8" in length	60	Oreo	1 cookie	8
Rice	1 cup, cooked	45	Toaster pastry, blueberry	1	35
Sweet potato	1 large	37	Maple syrup	2 tbsp	30
Spaghetti noodles	1 cup, cooked	45	Soft serve ice cream	1 cup	40

PROTEIN

Each food in the following table is listed in one-ounce portions which equal 7 grams of protein. To find out the amount of protein in your portion of any of the following foods, simply multiply your portion in ounces by 7.

Very Lean Meat (0-1 g fat; 35 calories)	Lean Meat (2-3 g fat; 55 calories)	Medium Fat Meat (4-5 g fat; 75 calories)	High Fat Meat (8 g fat; 100 calories)
Chicken or turkey (white meat, no skin)	Beef roast (rib, chuck, rump, round)	Prime grades of beef trimmed of fat	Pork spare rib
Cornish hen (no skin)	Steak (T-bone, porterhouse, cubed)	Meatloaf	Ground pork
Buffalo	Flank steak	Corned beef	Pork sausage
Venison	Tenderloin	Short rib	Bologna
Clams	Ground round beef	Ground beef	Salami
Crab	Sirloin	Top loin pork	Bratwurst
Shrimp	Lamb (roast, chop, leg)	Pork chop	Knockwurst
Scallops	Chicken or turkey (dark meat, no skin)	Lamb rib roast	Italian sausage
Lobster	Chicken (white meat with skin)	Ground lamb	Hot dog (unless otherwise noted)
Tuna (fresh or canned in water)	Herring	Veal cutlet	Bacon
Lox (smoked salmon)	Oysters (6 medium)	Chicken (dark meat, with skin)	Regular cheeses (American, Cheddar, Swiss, Monterey Jack)
Trout	Salmon* (fresh or canned)	Ground turkey or chicken	
Halibut	Sardines (canned)	Fried chicken (with skin)	
Cod	Tuna, fresh (canned in oil, drained)	Any fried fish product	
Flounder	Rabbit	Egg (1)	
Eggs whites (2)	Turkey pastrami	Soy Milk (1 cup)	
Cheeses, nonfat or low-fat cottage cheese, fat-free cheese (1/4 cup)	Low-fat cheese, 3 g fat/oz, 2 tbsp grated parmesan cheese	Tempeh* (1/4 cup)	
Beans, peas, and lentils, count as both protein and starch (1/2 cup)	Duck and pheasant (no skin)	Tofu* (4 oz or 1/2 cup)	
Haddock, whiting, Cornish hen		Cheeses, feta, mozzarella, ricotta or any with 5 grams or less per oz	

*Although the fat is a healthy fat

FAT

The quantity of each item in the following table provides approximately 5 grams of fat.

Monounsaturated fats	
Almonds	6
Avocado	2 Tablespoons or 1 ounce
Cashews	6
Macadamia nuts	3
Nut butters: peanut, almond, cashew	1 1/2 Tablespoons
Oils: canola, olive	1 teaspoon
Olives	8 black large or 10 green
Peanuts	10
Pecans	4 halves
Pistachios	16
Polyunsaturated fats	
Margarine, low fat	2 Tablespoons
Margarine: stick, tub	1 teaspoon
Mayonnaise	1 Tablespoon
Oil: corn, cottonseed, soybean, flaxseed, safflower, sunflower	1 Tablespoon
Salad dressing	1 Tablespoon
Salad dressing, low fat	2 Tablespoons
Seeds: flax, pumpkin, sunflower	1 Tablespoon
Walnuts	4 halves
Saturated fats	
Bacon	1 slice
Butter, stick	1 teaspoon
Butter, whipped	2 teaspoons
Cream cheese	1 Tablespoon
Cream, heavy	1 Tablespoon
Cream, half and half	2 Tablespoons
Cream, whipped	2 Tablespoons
Oil: coconut, palm	1 teaspoon
Sour cream	2 Tablespoons
Sour cream, reduced fat	3 Tablespoons

D

Meal and Snack Ideas

800- to 900-Calorie Meal Ideas

5 oz (150 g) grilled chicken dark meat/no skin	Tomato and cucumber salad, 1 cup
2 tbsp barbeque sauce	2 oz (60 g) biscuit + 1 pat butter
6 in (15 cm) corn on the cob	1/2 cup low-fat frozen yogurt
Approximately 820 calories (83 g carbohydrate, 50 g protein, 32 g fat)	

1 cup brown rice	4 oz (125 g) roast turkey breast
1 cup kidney beans	1/2 cup sauteed spinach
1 tbsp canola oil for cooking	Small strawberry tart
Approximately 880 calories (103 g carbohydrate, 57 g protein, 22 g fat)	

1 cup angel hair pasta	1 cup broccoli with 2 tbsp grated parmesan
1/4 cup pesto sauce	1/2 cup sorbet
6 oz (175 g) shrimp	
Approximately 815 calories (85 g carbohydrate, 58 g protein, 27 g fat)	

5 oz (150 g) lean beef for kebabs	3 tbsp grilling sauce
2 cups vegetables: mushrooms, peppers, zucchini, cherry tomatoes	2 small brownies, 2 in square
1 1/2 cups couscous	
Approximately 875 calories (109 g carbohydrate, 49 g protein, 27 g fat)	

5 oz (150 g) pork tenderloin	3 tbsp cheddar cheese sauce
6 oz (175 g) baked sweet potato	1/2 cup sweetened applesauce
1 cup cauliflower	2 oz (60 g) corn muffin
Approximately 840 calories (92 g carbohydrate, 45 g protein, 32 g fat)	

1/2 block firm tofu	1 1/2 cups rice
2 cups vegetables: peppers, water chestnuts, mushrooms, onion, celery, carrots, pea pods	1/2 cup fresh pineapple
1 tbsp peanut oil	
Approximately 825 calories (104 g carbohydrate, 39 g protein, 28 g fat)	

5 oz (150 g) broiled salmon	1 pat butter
1 cup wild rice	Baked apple with 1 T brown sugar
1 cup sugar snap peas	1/2 cup low-fat frozen yogurt
Approximately 850 calories (106 g carbohydrate, 47 g protein, 26 g fat)	

600- to 700-Calorie Meal Ideas

Bowl black bean soup/12 oz	1/4 cup hummus
6 in (15 cm) pita bread	1 cup raw vegetables: carrots, cucumber, tomato, peppers
Approximately 630 calories (104 g carbohydrate, 29 g protein, 11 g fat)	

12 oz (350 g) vegetarian chili	8 oz (250 g) baked potato
2 tbsp shredded cheddar cheese	Medium orange
Approximately 625 calories (116 g carbohydrate, 24 g protein, 7 g fat)	

10 in (25 cm) wrap	1 cup baby carrots
4 oz (125 g) tuna	1/2 cup sweetened applesauce
1 tbsp mayonnaise	4 oz (120 ml) grapefruit juice
Lettuce, tomato, sliced peppers (1 1/2 cups)	
Approximately 635 calories (86 g carbohydrate, 35 g protein, 16 g fat)	

Bowl chicken noodle soup, 12 oz + 4 saltines	2 slices rye bread
4 oz (125 g) ham	1 cup cucumber and tomato salad
1 oz (30 g) Swiss cheese	1 cup seedless grapes
Approximately 635 calories (75 g carbohydrate, 50 g protein, 15 g fat)	

1 1/2 cups vegetables: broccoli, carrots, peppers, pea pods, onion, mushroom	1 tbsp peanut oil
4 oz (125 g) chicken breast	1 cup brown rice
2 tbsp Thai peanut sauce	
Approximately 650 calories (62 g carbohydrate, 44 g protein, 25 g fat)	

1 1/2 cups pasta	Garden salad 2 cups
3/4 cup meat sauce	1 tbsp Italian salad dressing
2 tbsp grated Parmesan cheese	
Approximately 620 calories (79 g carbohydrate, 35 g protein, 18 g fat)	

Whole-wheat roll	Sauteed onions
4 oz (125 g) lean turkey burger	1 oz (30 g) Baked! Lay's potato chips
1 tbsp ketchup	8 dried apricot halves
Approximately 680 calories (107 g carbohydrate, 34 g protein, 13 g fat)	

500-Calorie Breakfast Ideas

1 cup cooked oatmeal	7 walnut halves
1 cup nonfat milk	8 oz (240 ml) orange juice
2 tbsp raisins	
Approximately 520 calories (85 g carbohydrate, 16 g protein, 13 g fat)	

1/2 cup Grape-Nuts cereal	7 pecan halves, chopped
6 oz (175 g) nonfat vanilla yogurt	4 oz (120 ml) apple juice
1/2 cup blueberries	
Approximately 520 calories (96 g carbohydrate, 16 g protein, 8 g fat)	

1 English muffin	large banana, 8 in
1 tbsp peanut butter	1 cup 1% chocolate milk
Approximately 510 calories (85 g carbohydrate, 16 g protein, 12 g fat)	

1 cup Kashi GoLean cereal	1 egg
1 cup nonfat milk	1 slice toast whole grain
Medium peach	1 tsp butter
Approximately 515 calories (72 g carbohydrate, 30 g protein, 12 g fat)	

3/4 cup granola	2 tbsp raisins
1 cup nonfat Greek yogurt	
Approximately 500 calories (78 g carbohydrate, 27 g protein, 9 g fat)	

1 scrambled egg	10 in (25 cm) tortilla
1/2 cup kidney beans	12 oz (240 ml) grapefruit juice
2 tbsp salsa	
Approximately 500 calories (83 g carbohydrate, 20 g protein, 10 g fat)	

2 toaster waffles	3/4 cup cottage cheese, low fat
2 tbsp syrup	1/2 cup blueberries
1 tsp butter	
Approximately 525 calories (75 g carbohydrate, 25 g protein, 14 g fat)	

300- to 400-Calorie Breakfast Ideas

2 eggs, scrambled	1 oz (30 g) cheddar cheese
2-3 tbsp salsa	4 oz (120 ml) apple juice
6-in (15 cm) flour tortilla	
Approximately 400 calories (29 g carbohydrate, 24 g protein, 21 g fat)	

1 cup cooked oatmeal	2 tbsp raisins
1 cup nonfat milk	2 tbsp chopped walnuts
Approximately 400 calories (61 g carbohydrate, 15 g protein, 13 g fat)	

1 English muffin	Small banana
1 tbsp peanut butter	1 cup nonfat milk
Approximately 400 calories (64 g carbohydrate, 16 g protein, 9 g fat)	

1/2 cup Grape-Nuts cereal	1/2 cup fresh blueberries
6 oz (175 g) nonfat vanilla yogurt	
Approximately 395 calories (83 g carbohydrate, 13 g protein, 1 g fat)	

1 cup 1% cottage cheese	2 toaster waffles
1 cup sliced strawberries	
Approximately 390 calories (48 g carbohydrate, 32 g protein, 8 g fat)	

6 oz (175 g) flavored nonfat Greek yogurt	2 granola bars (Nature Valley)
Approximately 320 calories (49 g carbohydrate, 18 g protein, 6 g fat)	

2 4-in (10 cm) pancakes	3 slices turkey bacon
1 tbsp maple syrup	4 oz (120 ml) orange juice
Approximately 350 calories (58 g carbohydrate, 12 g protein, 8 g fat)	

200- to 500-Calorie Snack Ideas

2 graham crackers	8 oz (240 ml) nonfat milk
2 tbsp peanut butter	
Approximately 405 calories (40 g carbohydrate, 18 g protein, 19 g fat)	
Mini bagel or 1/2 deli bagel (2 oz; 60 g)	1/4 cup shredded mozzarella cheese
1/4 cup marinara sauce	
Approximately 290 calories (37 g carbohydrate, 13 g protein, 10 g fat)	
Frozen burrito	8 oz (240 ml) cranberry juice
Approximately 405 calories (74 g carbohydrate, 9 g protein, 8 g fat)	
1/3 cup hummus	1 cup raw vegetables: carrots, peppers, celery
6-in (15 cm) pita, cut into pieces	
Approximately 325 calories (50 g carbohydrate, 16 g protein, 7 g fat)	
1/4 cup granola	6 oz (175 g) low-fat plain yogurt
Approximately 195 calories (30 g carbohydrate, 12 g protein, 3 g fat)	
1/4 cup guacamole	2 oz (60 g) baked tortilla chips
1/4 cup salsa	
Approximately 390 calories (57 g carbohydrate, 7 g protein, 15 g fat)	
1/2 cup chocolate pudding	8 Nilla wafer cookies
Approximately 280 calories (45 g carbohydrate, 2 g protein, 10 g fat)	
4-in (10 cm) oatmeal cookie	8 oz (240 ml) nonfat milk
Approximately 200 calories (29 g carbohydrate, 9 g protein, 5 g fat)	
1 cup Honey Bunches of Oats cereal	1 cup 1% milk
Approximately 225 calories (37 g carbohydrate, 10 g protein, 4 g fat)	
3 oz (90 g) can tuna	6 Triscuit crackers
2 tsp mayonnaise	
Approximately 230 calories (19 g carbohydrate, 23 g protein, 7 g fat)	
Large hard-boiled egg	Kashi TLC crackers, 15 pieces
Approximately 195 calories (22 g carbohydrate, 9 g protein, 8 g fat)	
Low-fat apple muffin (Dunkin' Donuts)	8 oz (240 ml) nonfat milk
Approximately 515 calories (106 g carbohydrate, 16 g protein, 3 g fat)	
Medium apple	2 oz (60 g) cheddar cheese
Approximately 320 calories (25 g carbohydrate, 14 g protein, 18 g fat)	
Large banana, 8 in	2 tbsp peanut butter
Approximately 320 calories (36 g carbohydrate, 8 g protein, 16 g fat)	
1/2 cup kidney beans	1 cup pasta
1/2 cup chopped raw carrots and peppers	1 tbsp Italian dressing
Approximately 390 calories (68 g carbohydrate, 16 g protein, 6 g fat)	

E

Preexercise and Recovery Fuel

PREEXERCISE FUEL

As a general rule, the closer food is taken to training, the purer in carbohydrate it should be. Given more time (1 hour or more), it's fine to include some protein and a small amount of fat, and the snack may be larger. These are suggestions for foods to have at the times indicated before training; you can substitute similar favorite foods. Athletes fueling 2-3 hours ahead may also need another snack immediately or 15-30 minutes before. For larger athletes or those needing more fuel than listed below (for heavy or extended workouts), timing of carbohydrate intake may also be as follows: 4 g/kg four hours before; 3 g/kg three hours before; 2 g/kg two hours before; and 1 g/kg one hour before the start of training. Remember to hydrate on schedule 3, 2, and 1 hour and 30 minutes before.

Time before	Amount of food and sources	Amount of fluid
2-3 hr	**300-400 calories; mixed sources** 2 slices bread + 2 slices turkey + 1 slice cheese 4 oz (125 g) bagel + 1 tbsp each cream cheese and jelly English muffin + 1 tbsp peanut butter + small banana 2 eggs + 2 slices toast with jam Frozen burrito + 6 oz (180 ml) juice 1/4 cup trail mix/+ 8 oz (240 ml) cranberry juice 2 slices reduced-fat cheese + tomato melted on 2 slices bread Low-fat muffin + 8 oz (240 ml) low-fat milk 2 toaster waffles + 2 tbsp maple syrup Larabar + 12 oz (360 ml) cranberry juice	12-20 oz (360-600 ml)
2 hr	**Up to 300 calories; mixed sources** 1 cup Low-fat fruit yogurt + 1 cup apple juice English muffin + 1 tbsp peanut butter 2 slices bread + 2 slices turkey + lettuce, tomato, mustard Low-fat muffin (e.g., blueberry, cranberry) 1/2 cup low-fat granola + 6 oz (175 g) nonfat vanilla yogurt 6 in (15 cm) pita + 1/3 cup hummus English muffin + 2 slices cheese 4 oz (125 g) cinnamon raisin bagel Clif Bar Large sweet potato topped with 1/2 cup Greek nonfat yogurt 10 oz (300 ml) yogurt smoothie (Stoneyfield Farm) 10 oz (300 ml) Carnation Breakfast Essentials	12-20 oz (360-600 ml)

Time before	Amount of food and sources	Amount of fluid
1-2 hr	**Up to 200 calories; carbohydrate (up to 50 g)** 1 small bowl low-fiber cereal + skim milk (e.g., Corn Flakes, Rice Krispies, Crispix, Corn Chex, Rice Chex) Homemade fruit smoothie: 1 cup low-fat yogurt + 1/2 cup berries 1 original PowerBar 1 cup of noodles + 1 tbsp grated Parmesan cheese 1/2 peanut butter and jelly sandwich Kashi TLC bar + 8 oz (240 ml) sports drink 2 Nature Valley granola bars Small boxes raisins + 8 oz (240 ml) sports drink 6 oz (175 g) low-fat fruited yogurt Mini bagel + 1 tbsp jam Apple + mozzarella stick 1 packet flavored oatmeal + 1 clementine 1 packet flavored cream of wheat + 1 cup nonfat milk	10-20 oz (300-600 ml)
15-30 min	**Up to 100 calories; carbohydrate (up to 25 g)** 1/2 cup applesauce 1 slice toast + 2 tsp jam 1 packet instant cream of wheat, plain 6 in (15 cm) banana Wedge of cantaloupe 3 tbsp raisins (small handful) 1 Nutri-Grain bar 1 Clif Kid ZBar Gatorade Prime 01* 1 sports gel 16 oz (480 ml) sports drink 2 fig bars 1 low-fat granola bar 3/4 cup dry cereal: cinnamon Life, flavored Cheerios, Crispix, Rice Chex, or Corn Chex 7-8 saltine crackers 7-10 pretzel twists	7-10 oz (210-300 ml)
Immediately before	**Up to 60 calories; carbohydrate (up to 15 g)** 1 slice bread 1 rice cake 7-8 mini rice cakes Medium orange 1 cup melon 10 animal crackers 6 large jelly beans 1/4 bagel 1/2 sports gel 1/2 cup canned peaches, fruit cocktail, or pineapple in juice 8 oz (240 ml) sports drink	

*For strength athletes, Gatorade Recover 03 works as a pretraining fuel (16 g protein; 14 g carbohydrate; 130 calories)

RECOVERY FUEL

Recovery beginning within 15 minutes to one hour after activity helps prepare you for your next workout. To meet your recovery needs, here are some steps to take:

1. See the following table to determine recovery needs based on your type of training and intensity.
2. Next, find your weight in the first column of the following table, and follow the row across to find the grams of protein and minimum carbohydrate you need.

lb (kg)	Protein (g)	Carbohydrate (g)			
	.1-.25 g/kg	.7 g/kg	1.0 g/kg	1.2 g/kg	1.5 g/kg
100 (45)	5-11	32	45	54	68
105 (48)	5-12	34	48	54	72
110 (50)	5-13	35	50	60	75
115 (52)	5-13	36	52	62	78
120 (55)	6-14	39	55	66	83
125 (57)	6-14	40	57	68	86
130 (59)	6-15	41	59	71	89
135 (61)	6-15	43	61	73	92
140 (64)	6-16	45	64	77	96
145 (66)	7-17	46	66	79	99
150 (68)	7-17	48	68	82	102
155 (70)	7-18	49	70	84	105
160 (73)	7-18	51	73	88	110
165 (75)	7-19	53	75	90	113
170 (77)	8-19	54	77	92	116
175 (80)	8-20	56	80	96	120
180 (82)	8-21	57	82	98	123
185 (84)	8-21	59	84	101	126
190 (86)	9-22	60	86	103	129
195 (89)	9-22	62	89	107	134
200 (91)	9-23	64	91	109	137
205 (93)	9-23	65	93	112	140
210 (95)	10-24	67	95	114	143
215 (98)	10-25	69	98	118	147
220 (100)	10-25	70	100	120	150
225 (102)	10-26	71	102	122	153
230 (105)	11-26	74	105	125	158
235 (107)	11-27	75	107	128	161
240 (109)	11-27	76	109	131	164
250 (114)	11-29	80	114	137	171
260 (118)	12-30	83	118	142	177
275 (125)	13-31	88	125	150	188
300 (136)	14-34	95	136	163	204

3. After you determine your protein and carbohydrate recovery needs, choose a recovery snack from our suggestions in the following table. This table contains beverages and foods that provide both protein and carbohydrate (we call this your base recovery snack), however, you may need to add more carbohydrates to meet your individual need (see step 4).

FOODS	MACRONUTRIENT AMOUNT		
	Carbohydrate (g)	Protein (g)	Fat (g)
Boost (8 oz; 240 ml)	40	10	4
Carnation Instant Breakfast Essentials	40	13	5
Cheribundi/CherryPharm Natural Recovery (8 oz; 240 ml)	30	8	0
Chocolate milk, low fat (12 oz) 16 oz 20 oz	39 52 65	12 16 20	4 5 7
Clif Bar (2.4 oz; 68 g)	45	10	3
Cold cuts: turkey, ham, roast beef, 1 oz 30 g	0	7	0-2
Cottage cheese, plain 1/2 cup low-fat	3	14	1
Cottage cheese, pineapple, low-fat 1 cup	32	24	2
Cheese, American, cheddar, Swiss 1 oz	0	7	8
Chicken breast, 1 oz. 30 g	0	7	1
Dannon Frusion Smoothie (10 oz; 300 ml)	35	5	2.5
EAS Whey Protein powder (1 scoop) and orange juice (8 oz; 240 ml)	32	23	2
Edensoy Vanilla soy milk (8.45 oz; 250 ml)	25	7	3
Egg, hard boiled	0	6	5
Egg, white only	0	4	0
Endurox (2 scoops)	53	13	1
Gatorade Nutrition Bar	47	10	5
Gatorade Nutrition Shake	54	20	8
Gatorade Recover 03	14	16	0
Greek yogurt, fruited non-fat (6 oz; 175 g)	21	14	0
Isopure Plus (8 oz; 240 ml)	33	15	0
Jerky, beef or turkey (1 oz)	0	14	1
Lactaid milk (8 oz)	13	8	2.5
Muscle Milk (11 oz; 330 ml)	9	21	11
Myoplex Lite Bar (1.9 oz; 54 g)	20	20	2
Myoplex Strength Formula RTD (14 oz; 420 ml)	23	25	2.5
Nonfat dry milk, 3 tbsp	13	9	0
Peanut butter and jelly sandwich	45	12	18
ProMax bar (2.5 oz; 75 g)	38	20	5
Soy milk, chocolate 8 oz; 240 ml)	23	5	3
Soy milk, plain 1 cup	8	7	4
Soy yogurt, fruit, (6 oz.; 175 g)	29	4	2
Stonyfield Farm Smoothie (10 oz; 300 ml)	44	10	3
Whey protein powder: EAS vanilla (1 scoop)	0	23	0
Whey protein powder: BiPro, unflavored (1 scoop)	0	20	0
Yogurt, fruit on bottom, low-fat (6 oz; 175 g)	28	6	1
Yogurt, plain, nonfat (6 oz; 175 g)	13	10	0
Yogurt, vanilla, nonfat (6 oz)	28	7	0

4. Add additional carbohydrates from quickly digested sources. The following list provides suggestions; you can choose similar favorite foods, just check food labels to be sure you are taking in sufficient carbohydrate along with your protein.

FOOD	CARBOHYDRATE (G)
Breads, cereals, starches	
Deli bagel, large	60
Pretzels (2 oz bag)	46
Quaker Oatmeal-To-Go, bar	43
Baked potato, medium (6 oz)	36
Super Pretzel	34
Honey Nut Cheerios (1 cup)	30
Nature's Valley granola bar (2)	29
Instant oatmeal (1 packet)	27
Fig Newton bar	26
Corn flakes (1 cup)	24
Animal crackers (12)	23
Rice cakes (8 mini)	15
Graham crackers (1 sheet)	11
Fruit and juices	
Grape juice (11 oz)	60
Orange juice (16 oz)	60
Fruit cocktail (1 cup)	36
Cranberry juice (8 oz)	34
Dried pineapple (1/3 cup)	34
Dried cranberries (1 oz)	25
Applesauce, sweetened (1/2 cup)	25
Orange, medium	20
Melon (1 cup)	15
ZICO coconut water (11 oz)	15
Kiwi, medium	11
Sports products and sugars	
Clif Nectar bar	48
Powerbar gel	27
Jelly beans (10)	26
Clif Shot Bloks	24
Edy's Fruit Bars	21
Honey (1 tbsp)	17
Popsicle Big Stick ice pops (1)	15
Jam (1 tbsp)	13
Fruit leather	12
Honey sticks or straws	5

If you prefer, you can make up your own combination of foods for your recovery snack. Just choose adequate protein based on your needs and then add the appropriate amount of carbohydrate you need:

Endurance	Strength and power	Stop and go
Light: not necessary **Moderate:** 0.7-1.0 g/kg carb; 0.1-0.2 g/kg protein **Heavy:** 1.0-1.5 g/kg carb; 0.1-0.2 g protein	**Light:** not necessary **Moderate:** 0.7 g/kg carb; 0.1-0.2 g/kg protein **Heavy:** 1.0 1.2 g/kg carb; 0.1-0.25 g/kg protein	**Light:** not necessary **Moderate:** 0.7-1g/kg carb; 0.2-0.2 g/kg protein **Heavy:** 1.0-1.5 g/kg carb; 0.1-0.2 g/kg protein

For example, a 200-lb (91 kg) strength and power athlete who trains moderately would need 0.1-0.2 g/kg protein and .7 g/kg carb, which equates to 9-18 g protein and at least 64 g carbohydrate. This athlete could have a Gatorade Recover 03 drink (14 g carbohydrate + 16 g protein) and a large bagel (60 g carbohydrate) for a total of 16 g protein and 74 g carb. Or, the athlete could have 16 oz chocolate milk (52 g carbohydrate + 16 g protein) and a small granola bar (18 g carbohydrate) for a total of 16 g protein and 70 g carbohydrate. Recovery doesn't end with one snack: In two hours, repeat or have a larger meal. Be sure to take in adequate protein and carbohydrate to meet your needs throughout the day.

Bibliography

Aagaard P. Making muscles "stronger": Exercise, nutrition, drugs. *J Musculoskel Neuron Interact* 2004; 4(2):165-174.

Achten J, Gleeson M, Jeukendrup AE. Determination of the exercise intensity that elicits maximal fat oxidation. *Med Sci. Sports Exerc*, 2002 34, (1):92-97.

Achten J, Halson SL , Moseley L, Rayson MP, Casey A, Jeukendrup AE. Higher dietary carbohydrate content during intensified running training results in better maintenance of performance and mood state. *J Appl Physiol* 2004; 96: 1331-1340.

Ainsworth B, Haskell A, Jacobs J, Montoye H, Sallis J, Paffenbarger R. Compendium of physical activities: classification of energy costs of human physical activities. *Med Sci Sports Exerc* 1993;25(1): 71-80.

Allen NE, Appleby PN, Davey GK, Kaaks R, Sabina Rinaldi S, Timothy J. Key T. The associations of diet with serum insulin-like growth factor and its main binding proteins in 292 women meat-eaters, vegetarians, and vegans. *Cancer Epidemiology, Biomarkers & Prevention* 2002;(.11) 1441-1448.

American College of Sports Medicine Roundtable on the physiological and health effects of oral creatine supplementation. *Med. Sci. Sports Exerc* 2000; 32(3): 706-717, 2000.

American Dietetic Association. 2006. *Sports nutrition: A practice manual for professionals*. 4th ed. Chicago: American Dietetic Association.

American Dietetic Association; Dietitians of Canada; American College of Sports medicine, Rodriguez NR, Di Marco NM, Langley S. American College of Sports Medicine position stand. Nutrition and athletic performance. *Med Sci Sports Exer* 2009 Mar; 41(3):709-31.

Anastasiou CA, Kavouras SA, Arnaoutis G, Gioxari A , Kollia M, Botoula E, Sidossis LS, Sodium replacement and plasma sodium drop during exercise in the heat when fluid intake matches fluid loss. *Journal of Athletic Training* 2009; 44(2):117-123.

Armstrong LE, Maresh CM, Gabaree CV, Hoffman JR, Kavouras SA, Kenefick RW, Castellani JW, Ahlquist LE. Thermal and circulatory responses during exercise: Effects of hypohydration, dehydration, and water Intake. *J Appl Physiol* 1997; 82(6): 2028-2035.

Aoi W, NaitoY, Yoshikawa T. Exercise and functional foods. *Nutrition Journal* 2006, 5:15.

Azevedo JL Jr, Tietz E, Two-Feathers T, Paull J, Chapman K. Lactate, fructose and glucose oxidation profiles in sports drinks and the effect on exercise performance. *PLoS One* 2007;2(9): e927.

Beelen M, Koopman R, Gijsen AP, Vandereyt H, Kies AK, Kuipers H, Saris WH, van Loon LJ. Protein coingestion stimulates-muscle protein synthesis during resistance-type exercise. *Am J Physiol Endocrinol Metab* 2008; 295: E70-E77.

Beelen M, Tieland M, Gijsen A, Vandereyt H, Kies A, Kuipers H, Saris W, Koopman R, vanLoon L. Coingestion of carbohydrate and protein hydrolysate during exercise in young men with no further increase In overnight recovery. *J of Nutrition;* Nov 2008; 138 (11) 2198-2204.

Beltrami FG, Hew-Butler T, Noakes TD. Drinking policies and exercise-associated hyponatraemia: Is anyone still promoting overdrinking? *Br J Sports Med* 2008;42;796-801;

Berardi JM, Price TB, Noreen EE, Lemon PW. Postexercise muscle glycogen recovery enhanced with a carbohydrate-protein supplement. *Med Sci Sports Exerc* 2006; (38) 6: 1106-1113.

Bergeron MF. Muscle cramps during exercise: Is it fatigue or electrolyte deficit? *Curr Sports Med Rep* 2008;(7) 4:S50-S55.

Bergeron M. Dehydration and thermal strain in junior tennis. *Amer J Lifestyle Med Lifestyle Medicine* 2009; 3(4): 320-325.

Berneis K, Ninnis R, Haüssinger D, Keller U. Effects of hyper- and hypoosmolality on whole body protein and glucose kinetics in humans. *Am J Physiol* 276 (*Endocrinol Metab* 1999; (39): E188-E195.

Berning J. The role of medium-chain triglycerides in exercise. *Intl J Sports Nutr* 1996; (6): 121-133.

Betts JA, Stevenson E, Williams C, Sheppard C, Grey E, Griffin J. Recovery of endurance running capacity: Effect of carbohydrate- protein mixtures. *IJSNEM* 2005; (15): 590-609.

Bilsborough S, Mann N. A review of issues of dietary protein intake in humans. *Intl J Sport Nutr and Exer Metab* 2006, 16, 129-152.

Binnert C, Pachiaudi C, Beylot M, Croset M, Cohen R, Riou JP, Laville M. Metabolic fate of an oral long-chain triglyceride load in humans. *Am J Physiol* 270 (Endocrinol. Metab. 33): E445-E450, 1996.

Biolo G, Williams BD, Fleming RYD. Wolfe RR. Insulin action on muscle protein kinetics and amino acid transport during recovery after resistance exercise. *Diabetes* 1999;48:949-957.

Bird SP, Tarpenning KM, Marino FE. Liquid carbohydrate/essential amino acid ingestion during a short-term bout of resistance exercise suppresses myofibrillar protein degradation. *Metabolsim* 2006; 55(5):570-7.

Bjelakovic G, Nikolova D, Gluud LL, Simonetti RG, Gluud C. Mortality in randomized trials of antioxidant supplements for primary and secondary prevention systematic review and meta-analysis. *JAMA* 2007;297(8):842-857.

Bjorclc I, Granfeldt Y, Liljeberg H, Tovar J, Asp NG. Food properties affecting the digestion and absorption of carbohydrates. *Amer J Clin Nutr* 1994; 59 (suppl) 699S-705S.

Bloom SR, Johnson RH, Park DM, Rennie MJ, Sulaiman WR. Differences in the metabolic and hormonal response to exercise between racing cyclists and untrained individuals *J Physiol* 1976; 258: 1-18.

Blomstrand E, Eliasson J, Karlsson HKR, Köhnke R. Branched-chain amino acids activate key enzymes in protein synthesis after physical exercise. *J Nutr* 2006;136: 269S-273S.

Boirie Y, Dangin M, Gachon P, Vasson MP, Maubois JL, Beaufrere B. Slow and fast dietary proteins differently modulate postprandial protein accretion. *Proc Natl Acad Sci USA* 1997;(94): 14930-14935.

Bolster DR, Pikosky MA, Gaine PC, Martin W, Wolfe RR, Tipton KD, Maclean D, Maresh CM, Rodriguez NR. Dietary protein intake impacts human skeletal muscle protein fractional synthetic rates after endurance exercise. *Am J Physiol Endocrinol Metab* 2005;(289): E678-E683.

Børsheim E, Aarsland A, Wolfe RR. Effect of an amino acid, protein, and carbohydrate mixture on net muscle protein balance after resistance exercise. *Intl J of Sport Nutr and Exer Metab* 2004;(14):249-265.

Bos C, Metges CC, Gaudichon C, Petzke KJ, Pueyo ME, Morens C, Everwand J, Benamouzig R, Tome D. Postprandial kinetics of dietary amino acids are the main determinant of their metabolism after soy or milk protein ingestion in humans. *J Nutr* 2006;(133): 1308-1315.

Bradley NS, Heigenhauser GJ, Roy BD, Staples EM, Inglis JG, LeBlanc PJ, Peters SJ. The acute effects of differential dietary fatty acids on human skeletal muscle pyruvate dehydrogenase activity. *J Appl Physiol* 2008;(104): 1-9.

Branch JD. Effect of creatine supplementation on body composition and performance: A meta-analysis. *Intnl J Sp Nutr Exerc Metab* 2003, (13):198-226.

Brown EC, DiSilvestro RA, Babaknia A, Devor ST. Soy versus whey protein bars: Effects on exercise training impact on lean body mass and antioxidant status. *Nutrition Journal* 2004, (3):22.

Buford TW, Kreider RB, Stout JR, Greenwood M, Campbell B, Spano M, Ziegenfuss T, Lopez H, Landis J, Antonio J. International Society of Sports Nutrition position stand: Creatine supplementation and exercise. *Journal of the International Society of Sports Nutrition* 2007;4:6.

Burd NA, Tang JE, Moore DR, Phillips SM. Exercise training and protein metabolism: influences of contraction, protein intake, sex-based differences. *J Appl Physiol* 2009;106: 1692-1701.

Burke LM. Caffeine and sports performance. *Appl Physiol Nutr Metab* 2008;(33): 1319-1334.

Burke LM, Kiens B. "Fat adaptation" for athletic performance: the nail in the coffin? *J Appl Physiol* 2006 (100): 7-8.

Burke LM, Angus DJ, Cox GR, Cummings NK, Febbraio MA, Gawthorn K, Hawley JA, Minehan M, Martin DT, Hargreaves M. Effect of fat adaptation and carbohydrate restoration on metabolism and performance during prolonged cycling. *J Appl Physiol* 2000;(89): 2413-2421.

Burke LM, Hawley JA. Effects of short-term fat adaptation on metabolism and performance of prolonged exercise. *Med. Sci. Sports Exerc* 2002;(34) 9: 1492-1498.

Burke LM, Kiens B, Ivy JL. Carbohydrates and fat for training and recovery. *Journal of Sports Sciences* 2004;(22):1:15-30.

Burke LM, Loucks AB, Broad N. Energy and carbohydrate for training and recovery. *Journal of Sports Sciences* 2006;(24):7:675-685.

Cameron-Smith D, Burke LM, Angus DJ, Tunstall RJ, Cox GR, Bonen A, Hawley JA, Hargreaves M. A short-term, high-fat diet up-regulates lipid metabolism and gene expression in human skeletal muscle. *Am J Clin Nutr* 2003;77:313-8.

Candow DG, Burke NC, Smith-Palmer T, Burke DG. Effect of whey and soy protein supplementation combined with resistance training in young adults. *Intl J Sport Nutr and Exer Metab* 2006; (16): 233-244.

Carey AL, Staudacher HM, Cummings NK, Stepto NK, Vasilis Nikolopoulos V, Burke LM, Hawley JA. Effects of fat adaptation and carbohydrate restoration on prolonged endurance exercise. *J Appl Physiol* 2001;(91): 115-122.

Casa DJ, Armstrong LE, Hillman SK, Montain SJ, Reiff RV Rich BSE, Roberts WO, Stone JA. National Athletic Trainers' Association position statement: Fluid replacement for athletes. *Journal of Athletic Training* 2000;35(2):212-224.

Casey A, Mann R, Banister K, Fox J, Morris PG, Macdonald IA, Greenhaff PL. Effect of carbohydrate ingestion on glycogen resynthesis in human liver and skeletal muscle, measured by 13C MRS. *Am J Physiol Endocrinol Metab* 2000;(278): E65-E75.

Casey A, Short AH, Hultman E, Greenhaff PL. Glycogen resynthesis in human muscle fibre types following exercise-induced glycogen depletion. *Journal of Physiology* 1995; 483(1): 265-271

Chandra R. Nutrition and the immune system: an introduction. *Amer J Clin Nutr* 1997: (66)460s-03S.

Chen Y, Wong HS, Wong C, LaM CW, Huanga Y, Siu MP. The effect of pre-exercise carbohydrate meal on immune responses to an endurance performance run *British Journal of Nutrition* 2008; (100): 1260-1268.

Christ ER, Zehnder M, Boesch C, Trepp R, Mullis PE, Diem P, De´combaz J. The effect of increased lipid intake on hormonal responses during aerobic exercise in endurance-trained men. *European Journal of Endocrinology* 2006;154(3) 397-403.

Civitarese AE, Hesselink MKC, Russell AP, Ravussin E, Schrauwen P. Glucose ingestion during exercise blunts exercise-induced gene expression of skeletal muscle fat oxidative genes. *Am J Physiol Endocrinol Metab* 2005;289: E1023-E1029.

Chambers E, Bridge M, Jones D. Carbohydrate sensing in the human mouth: Effects on exercise performance and brain activity. *J Physiol* 2009;587(8): 1779-1794.

Cheuvront SN, Sawka MN. Hydration assessment of athletes *Sports Science Exchange* Gatorade Sports Science Institute. 2005;(18) 2.

Christ ER, Zehnder M, Boesch C, Trepp R, Mullis PE, Diem P and De´combaz J. The effect of increased lipid intake on hormonal responses during aerobic exercise in endurance-trained men. *European Journal of Endocrinology* 2006; (154) 397-403.

Clark N. *Nancy Clark's food guide for marathoners.* 2007. Oxford: Meyer & Meyer.

Clark N. *Nancy Clark's food guide for new runners.* 2007. Maidenhead: Meyer & Myer.

Clarkson P, Thompson H. Antioxidants: What role do they play in physical activity and health? *Am J Clin Nutr* 2000;72(suppl):637S-46S.

Clarkson PM, Haymes EM. Exercise and mineral status of athletes: Calcium, magnesium, phosphorous and iron. *Med Sci Sport Exer* 1995; 27(6) 831-43.

Clarkson PM, Haymes EM. Trace mineral requirements for Athletes. *IJSN* 1994;4:104-119.

Collier G, McLean A, O'Dea K. Effect of co-ingestion of fat on the metabolic responses to slowly and rapidly absorbed carbohydrates. *Diabetologia* 1984; 26: 50-54.

Connolly DA, McHugh MP, Padilla-Zakour OI. Efficacy of a tart cherry juice blend in preventing the symptoms of muscle damage. *Br J Sports Med* 2006; 40:679-83.

Cooke MB, Rybalk E, Andrew D. Williams AD, Cribb PJ, Hayes A. Creatine supplementation enhances muscle force recovery after eccentrically-induced muscle damage in healthy individuals. *J Internl Soci of Sports Nutri* 2009; 6:13.

Costa RJS, Oliver SJ, Laing SJ, Walters R, Bilzon JLJ, Nel P, Walsh NP. Influence of timing of postexercise carbohydrate-protein ingestion on selected immune indices. *Intl J of Sport Nutri and Exer Metab* 2009; (19): 366-384.

Costill DL, Bowers R, Branam G, Sparks K. Muscle glycogen utilization during prolonged exerciseon successive days. *J Appl Physiol* 1971;31(6) : 834-838.

Costill DL, Sherman WM, Fink WJ, Maresh C, Witten M, Miller JM. The role of dietary carbohydrates in muscle glycogen resynthesis after strenuous running. *Amer J Clin Nutri* 1981;34: 1831-1836.

Cox GR, Desbrow B, Montgomery PG, Anderson ME, Bruce CR, Macrides TA, Martin DT, Moquin A, Roberts A, Hawley JA, Burke LM. Effect of different protocols of caffeine intake on metabolism and endurance performance. *J Appl Physiol* 2002;(93): 990-999.

Coyle EF. Substrate utilization during exercise in active people *Amer J Clin Nutr* 1995; 61 (Suppl) 968-79.

Coyle EF. Fat oxidation during whole body exercise appears to be a good example of regulation by the interaction of physiological systems. *J Physiol* 2007;581(3): 886

Coyle EF Physical activity as a metabolic stressor *Am J Clin Nutr* 2000;72(suppl):512S-20S.

Coyle EF. Fluid and fuel intake during exercise. *J Sports Sci* 2004, 22, 39-55.

Cribb PJ, Hayes A. Effects of supplement timing and resistance exercise on skeletal muscle hypertrophy. *Med Sci Sports Exerc* 2006; 38 (11): 1918-1925.

Cribb PJ, Williams AD, Carey MF, Hayes A. The effect of whey isolate and resistance training on strength, body composition, plasma glutamine. *Intern J Sport Nutrin and Exer Metab* 2006;16,:494-509.

Cribb PJ, Williams AD, Stathis CG, Carey MF, Hayes A. Effects of whey isolate, creatine, resistance training on muscle hypertrophy. *Med Sci Sports Exerc* 2007; 39 (2): 298-307.

Crozier PG, Cordain L, Sampson DA. Exercise induced changes in plasma vitamin B-6 concentrations do not vary with exercise intensity. *Amer J Clin Nutr* 1994;60:552-8.

Dangin M, Boirie Y, Guillet C, Beaufrere B. Influence of the protein digestion rate on protein turnover in young and elderly subjects. *J Nutr* 2002;(132):3228S-3233S.

Dangin M, Boirie Y, Garcia-Rodenas C, Gachon P, Fauquant J, Callier P, Ballvre O, Beaufrere B. The digestion rate of protein is an independent regulating factor of postprandial protein retention. *Am J Physiol Endocrinol Metab* 2001;280: E340-E348, 2001.

Davidson G, Gleeson M, Phillips S. Antioxidant Supplementation and Immunoendocrine Responses to Prolonged Exercise *Med Sci Sports Exer* 2007; 39(4): 645-652.

De Bock K, Derave W, Eijnde BO, Hesselink MK, Koninckx E, Rose AJ, Schrauwen P, Bonen A, Richter EA, Hespel P. Effect of training in the fasted state on metabolic responses during exercise with carbohydrate intake. *J Appl Physiol* 2008;104: 1045-1055.

De Bock K, Derave W, Ramaekers M, Richter EA, Hespel P. Fiber type-specific muscle glycogen sparing due to carbohydrate intake before and during exercise. *J Appl Physiol* 2007;102: 183-188.

DeMarco H, Sucher K, Cisar C, Butterfield, G. Pre-exercise carbohydrate meals: Application of glycemic index. *Med Sci Sports Exerc* 1999;31(1):164-170.

Dorgan JF, Judd JT, Longcope C, Brown C, Schatzkin A, Clevidence BA, Campbell WS, Nair PP, Franz C, Kahie L, Taylor PR. Effects of dietary fat and fiber on plasma and urine androgens and estrogens in men: A controlled feeding study. *Am J Clin Nutr* 1996;64:850-54.

Dougherty KA, Baker LB, Chow M, Kenney WL. Two percent dehydration impairs and six percent carbohydrate drink improves boys basketball skills. *Med Sci Sports Exerc* 2006; 38, (9);1650-1658.

Eberle SG. *Endurance Sports Nutrition* 2nd ed. 2007. Champaign, IL: Human Kinetics.

Erlenbusch M, Haub M, Munoz K, MacConnie, S, Stillwell B. Effect of high-fat or high-carbohydrate diets on endurance exercise: A meta-analysis. *Intl Journal Sport Nutrition and Exercise Metabolism* 2005; 15, 1-14.

Falk B, Bar-Or O, MacDougall JD. Thermoregulatory responses of pre-, mid-, and late pubertal boys to exercise in dry heat. *Med Sci Sports Exerc* 1992; 24(6): 688-694.

Febbraio MA, Stewart KL. CHO feeding before prolonged exercise: effect of glycemic index on muscle glycogenolysis and exercise performance. *J Appl Physiol* 1996;81(3): 1115-1120.

Fink HH, Burgoon LA, Mikesky AE. 2009. *Practical applications in sports nutrition*. 2nd ed. Sudbury, MA: Jones and Bartlett, 359.

Fitchett MA. Predictability of VO2 max from submaximal cycle ergometer and bench stepping tests. *Br J Sports Med* 1985;19;85-88.

Fontana L, Klein S, Holloszy JO. Long-term low-protein, low-calorie diet and endurance exercise modulate metabolic factors associated with cancer risk *Am J Clin Nutr* 2006;84:1456-62.

Foss ME and Keteyian SJ. 2005. *Fox's physiological basis for exercise and sport*. 6th ed. New York: McGraw-Hill.

Fujita S, Dreyer HC, Drummond MJ, Glynn EL, Volpi E, Rasmussen BB. Essential amino acid and carbohydrate ingestion before resistance exercise does not enhance postexercise muscle protein synthesis. *J Appl Physiol* 2009;106: 1730-1739.

Gaine PC, Pikosky MA, Bolster DR, Martin WF, Maresh CM, Rodriguez NR. Postexercise whole-body protein turnover response to three levels of protein intake. *Med Sci Sports Exerc* 2007; 39(3):480-486, 2007.

Galbo H. The hormonal response to exercise. *Proceedings of the Nutrition Society* 1985; 44: 257-266.

Gallagher PM, Carrithers JA, Godard MP, Schulze KE, Trappe SW. β-hydroxy-β-methylbutyrate ingestion, part I: Effects of strength and fat free mass. *Med Sc. Sports Exerc* 2000; 32(12): 2109-2115.

Ganio MS, Casa DJ, Armstrong LE, Maresh C. Evidence-based approach to lingering hydration questions. *Clin Sports Med* 2007;26: 1-16.

Garlick P. Assessment of the safety of glutamine and other amino acids. *J Nutr* 2001;131: 2556S-2561S.

Gellish RL, Goslin BR, Olson RE, McDonald A, Russi GD, Moudgil VK. Longitudinal modeling of the relationship between age and maximal heart rate. *Med Sci Sports Exerc* 2007;39(5): 822-829.

Gibala M. Protein metabolism and endurance exercise. *Sports Med* 2007;37 (4-5): 337-340.

Gibala M. Regulation of skeletal muscle amino acid metabolism during exercise. *IJSNEM* 2001;11: 87-108.

Gisolfi CV, Duchman SM. Guidelines for optimal replacement beverages for different athletic events. *Med Sci Sports Exerc* 1992;24(6); 679-687.

Glace BW, Murphy CA, McHugh MP. Food intake and electrolyte status of ultramarathoners competing in extreme heat. *J Amer Coll Nutr*, 2002;21(6): 553-559.

Gleeson M. Immune function in sport and exercise. *J Appl Physiol* 2007;103:693-699.

Gleeson M. Interrelationship between physical activity and branched-chain amino acids *J Nutr* 2005;35:1591S-1595S.

Gleeson M, Nieman DC, Pedersen, BK. Exercise, nutrition and immune function. *J Sport Sci* 2004;22(1):115-125.

Goedecke JH, Elmer-English R, Dennis SC, Schloss I, Noakes TD, Lambert EV. Effects of medium-chain triacylglycerol ingested with carbohydrate on metabolism and exercise performance. *Intl J Sports Nutr* 1999 (9) 35-47.

Gomez-Cabrera MC, Domenech E, Romagnoli M, Arduini A, Borras C, Pallardo FV, Juan Sastre, Vina J. Oral administration of vitamin C decreases muscle mitochondrial biogenesis and hampers training-induced adaptations in endurance performance *Am J Clin Nutr* 2008;87:142-9.

Graham T, Battram D, Dela F, El-Sohemy A, Thong F. Does caffeine alter muscle fat and carbohydrate metabolism during exercise? *Appl Phys Nutr Metab* 2008;33:1311-18.

Greenleaf JE. Problem: Thirst, drinking behavior, and involuntary dehydration. *Med Sci Sports Exerc* 1992; 24(6): 645-656.

Greenwood M, Kreider RB, Greenwood L, Byars A. Cramping and injury incidence in collegiate football players are reduced by creatine supplementation. *Journal of Athletic Training* 2003;38(3):216-219.

Greer BK, Woodard JL, White JP, Arguello EM, Haymes EM. Branched-chain amino acid supplementation and indicators of muscle damage after endurance exercise. *Intl J Sport Nutr and Exer Metab* 2007; (s17): 595-607.

Gropper SS, Smith JL, Groff JL. *Advanced Nutrition and Human Metabolism* 5th ed. 2009. Belmont, CA: Wadsworth.

Haff G, Koch A, Potteiger J, Kuphal K, Magee I, Green S, Jakicic J. Carbohydrate supplement attenuates muscle glycogen los during acute bouts of resistance exercise. *Intl J Sports Nutr Exer Metab* 2000; (10): 326-339.

Halson SL, Lancaster GI, Achten J, Gleeson M, Jeukendrup AE. Effects of carbohydrate supplementation on performance and carbohydrate oxidation after intensified cycling training. *J Appl Physiol* 2004;97: 1245-1253.

Hansen KC, Zhang Z, Gomez T, Adams AK, Schoeller DA. Exercise increases the proportion of fat utilization during short-term consumption of a high-fat diet. *Am J Clin Nutr* 2007;85:109 -16.

Harkey MR, Henderson GL, Gershwin ME, Stern JS, Hackman RM. Variability in commercial ginseng products: an analysis of 25 preparations. *Am J Clin Nutr* 2001;73:1101-6.

Hargreaves M, Costill D, Katz A, Fink W. Effect of fructose ingestion on muscle glycogen usage during exercise. *Med Sci. Sports Exer* 1985;17(3): 360-363.

Hargreaves M, Costill D, Fink W, King D, Fielding R. Effect of pre-exercise carbohydrate feedings on endurance cycling performance. *Med Sci. Sports Exer* 1987;19(1): 33-36.

Hargreaves M, Snow R. Amino acids and endurance exercise. *Intl J Sports Nutr & Exer Metab* 2001;(11):133-145.

Harrison M, Gorman DJ, McCaffrey N, Hamilton MT, Zderic TW, Carson BP, Moyna NM. Influence of acute exercise with and without carbohydrate replacement on postprandial lipid metabolism *J Appl Physiol* 2009;106(3):943-9.

Hartman J, Tang J, Wilkinson S, Tarnopolsky M, Lawrence R, Fullerton A, Phillips S. Consumption of fat-free fluid milk after resistance exercise promotes greater lean mass accretion than does consumption of soy or carbohydrate in young, novice, male weightlifters. *Am J Clin Nutr* 2007;86:373- 81.

Havemann L, West SJ, Goedecke JH, Macdonald IA, St Clair Gibson A, Noakes TD, Lambert EV. Fat adaptation followed by carbohydrate loading compromised high-intensity sprint performance. *J Appl Physiol* 2006;100: 194-202.

Hawley JA. Effect of increased fat availability on metabolism and exercise capacity. *Med. Sci. Sports Exerc* 2002; 34(9):1485-1491.

Hawley J, Dennis S, Noakes T. Carbohydrate, fluid, electrolyte requirements of the soccer player: A review. *Intl J Sports Nutr Exer Metab* 1994;(4): 221-236.

Heaney RP. Vitamin D in health and disease. *Clin J Am Soc Nephrol* 3 2008: 1535-1541.

Heath EM, Wilcox AR, Quinn CM. Effects of nicotinic acid on respiratory exchange ratio and substrate levels during exercise. *Med Sci Sports Exer* 1993; 25(9):1018-1023.

Helge JW. Long-term fat diet adaptation effects on performance, training capacity, and fat utilization. *Med Sci Sports Exerc* 2002; 34(9): 1499-1504.

Helge JW, Stallknecht B, Richter EA, Galbo H, Bente, Kien B. Muscle metabolism during graded quadriceps exercise in man *J Physiol* 2007;581(3): 1247-1258.

Hellsten Y, Skadhauge L, Bangsbo J. Effect of ribose supplementation on resynthesis of adenine nucleotides after intense intermittent training in humans. *Am J Physiol Regul Integr Comp Physiol* 2004;286: R182-R188.

Hew-Butler T, Almond CJ, Ayus C, Dugas J, Meeuwisse W, Noakes T, Reid S, Siegel A, Speedy D, Stuempfle K, Verbalis J, Weschler L. Consensus statement of the 1st International Exercise-Associated Hyponatremia Consensus Development Conference, Cape Town, South Africa 2005 *Clin J Sport Med* 2005;15(4);208-213.

Hew-Butler T, Verbalis JG, Noakes TD. Updated fluid recommendation: Position statement from the International Marathon Medical Directors Association (IMMDA). *Clin J Sport Med* 2006;16:283-292.

Hill AM, Worthley C, Murphy KJ, Buckley JD, Ferrante A, Howe PR. n-3 Fatty acid supplementation and regular moderate exercise: differential effects of a combined intervention on neutrophil function. *Br J Nutr.* 2007; 98(2):300-9.

Hoffman JR, Falvo MJ. Protein: Which is best? *Journal of Sports Science and Medicine* 2004;(3): 118-130.

Hoffman JR, Ratamess NA, Kang J, Falvo MJ, Faigenbaum AD. Effect of protein intake on strength, body composition and endocrine changes in strength/power athletes. *Journal of the International Society of Sports Nutrition* 2006;3(2): 12-18.

Hoffman JR, Ratamess NA, Kang J, Falvo MJ and Faigenbaum AD. Effects of protein supplementation on muscular performance and resting hormonal changes in college football players. *J of Sports Sci and Med* 2007;(6): 85-92

Hoffman JR, Ratamess NA, Tranchina CP, Stefanie L. Rashti SL Kang J, Faigenbaum AD. Effect of protein supplement timing on strength, power and body compositional changes in resistance-trained men. *IJSNEM* 2009;19(2):172-185.

Horton TJ, Grunwald GK, Lavely J, Donahoo WT. Glucose kinetics differ between women and men, during and after exercise. *J Appl Physiol* 2006;100: 1883-1894.

Horowitz JF, Coyle EF Metabolic responses to pre exercise meals containing various carbohydrates and fat. *Amer J Clin Nutr* 1993; (58): 235-41.

Horowitz JF, Klein S. Lipid metabolism during endurance exercise *Am J Clin Nutr* 2000;72(suppl):558S-63S

Horowitz JF, Mora-Rodriguez R, Byerley LO, Coyle EF. Substrate metabolism when subjects are fed carbohydrate during exercise. *Am J Physiol* 1999; 276 (*Endocrinol. Metab.* 39): E828-E835.

Horvath PJ, Eagen CK, Ryer-Calvin SD, B. Pendergast DR. The effects of varying dietary fat on the nutrient intake in male and female runners. *Journal of the American College of Nutrition* 2000; 19(1): 42-51.

Horvath PJ, Eagen CK, Fisher NM,. Leddy JJ, Pendergast DR. The effects of varying dietary fat on performance and metabolism in trained male and female runners. *Journal of the American College of Nutrition* 2000; 19(1):52-60.

Howarth KR, Moreau NA, Phillips SM, Gibala MJ. Co-ingestion of protein with carbohydrate during recovery from endurance exercise stimulates skeletal muscle protein synthesis in humans *J Appl Physiol* Apr 2009; 106: 1394-1402.

Howlett K, Febbraio M, Hargreaves M. Glucose production during strenuous exercise in humans: role of epinephrine. *Am J Physiol* 1999;276 (*Endocrinol Metab* 39): E1130-E1135.

Hulston CJ, Jeukendrup AE. Substrate metabolism and exercise performance with caffeine and carbohydrate intake. *Med. Sci. Sports Exerc* 2008; 40(12): 2096-2104.

Institute of Medicine of the National Academies. (Eds Otten JJ, Hellwig JP, Meyers LD). *Dietary reference intakes: The essential guide to nutrient requirements.* 2006. Washington, DC: National Academies Press.

International Ski Federation. The role of adequate nutrition for performance and health for female cross-country skiers. 2006-2007. www.fis-ski.com.

Isley W, Underwood L, Clemmons D. Dietary components that regulate serum somatomedin-C concentrations in humans. *J Clin Invest* 1983; 71 February 175-182.

Ivy JL, Portman R. *Nutrient timing.* 2004. Laguna Beach, CA: Basic Health.

Ivy JL, Res PT, Sprague RC, Widzer MO. Effect of a carbohydrate-protein supplement on endurance performance during exercise of varying intensity. *Intl J Sport Nutr and Exer Metab* 2003;(13): 382-395.

Jacobs KA, Paul DR, Geor RJ, Hinchcliff, KW, Sherman WM. Dietary composition influences short-term endurance training-induced adaptations of substrate partitioning during exercise. *Intl J of Sport Nutr and Exer Metab,* 2004;(14): 38-61.

Jacobson BH, Weber MD, Claypool L, Hunt LE. Effect of caffeine on maximal strength and power in elite male athletes. *Br J Sports Med* 1992;26:276-280.

Jeukendrup AE. Lipids and insulin resistance: The role of fatty acid metabolism and fuel partitioning: Part vi. skeletal muscle lipid metabolism at rest and during exercise. *Annals of The New York Academy of Sciences* 2002;967: 217-235.

Jeukendrup AE, Thielen J, Wagenmakers, A, Brouns F, Saris W. Effect of medium-chain triacylglycerol and carbohydrate ingestion during exercise on substrate utilization and subsequent cycling performance. *Am J Clin Nutr* 1998;67:397-404.

Jenkins DG, Hutchins CA, Spillman D. The influence of dietary carbohydrate and pre-exercise glucose consumption on supramaximal intermittent exercise performance. *Br J Sp Med* 1994; 28(3):171-6.

Jentjens RLPG., Achten J, Jeukendrup AE. High oxidation rates from combined carbohydrates ingested during exercise. *Med Sci Sports Exerc* 2004: 36(9): 1551-1558.

Jentjens R LPG, Moseley L, Waring RH, Harding LK, Jeukendrup AE. Oxidation of combined ingestion of glucose and fructose during exercise. *J Appl Physiol* 2004;96: 1277-1284.

Jentjens RLPG., Venables MC, Jeukendrup AE. Oxidation of exogenous glucose, sucrose, and maltose during prolonged cycling exercise. *J Appl Physiol* 2004;96: 1285-1291.

Jentjens RL PG, Underwood K, Achten J, Currell K, Mann CH, Asker E. Jeukendrup AE. Exogenous carbohydrate oxidation rates are elevated after combined ingestion of glucose and fructose during exercise in theheat. *J Appl Physiol* 2006;100: 807-816.

Judelson DA, Maresh CM, Farrell MJ, Yamamoto LM, Armstrong LE, Kraemer WJ Volek JS, Spiering BA, Casa DJ, Anderson JM. Effect of hydration state on strength, power, and resistance exercise performance. *Med Sci Sports Exerc* 2007; 39(10): 1817-1824.

Judelson DA, Maresh CM, Yamamoto LM, Farrell MJ, Armstrong LE, Kraemer WJ, Volek JS, Spiering BA, Casa DJ, Anderson JM. Effect of hydration state on resistance exercise induced endocrine markers of anabolism, catabolism, and metabolism. *J Appl Physiol* 2008;105: 816 -824.

Jurczak MJ, Danos AM, Rehrmann VR, Allison MB, Greenberg CC, Brady MJ. Transgenic overexpression of protein targeting to glycogen markedly increases adipocytic glycogen storage in mice. *Am J Physiol Endocrinol Metab* 2007;292: E952-E963.

Juzwiak CR, Paschoal VCP, Lopez FA. Nutrition and physical activity *J Pediatr (Rio J).* 2000; 76 (Supl.3): S349-S358.

Kaminogawa S, Nanno M. Modulation of immune functions by foods. eCAM 2004;1(3)241-250.

Kannisto K, Chibalin A, Glinghammar B, Zierath JR, Hamsten A, Ehrenborg E. Differential expression of peroxisomal proliferator activated receptors · and ‰ in skeletal muscle in response to changes in diet and exercise. *Interl J Molecular Med* 2006;17: 45-52, 2006.

Kerksick C, Harvey T, Stout J, Campbell B, Wilborn C, Kreider R, Kalman D, Ziegenfuss T, Lopez H, Landis J, Ivy JL and Antonio J. International Society of Sports Nutrition position stand: Nutrient timing. *Journal of the International Society of Sports Nutrition* 2008, 5:17.

Kerksick CM and Leutholtz, B. Nutrient Administration and Resistance Training. *Journal of the International Society of Sports Nutrition.* 2005;2(1):50-67.

Kerksick C, Rasmussen C, Bowden R, Leutholtz B,. Harvey T, Earnest C, Greenwood M, Almada A, Kreider R. Effects of ribose supplementation prior to and during intense exercise on anaerobic capacity and metabolic markers. *International J Sport Nutr Exer Metab,* 2005;15: 653-664.

Kew S, Mesa MD, Tricon S, Buckley R, Minihane AM, Yaqoob P. Effects of oils rich in eicosapentaenoic and docosahexaenoic acids on immune cell composition and function in healthy humans. *Am J Clin Nutr* 2004;79:674-81.

King RFGJ, Cooke C, Carroll S, O'Hara J. Estimating changes in hydration status from changes in body mass: Considerations regarding metabolic water and glycogen storage. *Journal of Sports Sciences* 2008;26(12):1361-1363.

Kirkendall DT. Effects of nutrition on performance in soccer. *Med Sci Sports Exer* 1993;25(12):1370-74.

Kirwan JP, O'Gorman DJ, Cyr-Campbell D, Campbell WW, Yarasheski KE, Evans WJ. Effects of a moderate glycemic meal on exercise duration and substrate utilization. *Med Sci Sports Exerc*, 2001; 33(9): 1517-1523.

Koopman R, Beelen M, Stellingwerff T, Pennings B, Saris WHM, Kies AK, Kuipers H, van Loon LJC. Coingestion of carbohydrate with protein does not further augment postexercise muscle protein synthesis. *Am J Physiol Endocrinol Metab* 2007;293: E833-E842.

Koopman R, Pannemans DLE, Jeukendrup AE, Gijsen AP, Senden JMG, Halliday D, Saris WHM, van Loon LJC, Wagenmakers AJM. Combined ingestion of protein and carbohydrate improves protein balance during ultra-endurance exercise. *Am J Physiol Endocrinol Metab* 2004;287: E712-E720.

Kotze HF, van der Walt WH, Rogers GG, Strydom NB. Effects of plasma ascorbic acid levels on heat acclimatization in man. *J Appl Physiol* 1977; 42(5): 711-716.

Kraemer WJ. Endocrine responses to resistance exercise. *Med Sci Sport Exer* 1988;20(5) S152-7.

Kraemer WJ, Fry AC, Rubin MR, Triplett-Mcbride T, Gordon SE, Koziris LP, Lynch JM, Volek JS, Meuffels DE, Newton RU, Fleck SJ. Physiological and performance responses to tournament wrestling. *Med Sci Sports Exerc*, 2001;33(8):1367-1378.

Kraemer WJ, Hatfield DL, Volek JS, Fragala MS, Vingren JL, Anderson JM, Spiering BA, Thomas GA, Ho JY, Quann EE, Izquierdo M, Hakkinen K, Maresh CM. Effects of amino acids supplement on physiological adaptations to resistance training. *Med Sci Sports Exerc* 2009; 41(5): 1111-1121.

Kraemer WJ, Volek JS, Bush JA, Putukian M, Sebastianelli WJ. Hormonal responses to consecutive days of heavy-resistance exercise with or without nutritional supplementation. *J Appl Physiol* 1998;85(4):1544-1555.

Kreider RB, Earnest CP, Lundberg J, Rasmussen C, Greenwood M, Cowan P, Almada AL. Effects of ingesting protein with various forms of carbohydrate following resistance-exercise on substrate availability and markers of anabolism, catabolism, and immunity. *Journal of the International Society Sports Nutr* 2007, 4:18

Kreider RB, Melton C, Greenwood M, Rasmussen C, Lundberg J, Earnest C, Almada A. Effects of oral D-ribose supplementation on anaerobic capacity and selected metabolic markers in healthy males. *IJSNEM* 2003 13, 76-86

Kreisman SH, Manzon A, Nessim SJ, Morais JA, Gougeon R, Fisher SJ, Vranic M, Marliss EB. Glucoregulatory responses to intense exercise performed in the post prandial state. *Am J Physiol Endocrinol Metab* 2000;278: E786-E793.

Lagranha CJ, Levada-Pires AC, Sellitti DF, Procopio J, Curi R, Pithon-Curi TC. The effect of glutamine supplementation and physical exercise on neutrophil function. *Amino Acids* 2008; 34: 337-346.

Lambert EV, Goedecke JH, van Zyl C, Murphy K,. Hawley JA,. Dennis SC, Noakes TD. High-Fat Diet Versus Habitual Diet Prior to Carbohydrate Loading: Effects on Exercise Metabolism and Cycling Performance *Intl J Sports Nutr Metab* 2001; 11: 209-225.

Lancaster GI, Khan Q, Drysdale PT, Wallace F, Jeukendrup AE, Drayson MT, Gleeson M. Effect of prolonged exercise and carbohydrate ingestion on type 1 and type 2 T lymphocyte distribution and intracellular cytokine production in humans. *J Appl Physiol* 2005;98: 565-571.

Laursen PB, Suriano R, Quod MJ, Lee H, Abbiss CR, Nosaka K, Martin DT, Bishop D. Core temperature and hydration status during an Ironman Triathlon. *Br J Sports Med* 2006;40:320-325.

Lavienja AJ, Braam LM, Knapen MHJ, Geusens P, Brouns F Vermeer C. Factors affecting bone loss in female endurance athletes. *Am J Sports Med* 2003 31: 889.

Lehmann M, Foster C, Keul J. Overtraining in endurance athletes; a brief review. *Med Sci Sports Exerc* 1993; 25 (7):854-862.

Lee JKW, Shirreffs SM, Maughan RJ. Cold drink ingestion improves exercise endurance capacity in the heat. *Med Sci Sports Exerc* 2008;40(9): 1637-1644.

Lemon P. Protein and amino acid needs of the strength athlete. *Intl J Sports Nutr* 1991, 1, 127-145.

Lemon P. Effects of exercise on protein requirements. *Intl J Sports Nutr* 1998 (8) 426-447.

Levenhagen DK, Carr C, Carlson MG, Maron DJ, Borel MJ, Flakoll PJ. Postexercise protein intake enhances whole-body and leg protein accretion in humans. *Med Sci Sports Exerc*, 2002; 34(5); 828-837.

Lopez RM, Casa DJ, McDermott BP, Ganio MS, Armstrong LE, Maresh CM. Does creatine supplementation hinder exercise heat tolerance or hydration status? A systematic review with meta-analyses. *J Athletic Training* 2009;44(2):215-223.

Lounana J, Campion F, Noakes TD, Medelli J. Relationship between %HRmax, %HR reserve, %VO2max, and %VO2 reserve in elite cyclists. *Med Sci Sports Exerc* 2007;39(2): 350-357.

Lukaski H. Magnesium, zinc, and chromium nutriture and physical activity. *Am J Clin Nutr* 2000;72(suppl):585S-93S.

Lukaski H. Vitamin and mineral status: Effects on physical performance. *Nutrition* 2004;20:632-644.

Maresh CM, Whittlesey MJ, Armstrong LE, Yamamoto LM, Judelson DA, Fish KE, Casa DJ, Kavouras SA, Castracane VD. Effect of hydration state on testosterone and cortisol responses to training-intensity in collegiate runners. *Int'l J Sports Med* 2006 Oct 27 (10) 765-70.

Marliss EB, Stuart H. Kreisman SH, Manzon A, Halter JB, Vranic M, Nessim SJ. Gender differences in glucoregulatory responses to intense exercise. *J Appl Physiol* 2000; 88: 457-466.

Mastorakos G, Pavlatou M, Diamanti-Kandarakis E, Chrousos GP. Exercise and the stress system. Hormones. *Intl J End and Metab* 2005 4(2):73-89.

Maughan RJ, Leiper JB McGaw BA. Effects of exercise intensity on absorption of ingested fluids in man. *Experimental Physiology* 1990; 75: 419-421.

Maughan RJ, Shirreffs SM. Development of individual hydration strategies for athletes. *Intl J Sport Nutr Exer Metab* 2008;18: 457-472.

McArdle WD, Katch FI, Katch VL. 2007. *Exercise physiology: Energy, nutrition, & human performance.* 6th ed. Baltimore: Lippincott, Williams and Wilkins.

McArdle WD, Katch FI, Katch VL. 2008. *Sports and Exercise Nutrition* 3rd ed. Philadelphia: Lippincott Williams & Wilkins.

McConell GK, Canny BJ, Daddo MC, Nance MJ, Snow RJ. Effect of carbohydrate ingestion on glucose kinetics and muscle metabolism during intense endurance exercise. *J Appl Physiol* 2000;89: 1690-1698.

McDowall JA. Supplement use by young athletes. *J Sports Sci Med* 2007; (6): 337-342.

McFarlin BK, Flynn MG, Stewart LK, Timmerman KL. Carbohydrate intake during endurance exercise increases natural killer cell responsiveness to IL-2. *J Appl Physiol* 2004; 96:271-275.

Meyer NL, Parker-Simmons S, Erbacher JM, n.d. *The role of adequate nutrition for performance and health for female cross-country skiers, 2006-07.* Thunersee, Switzerland: International Ski Federation.

Millard-Stafford M, Warren GL, Thomas LM, J. Doyle A, Snow T, Hitchcock K. Recovery from run training: Efficacy of a carbohydrate-protein beverage? *Intl J Sport Nutr Exer Metab*, 2005; 15, 610-624.

Miller SL, P. Gaine C, Maresh CM, Armstrong LE. Ebbeling CB, Lamont LS, Rodriguez NR. The effects of nutritional supplementation throughout an endurance run on leucine kinetics during recovery. *IJSNEM* 2007, 17, 456-467.

Mitchell JB, Pizza FX, Paquet A, Davis BJ, Forrest MB, Braun WA. Influence of carbohydrate status on immune responses before and after endurance exercise. *J Appl Physiol* 1998;84(6): 1917-1925.

Monro J. Redefining the glycemic index for dietary management of postprandial glycemia. *J Nutr* 2003;133: 4256-4258.

Monro J, Shaw M. Glycemic impact, glycemic glucose equivalents, glycemic index, and glycemic load: definitions, distinctions, and implications. *Am J Clin Nutr* 2008 87(suppl) 237S-43S.

Mora-Rodriguez R, Coyle EF. Effects of plasma epinephrine on fat metabolism during exercise: Interactions with exercise intensity. *Am J Physiol Endocrinol Metab* 2000;278: 669-E676.

Montain SJ. Hydration recommendations for sport. *Curr. Sports Med Rep* 2008; 7(4): 187-192.

Montain SJ, Cheuvront SN, Sawka MN. Exercise associated hyponatraemia: Quantitative analysis to understand the aetiology. *Br J Sports Med* 2006;40:98-106.

Moore DR, Robinson MJ, Fry JL, Tang JE, Glover EI, Wilkinson SB, Prior T, Tarnopolsky MA, Phillips SM. Ingested protein dose response of muscle and albumin protein synthesis after resistance exercise in young men. *Am J Clin Nutr* 2009;89: 161-168.

Morens C, Bos C,. Pueyo ME, Benamouzig R, Gaussere SN, Luengo C, Tome D, Gaudichon C. Increasing habitual protein intake accentuates differences in postprandial dietary nitrogen utilization between protein sources in humans. *J Nutr* 2003;133: 2733-2740.

Muckle DS. Glucose syrup ingestion and team performance in soccer. *Br J Sports Med* 1973; 7: 340-343.

Mündel T, King J, Collacott E, Jones DA. Drink temperature influences fluid intake and endurance capacity in men during exercise in a hot, dry environment. *Exp Physiol* 2006;91(5), 925-933.

Murray B. Hydration and physical performance. *J Am Coll Nutr* 2007 Oct; 26 (5 Suppl): 542S-548S.

Murray R, Bartoli WP, Eddy DE, Horn MK. Physiological and performance responses to nicotinic-acid ingestion during exercise. *Med Sci Sports Exer.* 1995. 27(7) 1057-62.

Murray R, Paul GL, Seifert JG, Eddy DE. Responses to varying rates of carbohydrate ingestion during exercise. *Med Sci. Sports Exerc.*, 1991;23(6) 713-8.

Nedergaard J, Bengtsson T, Cannon B. Unexpected evidence for active brown adipose tissue in adult humans. *Am J Physiol Endocrinol Metab* 2007;293: E444-E452.

Nichols C, Green P, Hawkins R, Williams C. Carbohydrate intake and recovery of intermittent running capacity. *Intl J Sport Nutr* 1997; (7): 251-260.

Nieman D. Upper respiratory tract infections and exercise. *Thorax* 1995;50;1229-1231.

Nieman DC. Immune response to heavy exertion. *J Appl Physiol* 1997;82(5): 1385-1394.

Nieman D. Immunonutrition support for athletes *Nutrition Reviews* 2008;66(6):310-320.

Nieman DC, Davis JM, Brown VA, Henson DA, Dumke CL, Utter AC, Vinci DM, Downs MF, Smith JC, Carson J, Brown A, McAnulty SR, McAnulty LS. Influence of carbohydrate ingestion on immune changes after 2 h of intensive resistance training. *J Appl Physiol* 2004;96: 1292-1298.

Nieman DC, Henson DA, Gross SJ, Jenkins DP, Davis JM, Murphy EA, Carmichael MD, Dumke CL, Utter AC, McAnulty SR, MCcAanulty LS, Mayer EP. Quercetin reduces illness but not immune perturbations after intensive exercise. *Med. Sci. Sports Exerc* 2007; 39(9):1561-1569.

Nieman DC, Henson DA, Maxwell KR, Williams AS, McAanulty SR, Jin F, Shanely RA, Lines TC. Effects of quercetin and EGCG on mitochondrial biogenesis and immunity. *Med Sci Sports Exerc* 2009; 41 (7): 1467-1475.

Nieman DC, Henson DA, Mcanulty SR, Mcanulty LS, Morrow JD, Ahmed A, Heward CB. Vitamin E and immunity after the Kona Triathlon World Championship. *Med Sci Sports Exerc* 2004; 36(8): 1328-1335.

Nissen SL, Sharp RL. Effect of dietary supplements on lean mass and strength gains with resistance exercise: A meta-analysis. *J Appl Physiol* 2003;94: 651-659.

Nissen S, Sharp R, Ray M, Rathmacher JA, Rice D, Fuller JC, Connelly AS, Abumrad N. Effect of leucine metabolite b-hydroxy-b-methylbutyrate on muscle metabolism during resistance-exercise training. *J Appl Physiol* 1996;81(5): 2095-2104.

Noakes TD, Rehrer NJ, Maughan RJ. The importance of volume in regulation gastric emptying. *Med Sci Sports Exerc* 1991; 23(3): 307-313.

Op 't Eijnde B, Van Leemputte M, Brouns F, Van der Vusse GJ, Labarque V, Ramaekers M, Van Schuylenberg R, Verbessem P, Wijnen H, Hespel P. No effects of oral ribose supplementation on repeated maximal exercise and de novo ATP resynthesis. *J Appl Physiol* 2001;91: 2275-2281.

Panel on Dietary Antioxidants and Related Compounds; Subcommittees on Upper Reference Levels of Nutrients and Interpretation and Uses of DRIs; Standing Committee on the Scientific Evaluation of Dietary Reference Intakes; Food and Nutrition Board; Institute of Medicine. *Dietary reference intakes for vitamin C, vitamin E, selenium, and carotenoids.* National Academies Press, 2000. www.nap.edu.

Panel on Dietary Reference Intakes for Electrolytes and Water; Standing Committee on the Scientific Evaluation of Dietary Reference Intakes. *Dietary reference intakes for water, potassium, sodium, chloride, and sulfate.* National Academies Press, 2005. www.nap.edu.

Panel on Micronutrients; Subcommittees on Upper Reference Levels of Nutrients and of Interpretation and Use of Dietary Reference Intakes; Standing Committee on the Scientific Evaluation of Dietary Reference Intakes. *Dietary reference intakes for vitamin A, vitamin K, arsenic, boron, chromium, copper, iodine, iron, manganese, molybdenum, nickel, silicon, vanadium, and zinc.* National Academies Press, 2000. www.nap.edu.

Pascoe D, Costill D, Fink W, Robergs R, Zachweija J. Glycogen resynthesis in skeletal muscle following resistive exercise *Med Sci Sports Exern* 1993; 25(2):349-354.

Passe D, Horn M, Stofan J, Horswill C, Murray R. Voluntary dehydration in runners despite favorable conditions for fluid intake. *IJSNEM* 2007; 17, 284-295.

Paul D, Jacobs KA, Geor RJ, Hinchcliff KW. No effect of pre-exercise meal on substrate metabolism and time trial performance during intense endurance exercise. *Intl J Sports Nutr Metab* 2003; (13): 489-503.

Peake JM. Vitamin C: Effects of exercise and requirements with training. *IJSNEM,* 2003; 13: 125-151.

Pedersen BK, Steensberg A, Schjerling P. Muscle-derived interleukin-6: possible biological effects *Journal of Physiology* 2001; 536(2):329-337.

Pedersen DJ, Lessard SJ, Coffey VG, Churchley EG, Wootton AM, Ng T, Watt MJ, Hawley JA. High rates of muscle glycogen resynthesis after exhaustive exercise when carbohydrate is coingested with caffeine. *J Appl Physiol* 2008; 105: 7-13.

Pedersen BK, Akerstrom TC, Nielsen AR, Fischer CP. Role of myokines in exercise and metabolism. *J Appl Physiol* 2007; 103: 1093-1098.

Peters EM, Goetzsche JM, Grobbelaar B, Noakes TD. Vitamin C supplementation reduces the incidence of post-race symptoms of upper respiratory tract infections in ultra-marathon runners. *Amer J Clin Nutr* 1993; 57:170-4.

Phillips T, Childs AC, Dreon DM, Phinney S, Leeuwenburgh C. A dietary supplement attenuates IL-6 and CRP after eccentric exercise in untrained males. *Med Sci Sports Exerc* 2003; 35(12): 2032-2037.

Phillips SM, Hartman JW, Wilkinson SB. Dietary protein to support anabolism with resistance exercise in young men. *J the Amer Coll Nutr,* 2005; 24(2): 134S-139S.

Pikosky MA, Smith TJ, Grediagin A, Castaneda-Sceppa C, Byerley L, Glickman EL, Young AJ. Increased protein maintains nitrogen balance during exercise-induced energy deficit. *Med Sci Sports Exerc* 2008; 40(3):505-512.

Raben A, Kiens B, Richter EA, Rasmussen LB, Svenstrup B, Micic S, Bennett P. Serum sex hormones and endurance performance after a lacto-ovo vegetarian and a mixed diet. *Med Sci. Sports Exerc.,* 1992; 24(11): 1290-97.

Rasmussen BB, Tipton KD, Miller SL, Wolf SE, Wolfe RR. An oral essential amino acid-carbohydrate supplement enhances muscle protein anabolism after resistance exercise *J Appl Physiol* 2000; 88:386-392.

Ratamess NA, Hoffman JR, Ross R, Shanklin M, Faigenbaum AD, Kang J. Effects of an amino acid/creatine energy supplement on the acute hormonal response to resistance exercise. *IJSNEM* 2007; 17:608-623.

Ristow M, Zarsea K, Oberbachc A, Klotingc N, Birringera M, Kiehntopfd M, Stumvollc M, Kahne CR, Bluher M. Antioxidants prevent health-promoting effects of physical exercise in humans. *Proc of Nat Acad Sci.* May 26, 2009; 106 (21): 8665-8670.

Rohde T, MacLean DA, Pedersen BK. Effect of glutamine supplementation on changes in the immune system induced by repeated exercise. *Med Sci Sports Exer* 1998; 30(6): 856-862.

Romano-Ely BC, Todd MK, Saunders MJ, St. Laurent T. Effect of an isocaloric carbohydrate-protein-antioxidant drink on cycling performance. *Med Sci Sports Exerc* 2006; 38 (9): 1608-1616.

Romijn JA, Coyle EF, Sidossis LS, Gastaldelli A, Horowitz JF, Endert E, Wolfe RR. Regulation of endogenous fat and carbohydrate metabolism in relation to exercise intensity and duration. *Am J Physiol* 1993; 265 (*Endocrinol. Metab.* 28): E380-E391.

Romijn JA, Coyle EF, Sidossis LS, Rosenblatt J, Wolfe RR. Substrate metabolism during different exercise intensities in endurance-trained women. *J Appl Physiol* 2000;88: 1707-1714.

Rosenbloom CA. 2000. *Sports nutrition: A guide for the professional working with active people.* Chicago: American Dietetic Association.

Rowlands DS, Thomson JS. Effects of ⊠-hydroxy-⊠-methylbutyrate supplementation during resistance training on strength, body composition and muscle damage in trained and untrained young men: A meta-analysis. *J Strenght Cond Res* 2009 May; 23(3):836-46.

Rowlands DS, Thorp RM, Rossler K, Graham DF, Rockell MJ. Effect of protein-rich feeding on recovery after intense exercise. *Intl J Sport Nutr and Exer Metab,* 2007, 17, 521-543.

Roy BD, Fowles JR, Hill R, Tarnopolsky MA. Macronutrient intake and whole body protein metabolism following resistance exercise. *Med Sci Sports Exerc* 2000; 32(8):1412-1418.

Roy LPG. Jentjens, van Loon LJC, Mann CH, Wagenmakers AJM and Jeukendrup AE. Addition of protein and amino acids to carbohydrates does not enhance postexercise muscle glycogen synthesis *J Appl Physiol* 2001;91:839-846.

Roy BD, Tarnopolsky MA. Influence of differing macronutrient intakes on muscle glycogen resynthesis after resistance exercise. *J Appl Physiol* 1998; 84(3): 890-896.

Satabin P, Portero P, Defer G, Bricout J, Guezennec CY. Metabolic and hormonal responses to lipid and carbohydrate diets during exercise in man. *Med Sci Sports Exerc* 1987; 19(3) 218-223.

Saunders MJ, Kane MD, Todd MK. Effects of a carbohydrate-protein beverage on cycling endurance and muscle damage. *Med Sci Sports Exerc* 2004; 36(7): 1233-1238.

Sawka MN. Physiological consequences of hypohydration: exercise performance and thermoregulation. *Med Sci Sports Exerc.,* 1992; 24(6):657-670.

Sawka MN, Burke L M, Eichner R E, Maughan R J, Montain S J, Nina S. Stachenfeld N S. Position stand of the American College of Sports Medicine: Exercise and fluid replacement. *Med Sci Sports Exerc.* 2007 Feb; 39(2):377-90.

Sawka MN, Noakes TD. Does dehydration impair exercise performance? *Med Sci Sports Exerc.* 2007; 39(8):1209-17.

SCAN. *Sports nutrition: A practice manual for professionals,* ed. M. Dunford. 2006. Chicago: American Dietetic Association.

SCAN. *Sports nutrition: A guide for the professional working with active people.* ed. C. Rosenbloom. 2000. Chicago: American Dietetic Association.

Schaafsma G. The protein digestibility-corrected amino acid score. *J Nutr* 2000; 130:1865S-1867S.

Schedl HP, Maughan RJ, Gisolfi CV. Intestinal absorption during rest and exercise: Implications for formulating an oral rehydration solution (ORS). *Med Sci Sports Exerc* 1994; 26 (3): 267-280.

Schumm SR, Triplett NT, McBride JM, Dumke CL. Hormonal response to carbohydrate supplementation at rest and after resistance exercise *IJSNEM.* 2008; 18: 260-280.

Schwenk TL, Costley CD. When food becomes a drug: Nonanabolic nutritional supplement use in athletes. *Am J Sports Med* 2002; 30(6): 907-16.

Sharp R. Role of whole foods in promoting hydration after exercise in humans. *J Am Coll Nutr* 2007 Oct; 26(5 Suppl): 592S-596S.

Sharp RL. Role of sodium in fluid homeostasis with exercise. *J Amer Coll of Nutr,* 2006; 25(3), 231S-239S.

Shimomura Y, Yamamoto Y, Bajotto G, Sato J, Murakami T, Shimomura N, Kobayashi H, Kazunori Mawatari K. Nutraceutical effects of branched-chain amino acids on skeletal muscle. *J Nutr* 2006;136: 529S-532S.

Shirreffs S. Conference on multidisciplinary approaches to nutritional problems. Symposium on performance, exercise and health. Hydration, fluids and performance. *Proceedings of the Nutrition Society* 2009; 68: 17-22.

Simopoulos AP. Omega-3 fatty acids and athletics. *Current Sports Medicine Reports* 2007; 6:230-236.

Simopoulos AP (ed). Nutrition and fitness: Cultural, genetic and metabolic aspects. *World Rev Nutr Diet.* 2008; 98:23-50.

Siu PM, Wong SHS, Morris JG, Lam CW, Chung PK, Chiung S. Effect of frequency of carbohydrate feedings on recovery and subsequent endurance run. *Med Sci Sports Exerc* 2004; 36(2): 315-323.

Slavin JL, Martini MC, Jacobs DR, Marquart L. Plausible mechanisms for the protectiveness of whole grains. *Am J Clin Nutr* 1999; 70(suppl):459S-63S.

Smith TJ, Montain SJ, Anderson D, Young AJ. Plasma amino acid responses after consumption of beverages with varying protein type. *International J of Sport Nutr and Exer Met,* 2009; 19: 1-17.

Sparks MJ, Selig SS, Febbraio MA. Pre-exercise carbohydrate ingestion: Effect of the glycemic index on endurance exercise performance. *Med. Sci. Sports Exerc.* 1998; Vol. 30, No. 6, 844-849.

Spriet LL. Regulation of skeletal muscle fat oxidation during exercise in humans. *Med. Sci. Sports Exerc.* 2002; 34(9): 1477-1484.

Standing Committee on the Scientific Evaluation of Dietary Reference Intakes and its Panel on Folate, Other B Vitamins, and Choline; Subcommittee on Upper Reference Levels of Nutrients; Food and Nutrition Board; Institute of Medicine. *Dietary reference intakes for thiamin, riboflavin, niacin, vitamin B6, folate, vitamin B12, pantothenic acid, biotin, and choline.* National Academies Press, 1998. www.nap.edu.

Standing Committee on the Scientific Evaluation of Dietary Reference Intakes; Food and Nutrition Board; Institute of Medicine. *Dietary reference intakes for calcium, phosphorus, magnesium, vitamin D, and fluoride.* National Academies Press, 1997. www.nap.edu.

Stellingwerff T, Spriet LL, Watt MJ, Kimber NE, Hargreaves, M, Hawley JA, Burke, LM. Decreased PDH activation and glycogenolysis during exercise following fat adaptation with carbohydrate restoration. *Am J Physiol Endocrinol Metab.* 2006; 290: E380-E388.

Stephens B, Braun B. Impact of nutrient intake timing on the metabolic response to exercise. *Nutrition Reviews* 2008; 66(8):473-476.

Stepto NK, Martin DT, Fallon KE, Hawley JA. Metabolic demands of intense aerobic interval training in competitive cyclists. *Med. Sci. Sports Exerc.* 2001; 33(2): 303-310.

Stover EA, Petrie HJ, Passe D, Horswill CA, Murray B, Wildman R. Urine specific gravity in exercisers prior to physical training. *Appl Physiol Nutr Metab.* 2006 Jun;31(3):320-7.

Sullo A, Brizzi G, Maffulli N. Triiodothyronine deiodinating activity in brown adipose tissue after short cold stimulation test in trained and untrained rats. *Physiol. Res.* 2004; 53: 69-75.

Tamura Y, Watadaa H, Igarashia Y, Nomiyamaa T, Onishib T, Takahashib K, Doib S, Katamotob S, Hirosea T, Tanakaa Y, Kawamoria R. Short-term effects of dietary fat on intramyocellular lipid in sprinters and endurance runners. *Metabolism Clinical and Experimental* 2008;57:373-379.

Tang JE, Perco JG, Moore DR, Wilkinson SB, Phillips SM. Resistance training alters the response of fed state mixed muscle protein synthesis in young men. *Am J Physiol Regul Integr Comp Physiol* 2008; 294: R172-R178.

Tang JE, Phillips SM. Maximizing muscle protein anabolism: The role of protein quality. *Curr Opin Clin Nutr Metab Care* 2009;12: 66-71.

Tarnopolsky M. A. Sex differences in exercise metabolism and the role of 17-beta estradiol. *Med Sci Sports Exerc* 2008;40(4):648-654.

Teixeira VH, Valente HF, Casal SI, Marques AF, Moreira PA. Antioxidants do not prevent postexercise peroxidation and may delay muscle recovery. *Med Sci Sports Exerc* 2009; 41(9): 1752-1760.

Timmons B, Bar-Or O, Riddell M. Influence of age and pubertal status on substrate utilization during exercise with and without carbohydrate intake in healthy boys. *J App Phys Nutr Metab* 2007;32:416-425.

Thorburn MS, Vistisen B, Thorp RM, Rockell MJ, Jeukendrup AE, Xu X, Rowlands DS. Attenuated gastric distress but no benefit to performance with adaptation to octanoate-rich esterified oils in well-trained male cyclists. *J Appl Physiol* 2006; 101: 1733-1743.

Tipton KD, Elliott TA, Cree MG, Wolf SE, Sanford AP, Wolfe RR. Ingestion of casein and whey proteins result in muscle anabolism after resistance exercise. *Med Sci Sports Exerc* 2004; 36(12): 2073-2081.

Tipton KD, Elliott TA, Cree MG, Aarsland AA, Sanford AP, Wolfe RR. Stimulation of net muscle protein synthesis by whey-protein ingestion before and after exercise. *Am J Physiol Endocrinol Metab* 2007; 292: E71-E76.

Tipton KD, Ferrando AA. Improving muscle mass: Response of muscle metabolism to exercise, nutrition and anabolic agents. *Essays Biochem* 2008; 44:85-98.

Tipton KD, Ferrando AA, Phillips SM, Doyle D, Wolfe RR. Postexercise net protein synthesis in human muscle from orally administered amino acids. *Am J Physiol* 1999; 276 (*Endocrinol. Metab*.39): E628-E634.

Tipton KD, Rasmussen BB, Miller SL, Wolf SE, Owens-Stovall SK, Petrini BE, Wolfe RR. Timing of amino acid-carbohydrate ingestion alters anabolic response of muscle to resistance exercise. *Am J Physiol Endocrinol Metab* 2001; 281:E197-E206.

Tipton KD, Wolfe RR. Exercise protein metabolism and muscle growth. *IJSNEM*. 2001; (11):109-132.

Tomakidis SP, Karamanolis IA. Effects of carbohydrate ingestion 15 min. before exercise on endurance running capacity. *Appl Physiol Nutr Metab.* 2008; 33(3): 441-9.

Tsintzas OK, Williams C, Boobis L, Greenhaff P. Carbohydrate ingestion and glycogen utilization in different muscle fibre types in man. *J of Phys* 1995; 489(1):243-250.

Tsintzas K, Williams C, Constantin-Teodosiu D, Hultman E, Boobis L, Clarys P, Greenhaff P. Phosphocreatine degradation in type I and type II muscle fibres during submaximal exercise in man: Effect of carbohydrate ingestion. *Journal of Physiology* 2001; 537(1): 305-311.

Valentine RJ, Saunders MJ, Todd MK, St. Laurent TG. Influence of carbohydrate-protein beverage on cycling endurance and indices of muscle disruption. *IJSNEM,* 2008; 18: 363-378.

Van Essen M, Gibala MJ. Failure of protein to improve time trial performance when added to a sports drink. *Med Sci Sports Exerc* 2006; 38(8): 1476-1483.

Van Loon LJC. Use of intramuscular triacylglycerol as a substrate source during exercise in humans. *J Appl Physiol* 2004; 97: 1170-1187.

Van Loon LJ, Greenhaff PL, Constantin-Teodosiu D, Saris WH, Wagenmakers AJ. The effects of increasing exercise intensity on muscle fuel utilisation in humans. *J of Phys* 2001; 536(1):295-304.

Van Loon LJC, Saris WHM, Kruijshoop M, Wagenmakers AJM. Maximizing postexercise muscle glycogen synthesis: Carbohydrate supplementation and the application of amino acid or protein hydrolysate mixtures. *Am J Clin Nutr* 2000; 72:106-11.

Vandenberghe K, Gillis N, Van Leemputte M, Van Hecke P, Vanstapel F, Hespel P. Caffeine counteracts the ergogenic action of muscle creatine loading. *J Appl Physio* 1996; 80(2): 452-457.

Venkatraman JT, Leddy J, Pendergast D. Dietary fats and immune status in athletes: Clinical implications. *Med Sci Sports Exerc* 2000; 32(7): Suppl. S389-S395.

Virk RS, Dunton NJ, Young JC, Leklem JE. Effect of vitamin B-6 supplementation on fuels, catecholamines and amino acids during exercise in men. *Med Sci Sports Exer* 1999: 31(3): 400-408.

Vogt M, Puntschart A, Howald H, Mueller B, Mannhart CH, Gfeller-Tuescher L, Mullis P, Hoppeler H. Effects of dietary fat on muscle substrates, metabolism, and performance in athletes. *Med. Sci. Sports Exerc* 2003; 35(6): 952-960.

Volek J. Influence of nutrition on responses to resistance training. *Med Sci Sport Exer* 2004; 36(4): 689-696.

Volek J. Strength nutrition. *Curr Sports Med Rep* 2003; 2:189-193.

Wallis GA, Dawson R, Achten J, Webber J, Jeukendrup AE. Metabolic response to carbohydrate ingestion during exercise in males and females. *Am J Physiol Endocrinol Metab* 2006; 290: E708-E715.

Walsh NP, Blannin AK, Bishop NC, Robson PJ, Gleeson MJ. Effect of oral glutamine supplementation on human neutrophil lipopolysaccharide-stimulated degranulation following prolonged exercise. *IJSNEM* 2000; (10): 39-50.

Wee SL, Williams C, Gray S, Horabin J. Influence of high and low glycemic index meals on endurance running capacity. *Med Sci Sports Exerc* 1999; 31(3): 393-399.

Wee SL, Williams C, Tsintzas K, Boobis L. Ingestion of a high-glycemic index meal increases muscle glycogen storage at rest but augments its utilization during subsequent exercise. *J Appl Physiol* 2005; 99: 707-714.

Whitley HA, Humphreys SM, Campbell IT, Keegan MA, Jayanetti TD, Sperry DA, MacLaren DP, Reilly T, Frayn KN. Metabolic and performance responses during endurance exercise after high fat and high-carbohydrate meals. *J Appl Physiol* 1998; 85(2): 418-424.

Wiles J, Woodward R, Bird SR. Effect of pre-exercise protein ingestion upon VO2, R and perceived exertion during treadmill running. *Br J Sports Med* 1991; 25:26-30.

Wilkinson SB, Tarnopolsky MA, MacDonald MJ, MacDonald JR, Armstrong D, Phillips SM. Consumption of fluid skim milk promotes greater muscle protein accretion after resistance exercise than does consumption of an isonitrogenous and isoenergetic soy-protein beverage *Am J Clin Nutr* 2007; 85:1031-40.

Williams MH. 2005. *Nutrition for health, fitness and sport*. 7th ed. New York: McGraw-Hill.

Williams MH. 2007. *Nutrition for health, fitness, & sport*. 8th ed. New York: McGraw Hill.

Williams MH, Branch JD. Creatine supplementation and exercise performance: An update. *Journal of the Amer Coll of Nutr* 1998; 17(3): 216-234.

Wilson JM, Kim J, Lee SR, Rathmacher JA, Dalmau B, Kingsley JD, Koch H, Manninen AH, Saadat R, Panton LB. Acute and timing effects of beta-hydroxy-beta-methylbutyrate (HMB) on indirect markers of skeletal muscle damage. *Nutrition & Metabolism* 2009; 6:6.

Wilson GJ, Wilson JM, Manninen AH. Effects of beta-hydroxy-beta-methylbutyrate (HMB) on exercise performance and body composition across varying levels of age, sex, and training experience: A review. *Nutrition & Metabolism* 2008, 5:1.

Woolf K, Manore MM. B-vitamins and exercise: Does exercise alter requirements? *International Journal of Sport Nutrition and Exercise Metabolism* 2006, 16, 453-484.

Yeo WK, Lessard SJ, Chen ZP, Garnham AP, Burke LM, Rivas DA, Kemp BE, Hawley JA. Fat adaptation followed by carbohydrate restoration increases AMPK activity in skeletal muscle from trained humans. *J Appl Physiol* 2008; 105: 1519-1526.

Yeo SE, Jentjens R, Wallis GA, Jeukendrup AE. Caffeine increases exogenous carbohydrate oxidation during exercise. *J Appl Physiol* 2005; 99: 844-850.

Zehnder M, Christ AR, Ith M, Acheson KJ, Pouteau E, Kreis R, Trepp R, Diem P, Boesch C, Decombaz J. Intramyocellular lipid stores increase markedly in athletes after 1.5 days lipid supplementation and are utilized during exercise in proportion to their content. *Eur J Appl Physiol* 2006;98:341-354.

Index

About the Authors

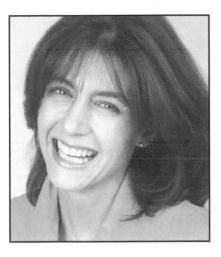

Heidi Skolnik, MS, CDN, FACSM, is the president of Nutrition Conditioning, Inc., a nutrition consulting practice. She has master's degrees in exercise science and human nutrition. She is also a New York State certified nutritionist, a fellow with the American College of Sports Medicine (ACSM), and a certified ACSM health fitness instructor.

Skolnik is the sports nutrition consultant to the New York Giants, the Juilliard School, and the School of American Ballet. She is a senior nutritionist at the Women's Sports Medicine Center at Hospital for Special Surgery and part of the New York Road Runners sports nutrition team. Previously, Skolnik spent 15 years working with the New York Mets. She has also worked with professional athletes in football, baseball, basketball, cycling, and soccer; Olympic-level athletes; marathoners; and collegiate wrestlers.

As an expert resource for national media, Skolnik has been referenced in newspapers and national magazines such as *Men's Health, Stack, Self, Glamour, GQ,* and *Real Simple.* She appears frequently on TV and has been seen on *CNN American Morning* and *Headline News,* the *Today Show, Good Morning America,* the *Early Show, Primetime, 20/20, Extra,* and the Food Network.

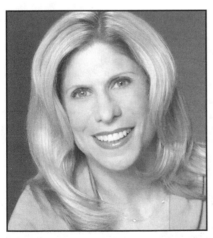

Andrea Chernus, MS, RD, CDE, is a registered dietitian and New York State certified dietitian and nutritionist. She holds a master's degree in nutrition and exercise physiology from Columbia University in New York. She maintains a full-time private practice on the upper west side in New York City, where she sees many athletes and performers.

Chernus consults with runners in the New York Road Runners Club and the New York City Marathon and is part of the New York Road Runners sports nutrition team. As part of Nutrition Conditioning, Inc., she also consults to the Juilliard School. Previously, she was the clinical nutritionist for Columbia University Health and Related Services. Chernus' articles have been published in *Training & Conditioning, Stack, Dance Spirit, Bottom Line,* and *Pointe.* She has been quoted in *Outdoors, Shape, Self, YM, Women's Day,* and *Bicycling.* She has also appeared on local and national TV.

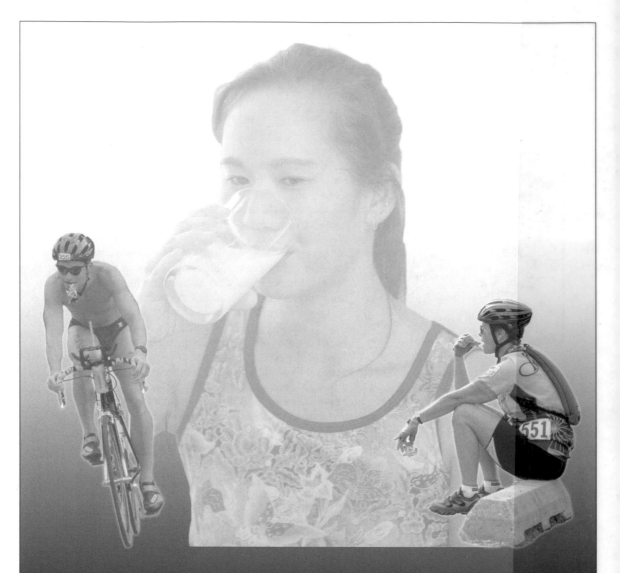
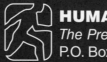